Modern Esthetics

A Scientific Source for Estheticians

Modern Esthetics

A Scientific Source for Estheticians

Henry J. Gambino, PhD

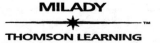

MILADY

THOMSON LEARNING

Africa • Australia • Canada • Denmark • Japan • Mexico • New Zealand • Philippines
Puerto Rico • Singapore • Spain • United Kingdom • United States

Cover Photograph: Michael A. Gallitelli

Milady Staff:

Administrative Editor: Catherine Frangie

Managing Editor: Susan Simpfenderfer

Editor Production Assistant: Lori McDonald

Production Manager: John Mickelbank

Art Supervisor: Judi Orozco

Photographs courtesy of:

Pibbs Laboratories; Proteus; Bucks County Beauty School; Nemectron; Rene Guinot; Amber Products; Bernard Jensen, PhD; Etablissements Doyer; *Les Nouvelles Esthetiques*—American Edition; Allergan Laboratories; Rohm and Haas Company

Library of Congress Cataloging-in-Publication Data

Gambino, Henry J.

Modern esthetics: a scientific source for estheticians / Henry J. Gambino.

       p.   cm.

       Includes index.

       1. Beauty culture. 2. Skin—Care and hygiene. 3. Cosmetics.
       I. Title.

TT957.G35   1992   92-7758

646.7'2—dc20   CIP

       ISBN-13: 978-1-5625-3043-3
       ISBN-10: 1-5625-3043-7

Contents

List of Illustrations

List of Tables

Foreword

Esthetics is the fastest growing segment of the beauty care field. More and more, men and women are realizing the value of proper skin care for their appearance and health. This is an exciting time for the esthetician. There is a tremendous opportunity for growth and prosperity for those who have the ability to perform the wide variety of services that fall under the label of esthetics, and who have the interest and the drive to keep learning as much as possible about their chosen profession.

For most estheticians, this means that specialized training will be necessary to enable them to practice this combination art and science effectively and to stay ahead of the competition.

This book is intended to help provide that specialized training. It is a tool estheticians can use to increase their knowledge about the art and the science of esthetics. Chapter 1, the introduction, gives a brief overview of the profession of esthetics and describes the qualities of a good esthetician. It also gives an idea of the breadth of knowledge required. Chapter 2 provides a review of the facial, the basic service the esthetician gives to clients. Chapter 3 reviews sanitation and safety, two subjects of vital interest in the conduct of business.

The balance of the book discusses the physical sciences—chemistry, physics and biology—that form the basic knowledge the esthetician needs to understand the principles behind the techniques and equipment used in the practice of skin care. It then expands upon those sciences to show how the information relates to the esthetician.

Appendix 1 is a glossary of the technical terms used throughout this book. Appendix 2 contains a list of suggested readings for further study.

The book is a resource manual meant to provide some of the basic information needed by the esthetician. It is not a "how-to" book, but a "why-to" study and reference work on esthetics. It makes no claim, however, to be the "last word" on any subject covered. All of the subjects are complex and could be expanded upon in volumes. The intent here is to present the basic information that will let the esthetician develop an efficient practice and to point the way toward additional knowledge.

Likewise, the techniques and data presented here are the culmination of the author's training and experience and are based on his philosophy of skin care. These techniques and data should be considered as guidelines and not as gospel. It is important that readers not learn the material by rote. Instead, they should understand it and develop a consistent and logical way of looking at the skin and of working with it.

There is no one right way to give a good facial. Each esthetician must draw upon training and experience to develop techniques and insights that fit individual work habits and philosophy.

Hopefully, this book will stimulate the reader to learn more. The professional esthetician never stops learning, reading as much as possible; taking courses whenever possible; attending seminars whenever possible; and taking part in professional organizations. The esthetician who works at increasing knowledge and understanding of the complex art and science of esthetics will reap the rewards and the satisfaction and pride that come with being a true professional.

H.J.G.
Doylestown, 1991

Acknowledgments

A book such as this may have only one author, but it is never the result of just one person's work. Many people have a hand in compiling, writing and illustrating a publication. I would like to thank all those people who have helped me in this endeavor. My appreciation and thanks go to Joan Poust and Diane Ripka, who spent hours posing as the subjects of many of the photographs in the work, and to Steve Wallin, owner of the Bucks County School of Beauty Culture and of Universal Techniques, who kindly let me use the school facilities to take the photographs. I would also like to thank Joni Lougheran and Geri Brooks of Columbia Pacific University, San Rafael, for their patient counsel as I developed the manuscript, and to Chris Pascal, of CD&P Products for providing background information about thalassotherapy techniques.

I would also like to extend my thanks to the people and companies who provided me with photographs and illustrations. These include Dr. Bernard Jensen, for letting me reprint his charts on iridology; *Les Nouvelles Esthetiques* (American Edition), for letting me use their electron microphotographs of the skin; the equipment manufacturers, Proteus, Etablissements Doyer, Pibbs Industries, Amber Products Co., Universal Techniques and Nemectron Skin Care Inc., for providing photographs and drawings of various pieces of equipment; to the makers of skin-care products, Lachman Imports, who market the Rene Guinot line of products; and Sothys USA, Ltd., for providing pictures of their product lines. Also, thanks go to Allergan Laboratories, for providing photographs of various skin disorders discussed in Chapter 7.

I wish to thank the following educators and professionals for reviewing my manuscript: Nancy Hall of International Academy of Cosmetology Arts and Science, Carmichael, CA; Johnell Baldwin of

Baldwin Beauty School, Austin, TX; Edwina Bogosian of Essex Agricultural and Technical Institute, Hathorne, MA; and Charles Mizelle of Charles for Total Image, Los Angeles, CA.

Last, but certainly not least, thanks go to a very special lady, Maureen Moore, for her patience and help in proofreading the manuscript and preparing the final copy.

1 Introduction to Esthetics

OBJECTIVES *After completing this chapter, you should be able to:*

❶ Define esthetics.

❷ Outline the historical significance of the subject, and discuss its importance.

❸ Understand the relationship between cleanliness, nutrition and attitude in modern skin care.

❹ Describe the role esthetics plays in the health and beauty care industry.

❺ Summarize the attributes an esthetician must possess to work in the field successfully.

INTRODUCTION

The profession of **esthetics** (es-THET-iks), the nonmedical care of the skin, is one of the fastest growing areas in the field of health and beauty care. The American public has, in the past few years, come to realize what Europeans and Asians have known for decades—our skin, that marvelous living fabric that covers and protects our bodies—requires on-going care to keep it healthy and beautiful.

A concern with health and beauty is not new to the human race. The earliest records of history chronicle many of the steps people have taken to beautify themselves through the ages. The ancient Egyptians valued cleanliness and used oils and lotions to anoint their skins. Cleopatra, for example, bathed in asses' milk as a method of keeping her skin soft and supple. The Old Testament contains numerous mentions of Hebrew health and beauty care practices.

The ancient Greeks, who gave us the word "cosmetics," from the Greek, "kosmetikos," believed in the value of cleanliness and used ointments and lotions widely. The Romans carried on those Greek traditions of health and beauty, constructing elaborate baths and also making extensive use of ointments and lotions.

The Dark Ages saw some lessening of the values of body care in western civilization, even though skin care was practiced to some extent. The Renaissance period, however, started the return to health and beauty care practice. The values of skin lotions and milk baths were well known and practiced by the wealthy through the seventeenth and eighteenth centuries, even though daily bathing was not commonplace. Fragrances were in wide use.

Personal hygiene came back into vogue from the middle of the nineteenth century, and has continued to the present time. Modern skin-care practices have been popular in Europe, especially in France and Germany, from the end of World War II. It is only in the last few years, however, that there has been increased interest in skin care in the United States, although there has long been a continuing emphasis on personal hygiene in modern America.

Modern skin care, as a cosmetics art and science, has moved away from its former position as a poor step-child of hair and nail care. It has become a full-fledged profession in its own right. And, like any profession, skin care will require more from its practitioners. The new esthetician will have to be more completely trained, more knowledgable about skin and its care than his or her beautician predecessor.

The growth of interest in skin care is shown by the increase in the promotional activities among the manufacturers of over-the-counter skin-care products. Almost every women's magazine runs a number of advertisements for skin-care products, along with many feature articles on various skin-care subjects. There are many commercials run on television and radio, as well. This promotional activity is an attempt to cash in on the ever increasing interest in skin care by the modern woman, who is better educated and more sophisticated than her sisters of a decade ago. This interest translates into annual retail sales of skin-care products amounting to billions of dollars. And this amount grows yearly.

There is also an increasing awareness that skin care is not just for women. Men, too, need to care for their skin, since it is just as subject to the effects of pollution, smoking and associated hazards.

ESTHETICS—A DEFINITION

Esthetics may be defined as the branch of cosmetology that treats the skin using nonmedical methods, for the purpose of beautifying the skin and keeping it healthy. As such, esthetics is a holistic endeavor because it recognizes that skin care is more than a superficial cleaning process. Rather, it takes into consideration the overall health of the individual because health affects the condition of the skin.

Under this view, skin care can be considered as a triad

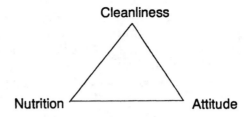

in which the three elements are at the corners of an equilateral triangle. No one element is more important than any other. They must all work equally together.

Cleanliness is vital to the external health of the skin. It is also necessary for the internal health of the body. Proper cleansing and normalization of the skin remove clogging and surface debris and help overcome problems caused by external factors.

Nutrition is important because the quality of the food consumed determines the quality of the energy produced and the efficiency of the various internal systems of the body, which in turn, affects the health of the skin and the body.

Attitude is important, because without the commitment of both the client and the esthetician to care for the skin and live in a manner that promotes well-being, the other two elements will be ineffectual.

THE ROLE OF ESTHETICS

Esthetics in the United States is a branch of cosmetology. As such, it is a licensed profession, under the jurisdiction of State Boards of Cosmetology. Licensing requirements vary from state to state, but generally, a practicing esthetician must hold a current cosmetologist's license. Some states recognize esthetics as a separate field.

Although esthetics is nonmedical in nature, it does interact, to a large extent, with the medical profession. It is a health care discipline as well as a cosmetological discipline and shares a commonality with **holistic** (ho-LIS-tik) medicine. It is a healing art rather than a healing science, as is modern **allopathic** (AL-o-path-ik) medicine.

The esthetician must recognize that he or she is not a physician and may not prescribe drugs, inject substances into the body, nor diagnose or treat disease conditions. This, properly, should be done only by a medical doctor, who is highly trained to do this work.

As a healing art, esthetics utilizes holistic health principles of wellness and disease prevention. The esthetician may treat certain skin conditions, apply topical lotions and creams—some of which are based on herbs and essential oils—and cleanse the skin to help remove blemishes. He or she may also suggest changes in dietary habits and offer nutrition guidelines that help the client achieve a more healthy state, which will be reflected in the skin.

Modern esthetics contains elements of both science and art. As a scientific discipline, it requires knowledge, study and an understanding of the basic principles of the physical sciences. As an art, it requires talent, experience, practice and an intuitive feel for the elements involved in the successful practice of skin care.

As a scientist, the esthetician tries to utilize the principles of physics and chemistry, along with an intimate knowledge of physiology to cleanse and normalize the skin so it performs its functions to the utmost efficiency. As an artist, the esthetician tries to prepare the perfect canvas for showing off the radiant glow of beauty.

BEAUTY AND HEALTH

As a practitioner of beauty care, the esthetician is concerned with the client's physical appearance. That "perfect canvas" the esthetician strives to create is not only for its own beauty, but also to prepare the face for the application of cosmetics to enhance the cultural reflection of beauty.

Beauty is largely a cultural phenomenon. What passes for beauty varies from age to age and from culture to culture. The adage that "beauty is in the eye of the beholder" is quite appropriate, since beauty is largely defined as what is pleasing to the eye of the receiver rather than as an absolute. In *The Sense of Beauty*, George Santayana defines beauty as "a value, that is, it is not a perception of a matter of fact or of a relation: it is an emotion, an affection of our volitional and appreciative nature."

The concept of beauty in western civilization stems from the ancient Greek concepts of symmetry and proportion, which were reflected in their art and writings. In "Timaeus," from *The Collected Dialogues of Plato*, Plato, for example, says "Everything that is good is fair, and the fair is not without proportion, and the animal which is to be fair must have due proportion" (Fig. 1.1).

The classical unit of proportion was the head length, and the well proportioned body was 7½ head lengths tall (Fig. 1.2). The head is trisected with one-third of the distance from the hairline to the eyebrows, one-third from the eyebrows to the tip of the nose, and the remaining one-third from the tip of the nose to the chin. The face is divided vertically into five equal parts, each being the width of an eye. With relatively minor variations, this sense of proportion has remained to the present day (Fig. 1.3), page 6.

As a holistic health practitioner, however, the esthetician is also concerned with the client's health, because beauty is health. One cannot be beautiful unless he or she feels beautiful. And one cannot feel beautiful unless he or she is healthy, both mentally and physically. Good health promotes well-being. Thus, today's esthetician also attempts to bring the inner being into balance to promote overall health.

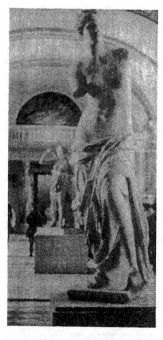

1.1—Venus de Milo

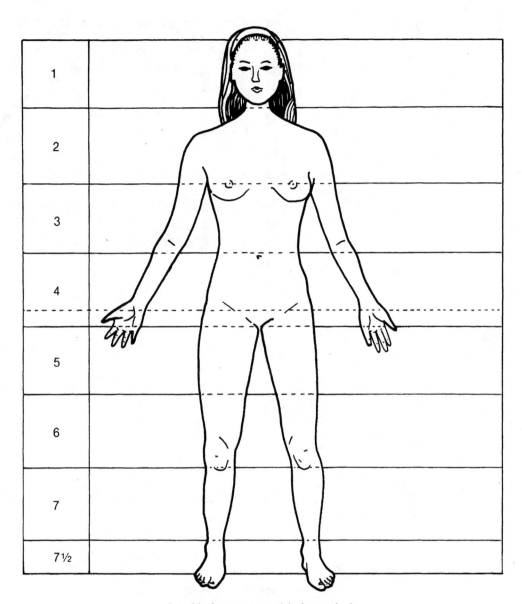

1
2
3
4
5
6
7
7½

1.2—Ideal proportions of the human body

Mental health is as important as physical health. State-of-mind can directly affect the health of the skin. Many organically caused skin disorders, such as acne, while not life-threatening, present profound psychological problems for the afflicted person. On the other hand, tension, aggravation and frustration can manifest externally as skin disorders. So, it is as important for the esthetician to be aware of the client's mental state and to encourage relaxation during the facial as it is to cleanse and normalize the skin.

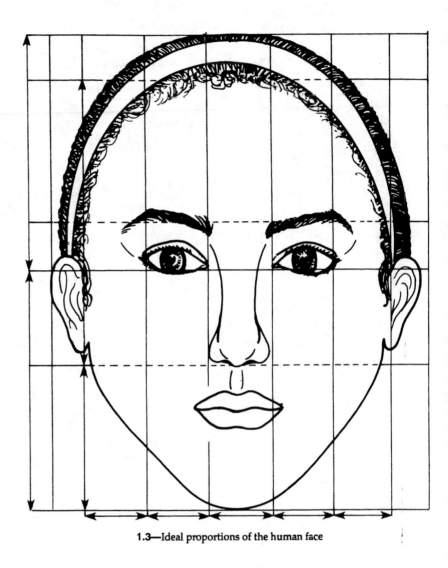

1.3—Ideal proportions of the human face

THE ESTHETICIAN

Esthetics is a multi-faceted discipline. Because of the breadth of subject matter relevant to the proper practice of esthetics, today's esthetician must be part chemist, part biologist, part therapist, part psychologist, part beautician and part salesperson, blending knowledge from all of these diverse elements into a coherent system for effective skin-care treatments.

The esthetician must have a well-rounded background, with basic training in the physical sciences and a thorough understanding of skin structure and function and of skin disorders and their causes. He or she must also be well versed in the use and composition of skin-care products and the proper use of machinery used in facials.

In addition, the esthetician must have a solid grasp of nutrition, human physiology and massage techniques. Not the least of the skills to be mastered is a grasp of psychology and of salesmanship.

The physical sciences—chemistry, physics and biology—are important because all aspects of skin care are based on the principles of these sciences. Chemistry, for example, explains the mechanisms that allow the various skin-care products to work effectively; physics explains the workings of much of the machinery; biology explains the effects of bacteria, the need for sanitation, and puts the human condition into its proper perspective.

The physical sciences contain all the elements of science—observation, measurement and experimentation. They also, however, contain many elements of philosophy—intuition, speculation and imagination. The scientist can afford to overlook the philosophical factors while discussing the purely physical factors—the measurable aspects—of science. The esthetician cannot afford to discount these factors. The effective esthetician is one who can transcend the purely physical aspects and utilize artistic sensitivities to meld the elements of the physical arts and the physical sciences, bringing both to bear on the profession.

Skin care cannot be practiced as a purely mechanical discipline. It must be practiced with sensitivity and empathy, as well.

The skin is the material with which the esthetician works, so knowledge of the structure and function of skin and about skin disorders is essential. By understanding how the skin works and by being able to recognize different disorders, the esthetician will be able to treat clients in the most effective manner.

And, since the skin-care products and machinery are the tools of the esthetician's profession, he or she must understand their use in order to utilize them most effectively.

An understanding of nutrition is important to the esthetician because diet directly affects the health of the skin. In addition, the esthetician should be able to counsel clients on their dietary habits to help their skin conditions.

Massage is an important part of skin-care treatment. Knowledge of the various techniques, coupled with a knowledge of human physiology, allows the esthetician to develop an effective style of massage that will most benefit clients.

A grasp of psychology is important to let the esthetician recognize the emotional states that may affect the client's skin and to help the client relax during the treatment. Psychology is also allied with salesmanship. The esthetician also must be a good salesperson to sell himself or herself to the client, so the client will have confidence in the services the esthetician will perform.

QUALITIES OF A PROFESSIONAL ESTHETICIAN

If a good esthetician could be summed up in one word, that word would be "professional." The overriding quality that sets the good esthetician apart from the others is a totally professional attitude and bearing in all aspects of skin care. A number of characteristics contribute to a professional attitude. These include:

- Appearance—The professional esthetician always presents a good appearance. He or she is clean and well-groomed, and is dressed in unwrinkled, clean clothes that are appropriate for the occasion. This may be a white uniform or white lab coat. Whether standing or sitting, posture is correct.

- Manner—The professional esthetician comports himself or herself with the proper demeanor. He or she is always courteous and friendly toward the client, but is never overly familiar. The esthetician must be cheerful at all times, must be attentive to the client's needs without being subservient and should feel good about the profession. Above all, the esthetician must have pride in the art and science of esthetics.

- Knowledge—The professional esthetician is intelligent and has a firm grasp of current techniques and practices of skin care. He or she has the background knowledge necessary to perform effectively. The esthetician is curious about the world and about people and recognizes that the learning process never ends. The professional esthetician keeps up-to-date by constantly reading books and magazines on skin care and related subjects, by attending trade shows devoted to the beauty industry, by attending seminars, and by taking an active part in professional skin-care organizations.

- Talent—The professional esthetician has a natural talent for and interest in the field of esthetics. As with most arts, the esthetician has not so much chosen to become a skin-care specialist as he or she has been chosen by the discipline. Talent alone, however, is not enough. The esthetician must also have adequate training and guidance.

- Confidence—The professional esthetician must have confidence in his or her judgment and ability. This confidence comes from focused talent; that is, ability sharpened through training, practice and knowledge.

- Creativity—The professional esthetician is innovative and has the ability to develop new techniques to fit the situation. Innovation is fueled by understanding and knowledge. Creativity, the ability to innovate, sets the professional esthetician apart from the competition.

- Empathy—The professional esthetician cares about other people and genuinely wants to help clients have better looking, healthier skin and feel better about themselves. The professional esthetician is a good listener and hears what the client has to say. The esthetician is observant as well, and can communicate so the client understands the processes involved. The professional esthetician is a giving person, capable of sharing knowledge with peers and with clients, giving back to the profession more than is taken away from it.

- Trustworthiness—Professional estheticians value their reputation and maintain a scrupulous honesty. They never lie to a client or misrepresent the services to be given or the results to be obtained.

Esthetics is a satisfying and rewarding profession. Those who have the talent and desire will become successful estheticians, far surpassing those who are content to merely give superficial salon facials.

REVIEW QUESTIONS

1. Define esthetics.
2. What are the three elements of a successful skin-care program?
3. Why is attitude important?
4. How does esthetics interact with the medical profession?
5. Is esthetics a science or an art?
6. What is beauty?
7. What is the classical measure of proportion in beauty?
8. Why is health important in beauty care?
9. What knowledge must the esthetician have to practice successfully?
10. What characteristics let the esthetician project a professional attitude?

2 Introduction to the Facial

OBJECTIVES   *After completing this chapter, you should be able to:*

❶ Describe the equipment used in the facial.
❷ Briefly discuss each step in the facial.
❸ Describe the subjects an esthetician must know to give a proper facial.
❹ Understand the machinery and the products involved.

INTRODUCTION   The facial is the cornerstone of esthetics. It is the key to effective skin care in the salon. More than any other aspect of the profession, the properly administered facial treatment will be the basis of the day-to-day work of the practicing esthetician.

The facial is a multi-step process designed to cleanse the client's skin, alleviate minor disorders, and normalize its function. Properly given, the facial will also make the client feel good. No matter what other services the esthetician performs, the facial will make or break a professional reputation.

To give a facial properly, the esthetician must know the procedures to use, the products to use, which equipment to use and how to use it. He or she must be able to identify skin types and skin problems and must know how to handle them. And the esthetician must know the theory of skin care to understand why a technique is performed in a certain way and to develop the capability to build on experience.

Estheticians must possess the licenses appropriate to the state in which they work. In addition, they must be aware of local ordinances and laws applicable in the state, especially with respect to health, sanitation practices, and safety requirements.

This chapter serves as an introduction to the chapters that follow. It gives an overview to the facial so the practitioner can get quickly into the practical aspects of esthetics. At the same time, the chapter sets the stage for the more detailed discussions to follow.

EQUIPMENT REQUIREMENTS

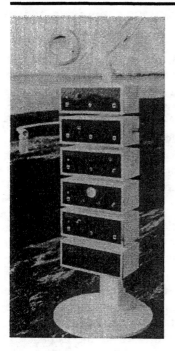

2.1—Typical rack of equipment (*Courtesy of Proteus, Inc.*)

Except for a suitable chair for the client, facials can be given without the use of equipment or machinery. The proper equipment, however, makes the procedure more efficient and more effective. There is a wide array of specialized machinery for the esthetician. Each type serves a particular purpose. The esthetician should know what equipment to use, when to use it, and how to use each to its maximum effectiveness.

There are a number of different manufacturers of skin-care machinery. As with the chemical products, it pays to use the best equipment available. Before choosing equipment, the esthetician should read the literature available from various manufacturers, and if possible, test the equipment.

It is not necessary to get all equipment at one time. If capital is limited, the esthetician can purchase the most important pieces first, then add other pieces as business warrants or the need arises.

Many manufacturers provide the equipment as a package in self-contained racks. These racks hold the equipment together and allow more efficient access to the various pieces during the facial treatment (Fig. 2.1). Skin-care equipment is discussed fully in Chapter 16.

While machinery may not be necessary for a facial, a chemical product is. The right product for the client's skin type—individually tailored—is extremely important. Just as it is important to use the best equipment, so is it important to use the best possible products. Skin-care products are discussed fully in Chapter 12.

THE FACIAL

In its simplest terms, a facial can be divided into two parts: deep pore cleansing, the process of removing impurities from the skin; and normalization and treatment, the process of putting nutrients back into the skin. The facial mask is a transition between the two parts—a bridge from one step to the other, since masks can perform both functions.

Before the facial is started, however, it is necessary to consult with clients and thoroughly analyze their skin to determine what problems may exist and to formulate the proper treatment.

Once the analysis is completed and the course of treatment developed, the facial can begin. In general, the facial consists of the following steps:

1. deep-pore cleansing, which includes application of cleanser with rotary brushing, removal of the cleanser, application of a toner or astringent, massage, steaming, disincrustation, vacuum application, and manual extraction;
2. the facial mask application;
3. normalization or treatment, which includes iontophoresis, use of high-frequency current, spray application of nutrients, and application of moisturizer or treatment products.

It is important to note that not all the steps described will be performed in every facial. Each skin type requires a different set of procedures, so the steps will vary from facial to facial. For example, a client with acne will require more emphasis on manual extraction; a client with dry skin would possibly skip manual extraction and vacuum but emphasize spray application and the facial mask.

After the facial is completed, a post-consultation step is necessary to assess the results of the treatment and to build the foundation for a good future relationship with the client.

Consultation and Analysis

In consultation and analysis, the esthetician gathers the information about the client necessary to determine the proper course of action. The esthetician asks the client a series of questions about health, dietary habits, lifestyle, and skin care.

Communication is the key to success during the consultation as the esthetician develops a rapport with the client. It is a two-way relationship. While the esthetician learns about the client, the client also learns about the esthetician and develops confidence in the esthetician's knowledge and ability. It is the esthetician's opportunity to educate the client about skin care and about what may be reasonably expected.

In the analysis phase, the esthetician examines the client's skin to determine its type and condition. After removing makeup or superficial dirt, the esthetician, using a magnifying lamp, checks for blemishes, pore size, texture and other obvious indications of condition (Fig. 2.2). After using the magnifying lamp, the esthetician may use a Wood's lamp as a further check on the client's skin condition (Fig. 2.3). The Wood's lamp utilizes black light, under which certain skin conditions fluoresce as different colors (Table 2.1).

Deep Pore Cleansing

In the deep pore cleansing step of the facial, dirt, excess sebum and other impurities are removed from the skin. In addition, ripe pimples and some other blemishes are extracted manually.

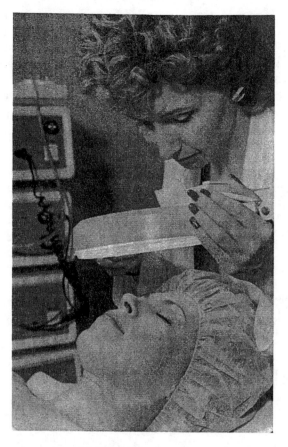

2.2—Magnifying lamp in use

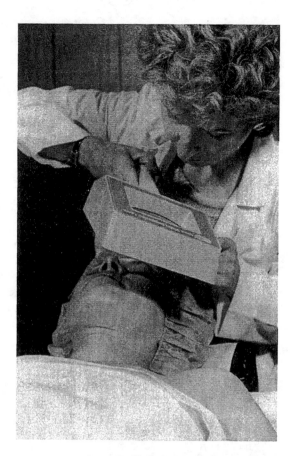

2.3—Wood's lamp in use

TABLE 2.1—Wood's Lamp Indications

FLUORESCENT COLOR	SKIN TYPE
Blue-white	Normal
Light to deep purple	Dry
Orange	Oily
White	Dead cells
Brown	Pigmentation
Orange	Clogged pores and comedones
White	Dandruff

Cleanser Application. The first step in cleansing is the application of a cleanser suitable for the client's skin type. The cleanser is applied with the hands or with viscous sponges and worked into the skin with a rotary brush (Fig. 2.4). If the rotary brush is not used, the cleanser should be worked into the skin thoroughly by hand.

After that, the cleanser is removed with tepid water, and a toner or astringent is applied to remove all traces of the cleanser. Once the cleanser has been removed, the massage step can begin.

Massage. The massage is probably the most pleasant stage of the facial. The facial massage relaxes the client and helps prepare the skin for the steps that follow. It both soothes and stimulates the skin and helps the skin rid itself of waste materials. Properly performed, the massage helps the body balance its energy. Good massage technique relies on a series of stroking, friction, kneading and tapping movements, done in a smooth, firm but gentle, rhythmic manner. The movements are performed in a logical sequence.

A small amount of warmed massage cream is applied to the face. The massage should begin with light contact, which gradually builds in pressure. Facial massage theory is covered in Chapter 9.

Steaming. Steaming loosens dead surface cells and softens embedded dirt and sebum. It also relaxes the pores and softens the skin (Fig. 2.5). Since the vaporizer requires some time to warm up, it

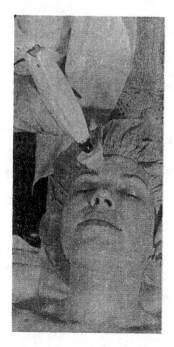

2.4—Use of rotary brush

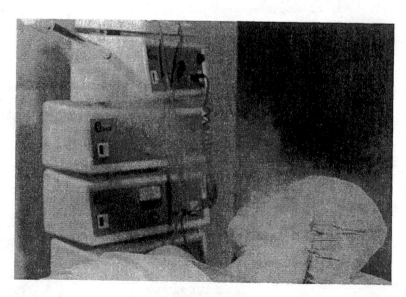

2.5—Use of steamer

should be turned on just before the massage is finished. After the massage, all traces of massage cream must be removed so the steam will penetrate. If a vaporizer is not used, the steaming can be accomplished with a series of hot towel compresses (Fig. 2.6).

Disincrustation. The disincrustation step utilizes the galvanic current machine to soften hardened sebum in the pores. An alkaline disincrustation solution is applied to the skin and the electric current helps it penetrate (Fig. 2.7). This step can be performed with a series of cotton compresses soaked in the solution, but it is not as effective as using the galvanic current. Disincrustation is only done on oily, blemished skin. It is not necessary on dry skin.

Vacuum. The vacuum side of the vacuum/spray machine is next used to remove excess oil and loose dirt from the skin (Fig. 2.8). As with disincrustation, this step is used only on oily or blemished skin. Before vacuuming, it is necessary to make sure the skin is free of cleansers or lotions that could clog the machine.

Manual Extraction. Everything done to this point has prepared the skin for manual extraction, the physical removal of blackheads, pimples and other blemishes from the skin. The degree of manual extraction necessary will vary according to the type of skin and the amount of blemishes to be removed. Manual extraction is the most unpleasant, but one of the most important, parts of the facial. Using

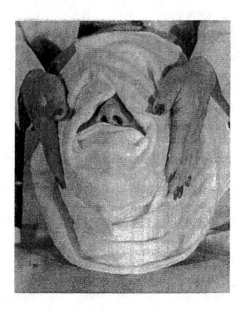

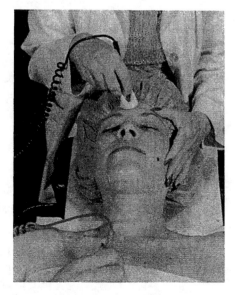

2.6—Steaming with hot towels   2.7—Disincrustation with galvanic current

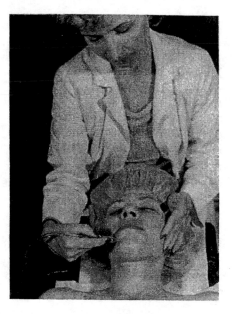

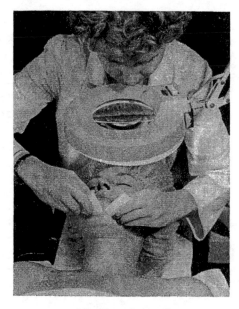

2.8—Use of vacuum

2.9—Manual extraction

the magnifying lamp, the esthetician gently removes blemishes with light to moderate pressure. Only the fingers, covered with cotton pads soaked in antiseptic, are used for this step (Fig. 2.9). Metal instruments should never be used. Once manual extraction is finished, a mild antiseptic should be applied to the skin.

Facial Mask The mask, which serves as a transition between the cleansing process and the normalization process, performs the functions of both processes. Depending on the type used, the mask can remove impurities from the skin, absorb excess oil, soothe or stimulate the skin, nourish the skin, or tighten the skin to remove small wrinkles temporarily.

Masks may be made from a wide variety of substances. Clays, muds, algaes, wax, creams, collagen and wheat germ are just some of the ingredients used. The wide variety gives the esthetician a considerable choice in picking a mask suited to the client's needs. Facial masks are discussed in detail in Chapter 13.

Normalization and Treatment In the normalization stage of the facial, the skin is nourished, revitalized and protected. Cleansing has opened the skin to the environment and removed its surface oils. This stage puts nutrients back into the skin.

Iontophoresis. Nutrients are put back into the skin through iontophoresis. This is done with the same galvanic current machine used for disincrustation, except now, the polarity of the current is reversed. A small amount, usually about two or three drops, of a water-soluble treatment product is lightly massaged into the skin. Then the working electrode of the galvanic current machine is gently moved over the client's face so the product will penetrate (Fig. 2.10). Iontophoresis can be used on any type of skin.

High-Frequency Application. The high-frequency machine increases circulation and helps the skin absorb treatment products and nutrients by stimulating the skin with high-frequency current. The ozone generated by the current also has germicidal properties and helps kill bacteria on the skin.

The current can be applied directly by placing the electrode on the client's face (Fig. 2.11). It may also be applied indirectly by having the client hold the electrode while the esthetician massages the treatment product into the skin (Fig. 2.12). In addition, the electrode can be held a short distance away from the skin, producing a spark that helps promote healing.

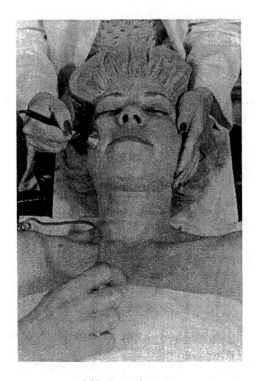

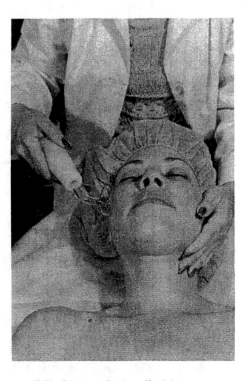

2.10—Iontophoresis   **2.11**—Direct application of high frequency

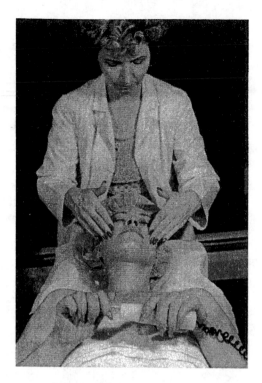

2.12—Indirect application of high frequency

Spray Application. The spray has a number of purposes during the facial. After cleansing, it helps remove cleanser or massage cream. After manual extraction, it helps soothe the skin. At the end of the facial, it nourishes and refreshes the skin. Toners, astringents, or liquid treatment products suitable for the client's skin and for the result required may be applied with the spray attachment of the vacuum/spray machine, the electric pulverisator, or with a hand pumped spray applicator (Fig. 2.13).

Treatment Product Application. At the end of the facial, a suitable treatment cream—such as a moisturizer, oil absorber, or pH balancer—is applied to the client's face. A small amount of the product is lightly massaged into the skin (Fig. 2.14). After this step, the client can change into street clothes and go through the posttreatment consultation.

Posttreatment Consultation   In many ways, the posttreatment consultation is as important as every step that preceded it. In this step, the esthetician has an opportunity to assess the treatment and to answer any questions the client may have. The esthetician may also use this time to outline a home treatment regimen for the client, suggest products for home use, and to set up an appointment for the next facial.

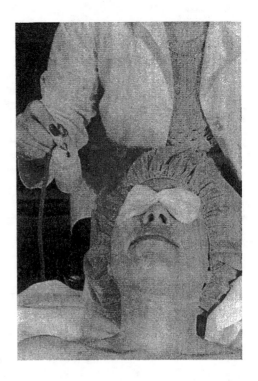

2.13—Spray with machine atomizer

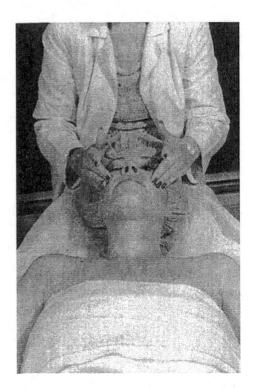

2.14—Application of treatment product

REVIEW
QUESTIONS

1. How important is the facial in esthetics?
2. What is a facial?
3. What must an esthetician know to give a facial properly?
4. Are equipment and products necessary for a facial?
5. What is the value of equipment in a facial?
6. What are the two basic parts of the facial?
7. What is the difference between the two parts?
8. What must the esthetician do before starting a facial?
9. What are the steps involved in a facial?
10. Are all of these steps necessary in every facial?

3 Bacteriology and Sanitation

OBJECTIVES   *After completing this chapter, you should be able to:*

❶ Discuss bacteriology and the microbes that cause disease.

❷ Discuss the body's immune system, which helps it fight disease.

❸ Describe sanitation measures, including waste disposal problems, and discuss the use of instruments such as lancets and comedone extractors.

❹ Discuss safety measures in the salon.

❺ Discuss government regulations and their effects on the salon.

INTRODUCTION

For the esthetician, cleanliness is of paramount importance. Sanitation prevents disease, an important consideration when working on the skin. To understand sanitation, it is necessary to understand bacteria and how they can affect health, and to be aware of the workings of the immune system in the body. The esthetician must be aware of the factors that cause and lead to the spread of disease, and how to control or eliminate those factors.

In the course of daily operations, estheticians come in contact with a variety of chemical substances, heat, and sharp implements. It is important that they know how to handle these materials effectively and safely. Also, many of the operations generate waste materials. So, it is important to know how to dispose of these waste products properly.

Many of the sanitation and safety procedures are mandated by a host of local, state and federal government rules and regulations. The esthetician must be aware of and comply with these various laws. Failure to obey these rules can result in a wide variety of penalties, ranging from fines to loss of licenses. And ignorance of the laws is not an excuse.

BACTERIOLOGY

Some bacteria are **saprophytes** (SAP-ro-fyts), that is, they take nourishment from dead organic matter; others are **parasites** (PAR-ah-syts), which take their nourishment from living organisms. The saprophytes are generally nonpathogenic, while the parasites are usually the causes of disease. Some bacteria are **motile** (MO-tyle), or capable of movement either through their own actions or through the action of flagella, hair-like appendages that move back and forth. Others are not capable of movement. These are said to be **nonmotile** (non-MO-tyle).

Most bacteria are reproduced asexually, multiplying by binary fission. When the cell reaches its maximum growth, it divides into two cells, which then continue to grow. Under ideal conditions, a single bacterium could multiply into more than 2 million bacteria in a day. A few bacteria reproduce sexually.

Bacteria thrive under warm, dark, damp and dirty conditions where there is an abundance of food. When conditions for growth are disrupted, some bacteria die, and others form **spores** (SPORZ), almost indestructible cells that are unaffected by boiling, freezing or treatment with disinfectants.

The smallest known form of life, bacteria belong to the phylum **Schizomycetes** (SKIZ-o-my-see-teez). There are five classes in this phylum, each consisting of a number of species. The classes are: eubacteria, myxobacteria, spirochetes, rickettsiae and actinomycetes.

The **myxobacteria** (MIKS-oh-bak-te-ree-ah) and **rickettsia** (ri-KET-see-ah) are the least important to the esthetician, since they play little or no part in skin function or disease. The myxobacteria, or **slime bacteria** (slym bak-TEER-i-ah), live in the soil in colonies. These motile, rod-shaped bacteria are saprophytic, taking nourishment from dead organic matter. The rickettsiae, the smallest of the bacteria, are nonmotile parasites that live in ticks and mites. They are responsible for such diseases as Rocky Mountain spotted fever and typhus.

The **actinomycetes** (ACK-tin-no-my-see-tes), like the slime bacteria, are saprophytes that live in the soil. They differ, however, in their structure and in that they are nonmotile. A few members of this class cause disease. **Mycobacterium tuberculosis** (MY-ko-bak-TEER-i-um tu-BER-ku-lo-sis), for example, causes tuberculosis in humans. The actinomycetes are of minor interest to the esthetician, however, because of their use in the commercial production of some antibiotics, especially tetracycline, used in the medical treatment of acne.

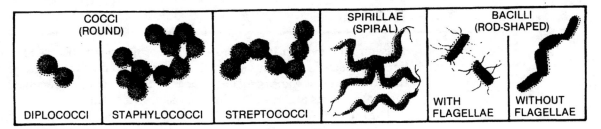

3.1—Bacterial shapes

The **spirochetes** (SPY-ro-keet-ees) are of importance since these microbes are mostly disease producers. These highly motile bacteria are long and curved, and move in a corkscrew motion. **Treponema pallidum** (trep-o-NE-mah PAL-i-dum) is the spirochete responsible for the disease, syphilis.

The esthetician, however, will be principally concerned with the class of **eubacteria** (U-bak-teer-i-ah), especially with the primary disease-causing species. These include the **bacilli** (ba-SIL-i), the **cocci** (KOK-si), and the **spirillae** (spi-RIL-a), which derive their names from their shapes. The bacilli, the most numerous, are rod shaped. Many have tail-like flagellae for locomotion. These bacteria are responsible for diseases such as tetanus and influenza (Fig. 3.1).

The cocci are round bacteria that grow in pairs, **diplococci** (dip-lo-KOK-si), in chains, **streptococci** (strep-to-KOK-si), or in clusters, **staphylococci** (staf-i-lo-KOK-si). They are largely nonmotile. Diplococci are responsible for diseases such as pneumonia; streptococci for infection, for example, the "strep throat;" and staphylococci for pus-forming infections, such as boils and abscesses. The spirilla are motile, spiral shaped bacteria.

Bacteria are not the only disease-causing organisms of concern to the esthetician. Like most pathogenic bacteria, viruses are infectious parasites. **Viruses** (VI-rus), however, are not living organisms and can only exist and reproduce inside living cells. **Virions** (VI-ree-ons), the name given to virus particles, are sub-microscopic, ranging from ¼ the size of a single bacterium to much smaller. They can be seen under the electron microscope. Each virion consists of a protein shell surrounding a core of nucleic acid, which may be either deoxyriboneucleic acid (DNA) or ribonucleic acid (RNA).

DNA-viruses are responsible for such diseases as herpes simplex, venereal herpes, shingles and some tumors. This type also causes warts. RNA-viruses are responsible for such diseases as measles, mumps, polio, and meningitis, as well as the common cold. DNA-viruses reproduce in the nuclei of living cells; RNA-viruses reproduce in the cell cytoplasm.

THE IMMUNE SYSTEM

The immune system is the body's watchdog against disease. The various specialized organs and cells that make up the system guard the body against the organisms that invade it, killing or repelling those organisms and keeping the body safe and healthy.

The immune system is not a physical system of organs in the same physiological sense of the nervous system, the circulatory system, or other systems of the body, as will be discussed in Chapter 5. Rather, it is a complex infrastructure of highly specialized organs and cells spread throughout and moving throughout the body as they are needed to counter invading organisms. Like watchdogs on patrol, they keep the entire inner body under surveillance, ready to attack on demand.

The basic units of the immune system are **lymphocytes** (LIM-fo-seyets), or white blood cells, based in the lymph nodes and spleen, but also moving freely throughout the body in the bloodstream. These cells start in the bone marrow and grow into specialized cells, such as the **T-lymphocytes** (T-LIM-fo-seyets), which help regulate the system, have the ability to recognize foreign bodies, and attack disease organisms, and the **B-lymphocytes** (B-LIM-fo-seyets), which produce **antibodies** (AN-tee-ba-dees), which fight **antigens** (AN-tee-jen), organisms that cause immune responses. The T-lymphocytes grow in the thymus gland; the B-lymphocytes grow in the tonsils and lymph nodes.

When a foreign organism enters the body, a complex series of events occurs. As the organism moves about, it will eventually encounter a T-lymphocyte, which will recognize it as an invader. The T-lymphocyte will alert the B-lymphocytes, which will start making antibodies that move through the bloodstream to fight the organism. At the same time, other T-lymphocytes will gather at the point of infection to coordinate the attack and help the antibodies kill or drive off the invader.

When the immune system does not work properly, the invading organism propagates and spreads and the body becomes sick. When this happens, outside agents, medicines, are used to suppress the infection and help the immune system get back into operation.

PREVENTION OF INFECTIOUS DISEASES

The prevention of infectious diseases should be at the top of the esthetician's mind. Infectious, or contagious, diseases are spread from one person to another through contact. The way to prevent the spread of these diseases is to avoid that contact and to maintain scrupulous cleanliness and sanitary procedures and standards. The esthetician will never work on a client who has an obvious infectious disease, but will refer that client to a physician. And as a matter of good professional practice, he or she will wash and sterilize all equipment used during a facial and will promptly place used materials in covered waste receptacles.

These days, however, the esthetician must be aware of diseases that may not be so evident. These include **AIDS** (AYDS), or Acquired Immune Deficiency Syndrome. The **HIV** (H-I-V) (the AIDS virus), the antibody that causes the disease, kills T-lymphocytes, rendering the immune system helpless and leaving the body prey to a wide variety of infections and diseases. The disease is always fatal. The AIDS virus is transmitted through blood or other body fluids, usually either through sexual contact or sharing of needles. The chance of transmission of AIDS by any other means, according to the Centers for Disease Control, is small.

Although the risk is small, there are some instances during the facial, especially during manual extraction, where the esthetician can come into contact with the client's blood. At these times, especially, the esthetician may want to consider using latex rubber gloves, even though the sense of touch may be slightly diminished. The esthetician may also consider wearing a surgical mask during many of the procedures.

Sanitation
The importance of sanitation to stopping the spread of disease was little understood, even by the medical profession, until the middle of the 19th century. In 1850, Ignatz Semmelweis, a German physician, was able to stop a series of fevers in his hospital by the simple expedient of having the doctors wash their hands before touching their next patients. In 1861, Louis Pasteur proved that germs cause disease and made a number of discoveries that helped prevent diseases. Since then, great advances have eliminated many serious diseases that were deadly scourges generations ago. Polio and diphtheria, for example, diseases that crippled or killed thousands of victims, have been virtually eradicated through the use of vaccines.

Even with these medical advances, however, sanitation is no less important today. The practice of proper sanitation procedures is vital to the success of the skin-care salon. The salon, itself, must be kept spotlessly clean, as must the implements used by the esthetician. The esthetician must wear clean clothing and make sure that hair and body are clean, also. Hands should be washed with soap and hot water and sanitized with alcohol before beginning work on a client.

Sanitation has two phases: sterilization, killing existing bacteria and viruses, and prevention, keeping new germs from growing. Towels and smocks, for example, must be washed in detergent and hot water and then be stored in a closed, dry area. Implements must be washed in hot, soapy water and rinsed or wiped with alcohol

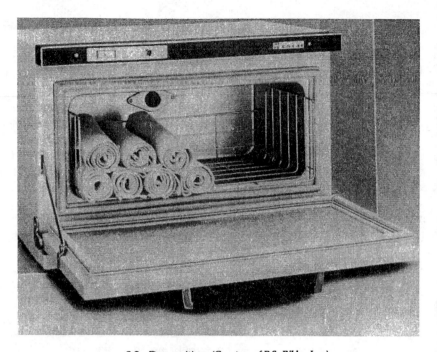

3.2—Dry sanitizer *(Courtesy of P.S. Pibbs, Inc.)*

after use and then be stored in a dry sanitizer, a closed cabinet containing a fumigant or an ultraviolet light source (Fig. 3.2 and Fig. 3.3).

Sterilization may be accomplished through the use of heat, ultraviolet light, gamma radiation, or with chemicals. Heat may be moist, as in boiling or steaming, or dry, as in baking. High heat is effective in killing germs, but it may have an adverse effect on many im-

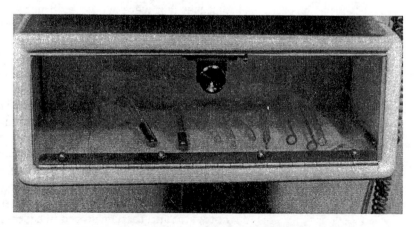

3.3—Dry sanitizer on rack *(Courtesy of Universal Techniques, Inc.)*

plements, especially those made of plastic. Steam sterilization is usually carried out in an **autoclave,** an instrument that combines steam with high pressure.

Short-wave ultraviolet light is effective in killing germs and is used in commercially available dry cabinet sanitizers and industrial germicidal lamps. Gamma radiation is also an effective germicide, but the equipment required is large and expensive, so its use is limited to the medical field.

Chemical sterilizing agents include fumigants, antiseptics, and disinfectants. **Fumigants** (FYOO-mi-gant) are chemical fumes that have the ability to kill germs. **Antiseptics** (an-ti-SEP-tik) and **disinfectants** (dis-in-FEK-tant) are liquid or dry chemical germicides. They differ only in degree. Antiseptics are generally milder than disinfectants and can be used safely on the skin. Isopropyl alcohol (99%), boric acid, hydrogen peroxide (3%), sodium hypochlorite (bleach), and some soaps are commonly used antiseptics. Quaternary ammonium compounds (quats), formaldehyde, ethyl alcohol (70%), cresol and phenol are commonly used disinfectants. Formaldehyde and formalin, a formaldehyde derivative, have been popular disinfectants for salon use. Formaldehyde has been suspected as a **carcinogen** (kar-SIN-o-gen), but recent studies have indicated that it is safe to use, as long as it is used carefully. When using any chemical product, read and follow the manufacturer's instructions.

State cosmetology boards and local health departments should be consulted for recommendations on safe and effective germicides for use in the salon. Manufacturers' instructions for commercial germicides should be followed.

Sanitary and Waste Disposal Procedures

Proper sanitary and waste disposal procedures are also important. During the course of a facial, the esthetician generates a considerable amount of waste, both reusable and disposable. These must be handled safely and efficiently, to avoid risk of contamination.

Reusable cloth items, such as towels and smocks, should be placed in a closed container after they are used. These items should be washed in hot water, dried with heat, folded and stored in a closed cabinet or dry sterilizer until used again. Reusable metal or plastic implements should be washed in hot soapy water and sterilized with alcohol or other disinfectant after use, then stored in a dry or fumigant sterilizer.

Where feasible, disposable rather than reusable items should be used. For example, it is more sanitary to use disposable bonnets, which are discarded after use on one client, than it is to wrap the client's head with towels (Fig. 3.4). Disposable items should be placed in a closed trash receptacle immediately after use. Trash should not be allowed to accumulate in the salon, but should be periodically bagged in heavy duty plastic trash bags, tightly sealed

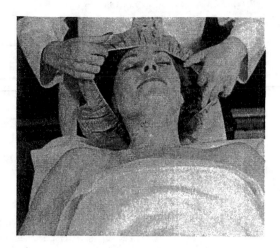

3.4—Use of the disposable bonnet

and disposed of according to local ordinances, either through municipal or private trash collection services or disposal in legal landfills. The waste products generated in the salon will rarely be considered as hazardous. However, the esthetician should be especially cautious when disposing of used lancets or other sharp implements. These should be wrapped so they can't become a danger to anyone handling the trash.

When it comes to sanitation procedures, common sense should prevail. Most measures are obvious. Clean and sanitize facial chairs and implements after each client. Don't put products back in their containers after taking them out. Wash and sanitize hands before and after each client. Sweep, scrub, and disinfect floors as needed. Keep the salon spotlessly clean. Establish a definite cleaning schedule. And follow it.

Sanitation and Safety in Manual Extraction

The manual extraction phase is one of the most important parts of the facial. It is the step that involves the physical removal of blackheads, milia, and ripe pimples from the skin. Though vital, this step is often the most unpleasant part of the facial for the client and the step that can cause the most trouble for the esthetician. It is the most invasive part of the facial and is the step during which the esthetician is most likely to come into contact with the client's blood and debris from the skin. Sanitation and cleanliness are especially critical at this juncture.

Before starting manual extraction, the hands must be clean and sterilized with alcohol. Protect the client's eyes from the bright light of the magnifying lamp by covering them with damp cotton pads. Only the index fingers should be used to remove blemishes. Metallic comedone extractors should never be used. They exert too much

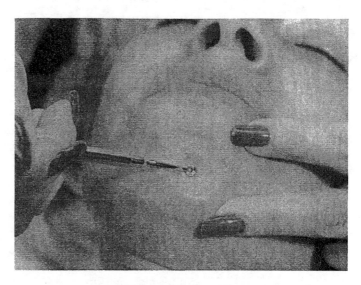

3.5—Misuse of comedone extractor

force and damage the skin easily (Fig. 3.5). Cover the index fingers with a thin layer of cotton dampened with an antiseptic such as witch hazel. If a stronger antiseptic is used, make sure the client is not sensitive to it.

Place the fingers on either side of the blemish and apply pressure toward the blemish. Don't force the issue. If the blemish doesn't come out with moderate pressure, it isn't ready for extraction. Don't give up too easily, but don't overdo it either. The object is to remove the blemish, not to cause pain or damage the skin (Fig. 3.6).

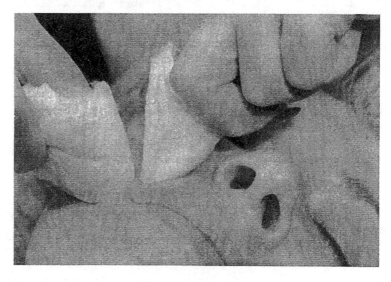

3.6—Manual extraction

In some cases, the wall of the blemish may be weakened by gently scraping the surface with a sterile **lancet** (LAN-set). A lancet is a small device that looks like a razor blade or like a needle. They are disposable implements, supplied in sterile packages. Although designed as medical devices, they may be used by estheticians in a limited fashion, as long as the skin is not penetrated.

The lancet should be opened, then applied to the blemish with the point parallel to the surface of the skin. Carefully scrape the point of the lancet against the blemish. Take care not to penetrate the skin. After using the lancet, dispose of it properly. Never reuse a lancet. Regulations governing the use of lancets vary from state to state. Check with the local State Board of Cosmetology for applicable regulations.

After finishing the manual extractions, discard the cotton on the fingers and the cotton eye pads and wash and sanitize the hands again. Then apply a mild antiseptic to the client's skin to kill germs and protect the skin.

SAFETY IN THE SALON

Safety should also be a key concern of the esthetician. During the course of a facial, the esthetician comes in contact with heat, water, steam, and electricity. He or she must be aware of the potential hazards involved with any of these. Heat and steam pose burn hazards; water can cause slipping, electricity can be a shock hazard. The esthetician must keep the client and himself or herself safe.

Safety is largely a matter of awareness—of being safety conscious and using common sense. It is a matter of good housekeeping. Spills should be wiped up as soon as they occur, before anyone can slip and fall. Trash and debris should not be allowed to accumulate, but should be disposed of promptly and properly. Vaporizers and other heat sources should be monitored closely when they are being used so the client doesn't get burned. Lights should be covered to cut glare and as protection if the bulb should break. Passageways should be uncluttered to prevent accidents. All equipment should be maintained in good working condition. Electrical circuits shouldn't be overloaded. Electrical machinery should be kept away from water to prevent short circuits.

Electrical circuits, whether in house wiring or in appliances, are protected against overloads by fuses or circuit breakers. When the current draw becomes too high for the circuit, the fuse blows before the wiring can overheat and cause a fire. Fuses are important safety devices. Don't use fuses that are too large for the circuit. Never bypass a fuse by inserting a metallic object into the fuse holder.

Before replacing a fuse, determine the cause of the overload. When replacing a fuse, use a new fuse of the proper rating for the circuit.

Circuit breakers (SUR-cut BRAY-kers) are resettable switches, designed to shut off when the permissible current draw is exceeded. Unlike fuses, which are destroyed in their function, circuit breakers are reusable.

Current can be either alternating or direct. **Alternating current** (ALL-ter-nay-ting KUR-ent) reverses polarity during a cycle. **Direct current** (dir-ECT KUR-ent) maintains the same polarity. Alternating current (AC) is usually developed by AC generators. Direct current (DC) is developed by batteries. Portable devices are usually powered by direct current. Because alternating current can be transmitted efficiently over long distances, it is the type of electricity used for house current. Alternating current, however, cannot be stored; direct current can. Most devices used in the skin-care salon rely on alternating current.

THE ESTHETICIAN AND THE LAW

In the course of conducting business, the esthetician is subject to a myriad of laws and regulations promulgated by agencies at the local, state and federal levels. Like it or not, these laws exist and must be obeyed. It is necessary for the esthetician to be aware of all of the laws and regulations that affect the profession.

The esthetician should not view the agencies that promulgate the regulations as adversaries. Rather, they should be considered allies. These agencies exist to protect the public. In this function, they can provide substantial help to the esthetician.

On the federal level, the two most important agencies for the esthetician are the Food and Drug Administration (FDA) and the Occupational Safety and Health Administration of the Department of Labor, who administer the Occupational Safety and Health Act (OSHA).

The FDA is a regulatory agency charged with making sure that a wide range of products, medical devices, drugs, and food as well as cosmetics, meet the standards of the Food, Drug and Cosmetic Act and are both safe and effective. The agency tests and approves products and has the authority to remove products that don't meet standards from the marketplace. It can also refer cases to the Justice Department for prosecution in cases of fraud.

The agency has the responsibility to challenge claims made for products under its jurisdiction and require substantiation for those claims. For example, the FDA is actively disputing the assertions some manufacturers of skin-care products are making about the antiaging capabilities of their products. If these manufacturers cannot prove their claims to the FDA's satisfaction, they will be forced to withdraw the products. The FDA also provides materials for consumer education, designed to keep consumers aware of the safety of the products they purchase.

OSHA is responsible for assuring safety in the workplace. It has jurisdiction over manufacturing and nonmanufacturing businesses of all sizes, including salons. The agency has the authority to conduct surprise inspections at any business location and to levy fines for noncompliance with safety regulations.

Salons are now covered under OSHA and are required by law to maintain a safe working environment for employees. Part of the law is the Hazard Communication Standard, which requires salons to make sure employees are aware of hazardous materials they may be required to use. This standard includes a written hazard communication program that outlines the salon's hazard communications efforts and is both available and understandable to all employees. The program must include a list of every hazardous chemical in use in the salon. This includes such chemicals as acetone, alcohol, and other solvents.

The salon must have on file Material Safety Data Sheets (MSDS) for all hazardous chemicals on site. These are available from the manufacturers of the products. In addition, any product that contains a hazardous chemical must so state on its label. The salon should maintain a roster of all products used, with complete ingredient information. In addition, the salon must establish an on-going training program for employees that teaches them the proper use and potential dangers of any products they utilize.

Both the FDA and OSHA maintain field offices around the country. The esthetician can call these offices and ask questions about the regulations or about products and get advice on compliance with the rules.

Many states have enacted "Right To Know" laws, which mandate that employers must inform employees about hazardous materials in the workplace. These regulations must be followed, as well. Additionally, on the state level, salons and estheticians are regulated by state Boards of Cosmetology, which establish standards for training, licensing, and the conduct of business.

REVIEW QUESTIONS

1. Why is cleanliness important in the salon?
2. What are two types of bacteria?
3. How are they different?
4. Under what conditions do bacteria thrive?
5. Which bacteria are of most interest to the esthetician?
6. What are three classes of eubacteria?
7. What kinds of disease do staphylococci cause?

8. How do viruses differ from bacteria?
9. Why are DNA-viruses important to the esthetician?
10. What is the immune system?
11. What are lymphocytes?
12. How can the esthetician prevent the spread of infectious diseases?
13. What is AIDS?
14. How can the esthetician help prevent the spread of AIDS?
15. Who was Louis Pasteur?
16. What are the two phases of sanitation?
17. What are four ways to sterilize implements?
18. How are antiseptics different from disinfectants?
19. Why must the esthetician handle waste materials properly?
20. What is the most important part of sanitation?
21. Why is sanitation especially critical during manual extraction?
22. Why should metallic comedone extractors never be used?
23. What is a lancet?
24. Why must the esthetician be aware of safety at all times?
25. Characterize safety.
26. How are electrical circuits protected?
27. What are the rules for safe use of fuses?
28. What are two kinds of electrical current?
29. What is the purpose of most government agencies?
30. What is the FDA?
31. What is OSHA?
32. What are Material Safety Data Sheets?

CHAPTER 4 Biology for the Esthetician

OBJECTIVES   *After completing this chapter, you should be able to:*

❶ Give a historical perspective to the science.
❷ Discuss the importance of biology to ecology.
❸ Describe the importance of biology.
❹ Discuss the various branches of biology as they relate to esthetics.

INTRODUCTION

Biology (By-OL-o-gee), like chemistry and physics, is one of the natural sciences. The domain of biology is the study of life and all things living, from single celled microscopic organisms to the largest plants and animals. The biologist, like his counterparts in the other sciences, seeks to uncover the laws that govern natural phenomena, in this case, the phenomena of life. And, like his colleagues, the biologist utilizes the scientific method of careful observation, measurement, and experimentation.

An understanding of biology is important to the esthetician because he or she works with living tissue, the client's skin. It is necessary to know, therefore, how that tissue works and what biological laws govern skin function. Similarly, nutrition is closely connected with biology, and the esthetician should understand how tissue utilizes food through the process of metabolism.

Sanitation is another concern of the esthetician. Biological principles govern the growth of bacteria. The esthetician should understand what bacteria are. It is important to recognize that some bacteria are harmful, that is, disease-causing or pathogenic. Others are beneficial, or nonpathogenic, such as the microflora that exist in the body. Bacteriology and sanitation were discussed in Chapter 3.

The study of biology also is important on a philosophical level. As Alexander Pope pointed out, "The proper study of mankind is man." To understand man, it is necessary to understand where man fits into the nature of things. A grasp of the basic fundamentals of biology will help the esthetician to keep the profession of esthetics in its proper perspective.

HISTORICAL PERSPECTIVE

Biology, like its sister sciences, has its genesis in prehistory as early man grappled with his environment for everyday survival. He used his observations of nature to help find and gather food, and later, to help grow his own food. It was the ancient Greeks who began the systematic study of life, just as they had begun the systematic study of matter. **Hippocrates** (hip-OK-rah-teez), the father of medicine, founded the first medical school around 400 B.C. **Aristotle** (ar-is-TOT-le), in the fourth century before Christ, began the systematic study of nature by grouping organisms by a single predominant feature. **Theophrastus** (the-o-FRAS-tus), a contemporary of Aristotle, organized the study of plants. The science of anatomy was begun by **Galen** (GAY-len) in the second century A.D.

During the Dark Ages, from about 200 to 1200 A.D., there was little exploration into the mysteries of the universe. Scientific inquiry was discouraged by the church hierarchy, which believed the church was the source of all knowledge. Scientific observation and experimentation that might refute church knowledge was considered dangerous to its authority.

From the fourteenth century on, however, as man expanded his horizons and began to break free of the barriers of ignorance, he made new discoveries about living organisms. **Andreas Vesalius**, early in the sixteenth century, was the first to dissect a human body and refute many of Galen's theories about anatomy. The seventeenth century brought much new knowledge about life. **William Harvey** showed that blood actually circulated throughout the body. **Anton Von Leeuwenhoek** developed the microscope and was the first to actually see living cells.

The pursuit of knowledge continued through the eighteenth century. **Carolus Linnaeus** developed the binomial naming system for species identification, which is still in use today. **Joseph Priestly** showed that air is replenished by green plants. The nineteenth century was no different. **Matthias Schleiden** and **Theodor Schwann**, early in that century, formulated the theory that all living organisms consist of cells. Later that century, **Louis Pasteur** proved that germs cause disease and **Joseph Lister** developed antiseptic techniques for combatting infection.

The invention of the electron microscope by **Max Knell** and **Ernst Ruska** and further refinements by **James Hillier** and **Albert Prebus** in the second quarter of the twentieth century enabled biologists to take giant steps in their breadth of knowledge about life and life processes. The discovery of the double helix structure of DNA in 1953 by **Francis Crick** and **James Watson** was the beginning of our understanding of the genetic code.

BIOLOGY AND ECOLOGY

One of man's concerns is the preservation of life in this fragile environment. As civilization grows more complex, the by-products of civilization have an increasingly harmful effect on the environment. Toxic wastes, nuclear waste, pesticide residues, industrial fumes, automotive exhausts, etc., are upsetting the delicate balance between the living, or **biotic** (by-OT-ik), factors and the nonliving, or **abiotic** (ahb-e-OT-ik), factors that make up the ecosystem. The abiotic factors are the physical and chemical conditions, such as temperature, light, minerals, soil, etc., that let life flourish in a given environment.

Pollution, whether in the form of acid rain, smog, or airborne dirt, changes the abiotic factors and, in turn, affects how we live. For the esthetician, pollution may be a factor in many skin conditions, from dirt embedded in the pores, to excessive dryness, to dermatitis.

An ecosystem is dependent on all of its parts. The sun provides the basic energy for the plant, called a **producer** (pro-DU-sir), because it takes the sun's energy, carbon dioxide, water, and nutrients from the soil to provide its own food for growth. The **herbivore** (her-BIF-or), or primary consumer, eats the plant. The secondary consumer, the **carnivore** (KAR-ni-vor), eats the herbivore. There may be a third consumer that eats the smaller carnivore as well as the herbivore. The **scavengers** (SKAV-en-gers) feed on the leavings of dead plants and animals. The **decomposers** (DEE-kom-po-sers), bacteria and fungi, break down dead organic matter and return compounds and minerals back to the soil (Fig. 4.1)

These members of the community—the plant, the herbivore, the carnivore, the scavenger, and the decomposer—are all vital to the balance of the ecosystem. They are all interdependent. They all take what they need from the ecosystem. And they all contribute to the ecosystem. The plant releases oxygen to the atmosphere as it consumes carbon dioxide through the process of photosynthesis. The consumers breathe in oxygen and exhale carbon diox-

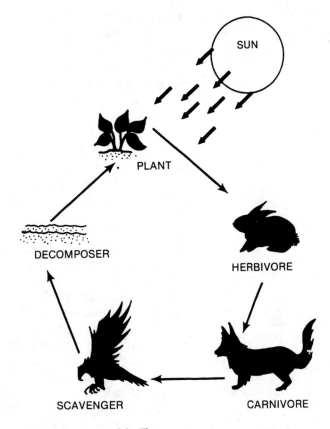

4.1—The ecosystem

ide, which is used by the plant. The consumers also release excess heat from their metabolic processes. This heat is absorbed back into the energy cycle. The scavengers keep the ecosystem clean by eating the scraps left by the consumers. The decomposers return minerals to the soil for reuse by the producers.

The environmental conditions under which any species can survive are limited. Life exists only within a relatively narrow range of temperatures, and requires appropriate water and light. Conditions outside of a certain range inhibit growth. Most species, for example, can survive only at temperatures between 32°F and 110°F. Temperatures above or below this range disrupt normal cell function, leading to the cessation of the ability to sustain life. Some species, however, have developed the ability to adapt to otherwise hostile environments. Man, for example, uses clothing to protect his body from the cold.

BIOLOGY AND LIFE

Biology is defined as the study of life. To study life, however, requires a definition of life, and that can be a difficult task. Simplistic definitions might include the ability to grow. And life forms do grow. But so can inanimate crystals grow. An adequate definition of life is complex and must be based on the functions of life. An organism, then, can be said to be alive if it supports the functions necessary to sustain life. These functions are: nutrition, transport, respiration, excretion, synthesis, regulation, growth, and reproduction.

Nutrition (new-TRI-shun) involves the complex process of **ingesting** (in-JES-ting) or taking in food, **digesting** (dy-JES-ting) it, that is, converting it to the materials needed by the cells, and **assimilating** (ah-SIM-i-lay-ting) it, changing it into cell matter or into energy. All living things take in nutrients from their surrounding environment, whether through direct absorption or through the process of eating.

The organism must have the ability to **transport** (trans-PORT) the nutrients throughout its body. It can do this by **diffusing** (di-FYOO-sing) them across cell membranes or by **circulating** (SUR-kyoo-lating) them through the bloodstream or through intercellular fluids.

Respiration (RES-pi-ray-shun) involves taking in oxygen from the outside air through the lungs, in the case of air-breathing animals, or through the gills, in the case of fish. The oxygen is converted by biochemical processes to provide energy at the cell level through **cellular respiration** (SELL-yoo-lar RES-pi-ray-shun). Carbon dioxide is released back to the outside environment. In the case of plants, respiration involves the absorption of carbon dioxide from the atmosphere and the expiration of oxygen back to the atmosphere. Waste products are removed from the organism by the process of **excretion** (eks-KRE-shun).

Through complex biochemical processes, the organism **synthesizes** (SIN-the-sizes) new tissues, enzymes, and hormones it needs for growth and regulation of the many activities that are occurring in the body at any given moment. In higher animals, **regulation** (reg-u-LAY-shun) is carried on by endocrine and nervous systems. In lower animals and plants, regulation is a function of the chemicals synthesized.

Finally, living organisms **grow** and **reproduce** (ree-pro-DYOOS). During growth, cells become larger or more numerous within the organism. The organism may reproduce either **asexually** (A-sek-shu-al), that is, with only one parent, or **sexually** (SEK-shyoo-al), through two parents. In either case, the end result is a new individual of the same kind.

These complex biochemical activities are referred to as the **metabolism** (meh-TAB-o-lis-em) of the organism. The metabolic processes can change nutrients into new tissue, that is, build tissue by **anabolism** (ah-NAB-o-lizm). Or they can convert tissue to energy, that is, break it down by **catabolism** (kah-TAB-o-liz-em).

To maintain life, the internal environment of the organism must stay essentially unchanged with respect to temperature, mineral content, acid-base balance, etc. The regulation of these processes that maintains the conditions unchanged is **homeostasis** (HO-me-oh-stay-sis).

BRANCHES OF BIOLOGY

Because of the vast numbers and types of known living organisms, the science of biology is broken into a number of different branches, each specializing in the study of a particular type of organism. Each branch may be further broken into sub-branches. **Botany** (BOT-n-ee) is the study of plants. Specialties within the field include **bryology** (bree-OL-o-jee), the study of mosses and liverworts; **pteridology** (ter-i-DOLL-ah-jee), the study of ferns; or **plant pathology** (PLANT pa-THOL-o-jee), the study of plant diseases.

Ecology (e-KOL-o-jee) is the study of the relationships between living organisms and their environment. An ecologist, for example, might specialize in a study of the effects of acid rain.

Embryology (EM-bree-ol-o-jee) is the study of the embryo, the period of early growth from the fertilization of the egg by the sperm to the formation of the complete body structure.

Genetics (jen-ET-iks) is the study of heredity and the gene structures of organisms. Genetic engineers, for example, have synthesized interferon, a potential cure for cancer, by the complex process of gene splicing.

Morphology (mor-FOL-o-jee) is the study of the structures of living organisms. The two major sub-branches are plant morphology and animal morphology. Animal morphology can be divided into **anatomy** (ah-NAHT-o-mee), the study of structures that can be seen with unaided vision; **histology** (hi-STOL-o-jee), the study of tissues at the microscopic level; and **cytology** (seye-TOL-o-jee), the study of cells at the microscopic level.

Paleontology (PAY-lee-on-tol-o-jee) is the study of ancient and extinct life forms through the examination of fossils. Our current knowledge of dinosaurs, for example, is a result of the work of paleontologists.

Physiology (fiz-i-OL-o-jee) is the study of the functioning of the parts of the organism. The divisions are plant physiology and animal physiology. The esthetician is most concerned with physiology, especially the functioning of the muscles and the bones of the face.

Taxonomy (tax-ON-o-mee) studies organisms as a whole, with the aim of classifying them into groups that are similar in structure.

Zoology (zew-OL-o-jee) is the study of animals. It, too, has several sub-branches including **entomology** (EN-to-mol-o-jee), the study of insects; **herpetology** (her-pet-OL-o-jee), the study of reptiles; **ornithology** (OR-ni-thol-o-jee), the study of birds; **ichthyology** (IK-thee-OL-o-jee), the study of fish; and **mammalogy** (mam-AL-o-jee), the study of mammals.

BIOLOGICAL CLASSIFICATION

Living organisms are classified by **species** (SPE-sheez), a group that can produce fertile young. Although two closely related species can sometimes produce young, the offspring will be sterile. Thus, a mule, the offspring of a horse and a donkey, two different species, will be sterile. The offspring of a German shepherd and a Doberman pinscher, however, will be able to reproduce since its parents are of the same species, although of different breeds.

The commonly used method of classification is the **binomial nomenclature system** (bye-NO-me-ahl NO-men-clay-ture SIS-tem), developed in the eighteenth century by Carolus Linnaeus, the "father of modern taxonomy." Under this system, each species is assigned a two-word Latin name. The first name is the **genus**, the next more general unit of classification. A genus is a group of related species. The second name is the specific name. The species is designated by the full two-word name. For example, man belongs to the genus **homo** (HO-mo). He is of the species **homo sapiens** (HO-mo SAY-pe-enz).

Since Latin is a "dead" language, that is, it is no longer the primary language of any country, it is ideal as a scientific language because it does not change. Its vocabulary and structure are fixed. Also, since it is not the language of any specific country, it can be used by all countries without offending national pride. Latin has long been accepted worldwide as a scientific language.

Living organisms are classified into a number of groups by virtue of significant biological characteristics. Each group, called a **taxon** (TAK-son), is established by related morphological details. The classification scheme currently used is in hierarchical order, from the largest grouping, the kingdom, to the most specific, the species. Each successive grouping becomes smaller and more specific than the previous grouping. These groupings are:

- Kingdom—e.g., animal.
- Phylum—e.g., chordate.
- Subphylum—e.g., vertebrate.

- Class—e.g., mammal.
- Order—e.g., primate.
- Family—e.g., hominid.
- Genus—e.g., homo.
- Species—e.g., homo sapiens.

In addition, species may be subdivided further. Man, for example, can be classified by race, as well. It is important to remember, however, that even though the species may be subdivided, it is still one species, of which all members can interbreed to produce fertile offspring.

There are five kingdoms currently recognized, based on the shared characteristics of the members of the group. These are:

Monera (mo-NAIR-ah)—single-celled organisms without an organized nucleus (e.g., bacteria). This kingdom is of major interest to the esthetician because of the ability of many bacteria to cause disease and because of the importance of sanitation and of the role of the skin as a barrier against bacterial invasion.

Protista (pro-TEES-ta)—single-celled organisms with an organized nucleus. Some ingest food; others produce nourishment by photosynthesis (e.g., amoebae). This kingdom is of little interest to the esthetician.

Fungi (FUN-jee)—plant-like organisms with a different cellular structure than plants. Most are parasites that absorb food from other living organisms (e.g., mushrooms). This kingdom is of minor interest to the esthetician, except for the ability of some fungi to cause infections manifesting themselves on the skin.

Plantae (plan-TEE)—multicellular organisms whose cells contain cellulose. They manufacture food by photosynthesis (e.g., moss). This kingdom is of considerable interest to the esthetician because of the role of plants as suppliers of nutrients and for the importance of herbs to skin care.

Animalia (an-i-MAL-ya)—multicellular organisms whose cells contain chromosomes. They ingest organic substances for food (e.g., dogs). This kingdom is of major interest to the esthetician, especially for the study of human physiology.

Kingdom Monera

Monerans include **bacteria** (bak-TEER-i-ah) and blue-green algae, known as **cyanobacteria** (SEE-an-o-bak-TEER-i-ah). They are microscopic, single-celled organisms whose cells do not contain nuclei. They live singly or in colonies.

For the esthetician, the bacteria are the most important members of kingdom monera. Some bacteria are harmful, or pathogenic. These cause disease and must be controlled. Control of pathogenic bacteria is a function of sanitation and sterilization. Most bacteria,

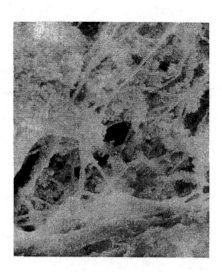

4.2—Electron microphotograph of bacteria *(Courtesy of Rohm and Haas Company)*

however, are helpful, or nonpathogenic. Intestinal microflora, bacteria that live in the intestines, help synthesize some vitamins and digestive enzymes. Other bacteria are responsible for the process of fermentation, by which wine is produced (Fig. 4.2). Bacteria were discussed in detail in Chapter 3.

Kingdom Protista   Like the monerans, the members of the protist kingdom are unicellular organisms. Their cellular structure, however, is significantly different. Although most protists live singly, some species live in colonies. The various species of this kingdom are among the oldest living organisms. It is thought that animals, fungi and plants evolved from the protists.

While not as important to the esthetician as the monerans, the protists do influence the quality of human life. Some species are pathogenic and are responsible for a number of debilitating diseases. One such disease is amoebic dysentery, caused by a parasitic amoeba that attacks the intestinal tract. Another type of protist, a red-colored dinoflagellate, is responsible for the condition known as the "red tide" that periodically infects East Coast beaches and kills fish.

Some species are beneficial. Plankton, for example, is an important food source for much marine life. Slime molds feed on dead organic matter and help maintain the ecological balance. There are three major groups of protists, the animal-like, the fungus-like and the plant-like.

The Animal-Like Protists. The animal-like protists, the protozoa, are divided into four phyla, according to their mode of movement. The **mastigophora** (MASS-ti-gof-o-ra), or **zooflagellates** (ZO-fla-jel-

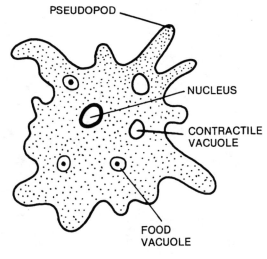

4.3—Amoeba

eyets), have one or more **flagella** (fla-JEL-ah), hair-like appendages that undulate, allowing movement. The zooflagellate, **trypanosoma gambiense** (TRI-pan-o-so-ma gam-be-EN-se), causes African sleeping sickness. The organism is carried by infected tse-tse flies.

The **sarcodina** (sar-ko-DEE-na), or **amoeboids** (ah-MEE-boyds), have flexible, amorphous bodies with pseudopods, extensions of their body that allow movement. **Entamoeba histolytica** (EN-ta-mee-ba HIS-toe-lick-ah) is the species responsible for amoebic dysentary (Fig. 4.3).

The **sporozoa** (SPOR-o-zo-ah) are parasitic spore formers. Although they may be capable of movement through the use of pseudopods when young, they have no means of motion in their adult stage. **Plasmodium vivax** (PLAZ-mo-dee-um VEE-vax) is the species responsible for malaria, transmitted through the anopheles mosquito.

The **ciliata** (SIL-ee-ah-ta), the most numerous of the protozoa, are surrounded by **cilia** (SIL-ee-ah), short hairs that are used for movement. The species in this phylum are characterized by the presence of two nuclei in their cells. The most well-known member of the ciliata is the **paramecium** (pair-ah-MEE-see-um) (Fig. 4.4).

The Fungus-Like Protists. There are two phyla of fungus-like protists: the **protomycota** (pro-toe-my-KOT-ah) and the **gymnomycota** (jim-no-my-KOT-ah). Some protomycota are parasites; others are saprophytes. They live in soil or on water plants. Some live in animals. The gymnomycota, or slime molds, live on rotting logs or decaying vegetation in forests.

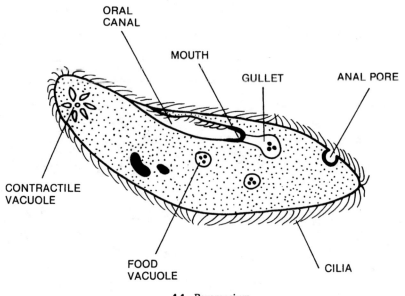

4.4—Paramecium

The Plant-Like Protists. The plant-like protists are divided into three phyla: the **euglenophyta** (yu-GLE-no-fi-ta), the **chrysophtya** (kris-e-FI-ta) and the **pyrrophyta** (pi-ro-FI-ta). The euglenophyta exhibit both plant and animal characteristics. They use flagella for locomotion and gather nutrients through photosynthesis.

The chrysophyta include diatoms as well as the golden-brown and yellow-green forms of algae. Most chrysophytes have flagella for locomotion. The diatoms have no flagella, but have shell-like cell walls. The remains of dead diatoms form **diatomaceous earth** (DI-ah-toe-may-shus URTH), used in air filters and abrasives, and sometimes used as an ingredient in facial masks.

The pyrrophyta, or dinoflagellates, usually have two unequal flagella. The dinoflagellate, **gonyaulax** (GON-ee-aw-laks), is responsible for the "red tide." Some species, such as the **noctiluca** (noc-ti-LU-ka), are bioluminescent and glow in the dark.

Kingdom Fungi

Fungi (FUN-gee) are multicellular organisms that are distinguished from other organisms by their method of obtaining nutrients. Unlike plants, they do not contain **chlorophyll** (KLOR-o-fil), so they can't manufacture food by photosynthesis. And, unlike animals, they have no means of ingesting food. Instead, they are saprophytic or parasitic organisms that absorb food either from dead organic matter or from living organisms. Fungi reproduce by releasing spores. **Yeasts** (YEESTS) are unicellular forms of fungi.

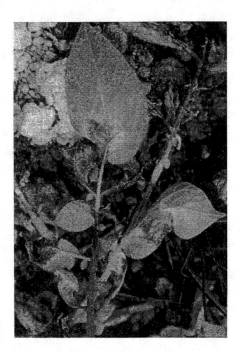

4.5—Potato blight fungus *(Courtesy of Rohm and Haas Company)*

Except for those fungi responsible for yeast infections and the contagious infection, ringworm, the members of this kingdom are of little importance to the esthetician. Nevertheless, many of the fungi are beneficial to humans. Some are important food materials. Some are used in making bread and in the fermentation process for making beer and wine. And some are important sources of antibiotics.

Not all fungi are beneficial, however. Although not generally pathogenic to humans, some are pathogenic to plant life and are responsible for a number of devastating plant diseases. The fungus **phytophthora infestans**, or **late blight**, for example, caused the nineteenth-century potato blight in Ireland (Fig. 4.5). Others are responsible for mildew, which can destroy clothing.

Kingdom fungi contains only one phylum, mycota. This phylum, however, is divided into five classes: oomycetes, ascomycetes, zygomycetes, basidiomycetes, and deuteromycetes.

The **oomycetes** (oo-MY-se-teez) have cell walls made of cellulose. They live mostly in water. Their spores have flagella, which are used for swimming. Most are saprophytes and live on dead organic matter. The **ascomycetes** (as-ko-MY-se-teez) are the largest class of fungi and get their name from the sac, or **ascus**, that contains the reproductive cells. Their cell walls are made of **chitin**, a tough polysaccharide. Truffles and morels, both gourmet delicacies, are members of this class, as is the mold **penicillium**, from which the antibiotic penicillin is made. Yeasts are also members of this class. Harmful ascomycetes include ceratosystis, which causes Dutch elm disease.

The **zygomycetes** (zy-go-MY-se-teez) are saprophytes that live in the soil. Like all fungi except the oomycetes, their cell walls are made of chiten. They are also called **thread fungi**, since they grow **rhizoids**, or thread-like appendages. The black bread mold, **rhizopus stolonifer** (sto-LON-i-fer), belongs to this class.

The **basidiomycetes** (ba-SID-ee-yo-MY-se-teez) get their name from the basidium, a club-like tip that forms on them. The common mushrooms are members of this class, as are the bracket fungi. Some mushrooms are edible; others are poisonous.

The **deuteromycetes** (DOO-ter-o-MY-se-teez) are also called the **fungi imperfecti**. This class is a "catch-all" class, since it contains species that cannot be readily classified into other groups. The members of this class include the fungi responsible for ringworm and athlete's foot.

Kingdom Plantae

The plant kingdom includes all of the green plants. Most members are multicellular, although a few are unicellular. Except for a very few lower species, the green plants are nonmotile; that is, they have no means of locomotion and spend their lives in one location. Some lower plant species live in water. Most higher plants, however, live on land.

All of the members contain **chlorophyll** (KLOR-o-fil), a green pigment that gives the plant its color and gathers light energy from the sun for the process of **photosynthesis** (fo-toe-SIN-the-sis). It is through photosynthesis that plants get nutrients. In this process, light energy is converted to chemical energy, reacting carbon dioxide from the atmosphere with water to yield sugar, which is absorbed by the plant, and oxygen, which is released back into the atmosphere.

The green plants are exceedingly important to human beings, serving as both a primary source of food and as the primary source of food for the animals they eat. The esthetician is concerned with the green plants because of the importance of nutrition to skin care and because the herbs that are used in skin-care products are members of this kingdom.

The plant kingdom contains two phyla: thallophyta and embryophyta. The thallophyta are lower aquatic species; the embryophyta are higher terrestrial species.

Thallophyta. **Thallophytes** (THAL-e-fyts) may be multicellular or unicellular. They are largely aquatic, although a few live on land. Most of the aquatic thallophytes are fresh water species, although a few grow in salt water. This group has a simple structure, without roots, stems, or leaves. The three divisions of thallophytes are the chlorophyta, or green **algae** (AL-jee); the phaeophyta, or brown algae; and the rhodophyta, or red algae.

The green **algae, chlorophyta** (KLOR-o-fy-ta), exist as unicellular organisms living singly, as unicellular organisms living in colonies, and as multicellular organisms. Most chlorophyta live in fresh or salt water. Some live on land. The chlorophyta are represented by the unicellular species, **chlamydomonas** (kla-MID-o-mo-nas); the colonial species, **volvox**; and the multicellular species, **ulva**, or **sea lettuce**. The green algae are an important source of food for small aquatic animals and insects.

The **brown algae, phaeophyta** (fay-o-FY-ta), are the multicellular organisms known as **seaweed** (SEE-weed). They live almost exclusively in the oceans. Some species, such as the **kelps**, are the largest of the algae, growing up to 150 feet long. The Sargasso Sea, in the middle of the North Atlantic, is so named because it contains large masses of the species sargassum. The phaeophytes contain a substance called **algin**, a commercially valuable gelatin-like material used in foods. The brown algaes are also a major ingredient in some skin-care preparations.

The **red algae, rhodophyta** (ro-do-FY-ta), are also multicellular marine organisms. These, however, live deeper in the oceans than the brown algae. **Chondrus**, or **Irish moss**, is a representative species. The red algae have considerable commercial value because they contain **agar**, which is used as a suspension agent in ice cream and in many other food stuffs.

Embryophyta. The **embryophytes** (EM-bree-o-fyts) are more structurally complex than the thallophytes. They live primarily on land and are generally of a higher order of plant life. There are two groups in this phylum, the bryophyta and the tracheophyta.

The **bryophyta** (bry-o-FY-ta) are small, primitive species and were the first green plants to live on land. They live under a wide variety of conditions, ranging from very wet to very dry. They do not have roots, stems, or leaves. They anchor themselves to the ground with **rhizomes**, simple structures that act like roots. The bryophytes include the hornworts, liverworts, and mosses.

The **tracheophyta** (TRAY-kee-o-FY-ta) range from primitive to highly developed plants. All species have a well-developed **vascular**, or water carrying, system along with roots, leaves and stems. The roots function to anchor the plant to the ground and to absorb moisture and nutrients from the soil. The leaves serve to capture light for the process of photosynthesis for manufacturing food, and the stems store food and transport it throughout the plant so it can be used.

There are five groups of tracheophytes: the **psilopsida**, the most primitive of the vascular plants, which are largely extinct; the **ycop-**

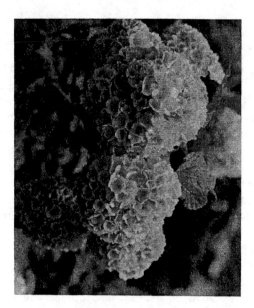

4.6—Flowering plant

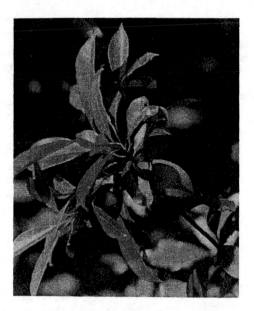

4.7—Woody plant

sida, or **club mosses**, which are also primitive; the **sphenopsida**, or **horsetails**; the **pteropsida**, or **ferns**; and the **seed plants**.

The seed plants are the most highly developed forms of plant life and include all of the flowers, trees, grasses, and agricultural crop plants. They are divided into two groups, the **gymnosperms**, or **cone bearing plants**, and the **angiosperms**, or **flowering plants**. The gymnosperms include the evergreen trees and other wood plants. All of the other higher plants belong to the angiosperm group (Figs. 4.6 and 4.7).

Kingdom Animalia

The animal kingdom includes all multicellular animal organisms, from the most primitive—**porifera**, or **sponges**—to the highest order—**homo sapiens**, that is, man—with a vast number of other species in between. Regardless of species, however, all animals share certain characteristics. They all must obtain food from other sources, either directly, from green plants, or indirectly, from other animals. **Herbivores** eat only plants; **carnivores** eat only other animals; and **omnivores** eat both plants and animals. No matter what the source, the food must be first ingested, then digested to a form the animal body can use.

Animals are more responsive to their environment than plants because they have nervous systems and contractile muscles. And most are motile for at least part of their life. In addition, all animals have some form of support for their body, whether in the form of an external skeleton, or **exoskeleton** (EK-sow-skel-e-ton) (e.g., a crab or a beetle); or in the form of an internal skeleton, or **endoskeleton** (EN-doh-skel-e-ton) (e.g., a dog or an ape).

The animal kingdom is important to humans since humans are, of course, part of that kingdom. In addition, animals are important as sources of food (e.g., fish, beef cattle, dairy animals, chickens as egg producers, etc.). And animals also serve to help man, (e.g., plowhorses, draft animals, seeing eye dogs, etc.). Some animals are harmful (e.g., insects that destroy crops or carry disease).

For the esthetician, the animal kingdom is of most interest because of human beings. Knowledge of human physiology, especially of the structure of the bones and muscles of the head, are important for the esthetician to practice the profession for the maximum benefit to the client.

The animal kingdom is divided into **invertebrates** (IN-ver-ti-brayt), animals without a backbone, and **vertebrates** (VER-ti-brayt), animals with a backbone. The invertebrates far outnumber the vertebrates. There are twenty-nine phyla in the animal kingdom. Twenty-eight phyla are of invertebrates; only one phylum is of vertebrates.

Since animal life is believed to have begun in the sea and evolved into terrestrial animal life, it is not surprising that the most primitive forms of animal life are marine creatures. **Sponges**, of the phylum **porifera**, are the most primitive species of animal, followed by the members of the phylum **coelenterata**, the jellyfish, **corals**, and **sea anemones**.

The next evolutionary plateau was reached by the **platyhelminthes**, the phylum of **flatworms**. These creatures, though still primi-

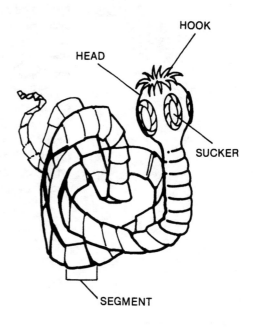

4.8—Tapeworm

tive, have more highly developed nervous systems. Some flatworms are aquatic; others live on land. Many species, for example, the **tapeworm,** are parasitic and are harmful to humans (Fig. 4.8). The phylum **aschelminthes,** or **roundworms,** are only slightly more advanced. These animals, which also may be either free-living or parasitic, are found in water or soil. The parasitic species, which live in human or animal hosts, include the **hookworm,** the **pinworm,** and the **filaria,** which causes the condition known as **elephantitis.**

The phylum **mollusca,** which includes clams, oysters, mussels, scallops and squid, contains more than 1,000 species, making it one of the largest phyla. The mollusks, most of which are marine animals, are the most advanced invertebrates, having well-developed disgestive and circulatory systems. The giant squid is the largest invertebrate. Many members of this phylum are important economically, as food sources and as the source of other products, such as polishing powders and mother-of-pearl.

The phylum **annelida,** or **segmented worms,** represents a large evolutionary advance. These creatures are the first to have a true **coelom** (SEE-lom), or body cavity developing from the **mesoderm,** the embryonic layer of middle skin. The segmented worms are both aquatic and terrestrial. A few species are parasitic. Classes include the sandworms, leeches, and earthworms.

There are more than 800,000 species in the phylum, **arthropoda,** making it the largest phylum of animal life. These animals are distinguished by the presence of jointed appendages and hard exoskeletons. They have well-developed nervous systems and circulatory systems. The arthropods are widely distributed in nature, living in fresh water, salt water, and on land. There are five major classes: **arachnids,** which include spiders, mites, and scorpions; **crustaceans,** which include crabs, shrimp, and lobsters; **insects,** which include flies, ants, and moths; **diplopods,** or millipedes; and **chilopods,** or centipedes.

The arthropods are important to humans. Some, such as crustaceans, are important sources of food. The insects, which are the most advanced of the arthropods, have a significant impact on human life. Bees, for example, provide honey and carry pollen from plant to plant, helping the plants reproduce. Caterpillars, however, destroy crops, causing great damage. Other insects, such as mosquitoes and flies, carry and transmit diseases (Fig. 4.9).

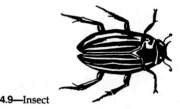

4.9—Insect

The phylum **echinodermata**, or **spiny-skinned** invertebrates, are relatively primitive, having a well-developed digestive system, but no execretory or reproductive system. Their embryonic stage, however, resembles that of the chordates, the next higher order of animals. The echinoderms are characterized by a pentaradial symmetry, in which five appendages radiate from a central core in a star-shaped pattern. Members of this phylum include the starfish, sand dollars, and sea urchins.

The members of the phylum **chordata** represent the highest stage of its development. They are characterized by the presence of a **notochord**, a gristly supporting structure running the length of the body. The chordates are divided into four subphyla. The first three are the prevertebrates, or invertebrate chordates. These are the **hemichordata**, worm-like marine animals; the **urochordata**, or **tunicates**, sac-like marine animals; and the **cephalochordata**, or lancets. The fourth subphylum is the **vertebrata**.

The vertebrates have a **segmented spinal column**, or **backbone**, made either of cartilage or bone. They also have an internal, jointed, supporting skeleton, which gives them great flexibility, and they have a brain protected by a **cranium**, a cavity in the head, protected by bony plates. In addition, vertebrates have a closed circulatory system. Most endoskeletons are made of bone, although a few species have an endoskeleton made of cartilage.

The vertebrates are divided into a number of classes. The **agnatha** are the most primitive and consist of the jawless fish, represented by the lamprey, a parasitic eel-like creature. The agnatha are fresh water fish. The **chondrichthyes**, or **cartilaginous fish**, are salt-water fish, and are represented by sharks and rays. This class is characterized by having endoskeletons made of cartilage and lacking air bladders like the bony fish.

The **osteichthyes**, or bony fish, have endoskeletons made of bone and have air bladders, which help them swim. They are found all over the world in almost all bodies of fresh and salt water. Many of the fish in this class have important commercial value and are valuable sources of food (Fig. 4.10).

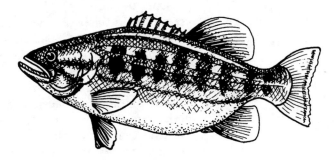

4.10—Bony fish

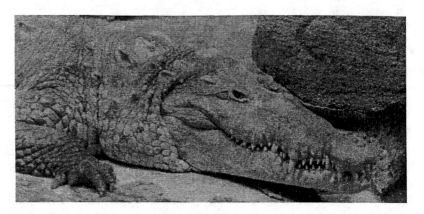

4.11—Crocodile

The **amphibia** represent a transition between the aquatic and the terrestrial vertebrates, since they begin life in the water and move to the land at some stage of their development. This class is represented by frogs, toads, and salamanders.

The **reptilia** were the first vertebrates to be totally adapted to life on land. They are all air breathers, even though a few species either live or spend some time in the water. Unlike other terrestrial vertebrates, the reptiles are cold blooded, that is, their body temperature varies with the temperature of the environment. The reptiles include snakes and lizards, turtles, crocodiles, and alligators (Fig. 4.11).

Birds, which belong to the class **aves**, are the only creatures to have a body covering of feathers. They are related to the reptiles in their bone structure, their horny beaks and the fact that they, like the reptiles, lay large eggs during the reproductive process. But birds are of a higher evolutionary order. The upper limbs of birds have developed as wings, even though not all birds are capable of flight. Birds are the first class of animals that show territorial instincts (Fig. 4.12).

The mammals, of the class, **mammalia** (me-MAYL-e-ya), are the most highly developed of the animals. They are characterized by the presence of mammary glands, which provide milk for feeding their young. In addition, all mammals have hair for at least part of their lives. They are found in all environments and vary in size from less than an inch in length, as is the shrew, to more than 90 feet in length, as is the great blue whale.

There are three major groups of mammals: the monotremes, the marsupials, and the placental, based on how they bear and/or nurse their young. The **monotremes**, represented by the duckbilled platypus and the spiny anteater, are primitive mammals that lay eggs. The **marsupials**, represented by the kangaroos and opossums, bear their young at an early stage of development, then place them in

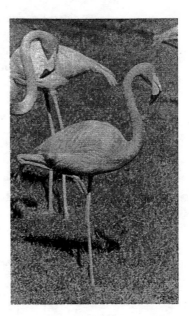

4.12—Flamingo

pouches, where they are nursed until they reach full development. The young of the **placental** mammals develop in the uterus and derive nourishment from the placenta. The placental mammals are the most highly developed animals.

There are a number of orders of placental mammals, including the **carnivora**, represented by dogs, cats and bears; the **rodentia**, represented by rats, squirrels and rabbits; the **chiroptera**, represented by bats; and the **primates** (preye-MAYTZ), represented by apes and humans. The primates, especially man, represent the highest evolutionary development to date (Fig. 4.13).

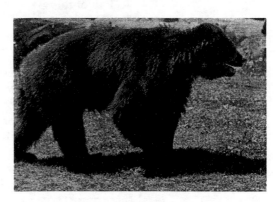

4.13—Bear

As stated earlier, many of the mammals are important to human beings. Some provide food. Others help with work. While many mammals are beneficial, some are harmful. Rats, for example, can spread disease; mice can destroy crops.

Of all the mammals, however, the primates are specially important, since that order includes humankind. And homo sapiens is the only order of animal, or any other creature, for that matter, who can study the other forms of life, learn about them, and, most importantly, learn from them.

REVIEW QUESTIONS

1. Why is an understanding of biology important to the esthetician?
2. Match each person with his contribution to biology.

   1. Hippocrates   a. blood circulation
   2. Aristotle   b. first medical school
   3. Theophrastus   c. DNA
   4. Galen   d. study of plants
   5. Andreas Vesalius   e. microscope
   6. William Harvey   f. germ theory of disease
   7. Von Leeuwenhoek   g. first dissection of human body
   8. Louis Pasteur   h. antiseptic techniques
   9. Joseph Lister   i. science of anatomy
   10. James Watson   j. grouping of organisms

3. Describe the food chain of the ecosystem.
4. Define biology.
5. What are the life functions?
6. Match the branch of biology with its specialty.

   1. Botany   a. study of living organisms
   2. Bryology   b. classification of organisms
   3. Ecology   c. study of the embryo
   4. Embryology   d. study of parts of organisms
   5. Genetics   e. study of the environment
   6. Morphology   f. study of heredity
   7. Paleontology   g. study of animals
   8. Physiology   h. study of plants
   9. Taxonomy   i. study of mosses
   10. Zoology   j. study of ancient life forms

7. How are living organisms classified?
8. What is the hierarchical order of the classification scheme?
9. What are the five kingdoms?
10. What do the remains of dead diatoms become, and why are they important to the esthetician?
11. What is chlorophyll?
12. What is photosynthesis?
13. Why are algaes important to the esthetician?
14. What characteristics do all species of animals share?

15. What are the two classifications of animals?
16. What is the largest phylum of animal life?
17. What is the most highly developed class of animals?
18. Biologically, how are human beings classified?

5 Physiology for the Esthetician

OBJECTIVES   *After completing this chapter, you should be able to:*

❶ Understand the importance of the bodily functions on the health and functioning of the skin.

❷ Discuss cellular structure and function, tissues and organs.

❸ Discuss the structure and functions of the various systems of the body.

INTRODUCTION

Physiology is that specific branch of biology that studies the functioning of living organisms. It includes anatomy, the study of the structure of the organism. Although the study of all types of living organisms is included in the science of physiology, the study of the human organism has been of paramount interest. Ever since Galen founded the science of anatomy in the second century A.D., men have been interested in studying man.

Human physiology and anatomy are important to the esthetician because it is important to understand the function of the various systems that affect the health of the skin. The esthetician must be familiar with the various bones that make up the skeletal structure, especially the bones of the head, face, and neck, as well as the muscles that cover and surround those bones, because of the effect massage has on these structures. The professional must know the blood vessels that carry blood through the body, especially those that bring blood to the skin, as well as the lymph vessels that carry off waste products. And the esthetician must understand the structure and function of the epithelial tissue, which includes the skin.

No less important to the esthetician is an understanding of the other systems—the digestive system, for example, and its role in nutrition; or the excretory system and its role in waste removal. In short, almost every organ, every system, plays a part of some importance to the health of the skin, either directly or indirectly.

The human animal, of the species homo sapiens, is a member of the animal kingdom. More specifically, he belongs to the sub-phylum of vertebrates, the class of mammals and the order of primates and represents the highest form of development. Human beings are set apart from their animal cousins by a number of distinct features, especially the brain development that allows speech and rational thought and the ability to walk upright, leaving the hands free for working.

Humans are multicellular organisms. Their bodies consist of millions of individual cells that show a high degree of specialization. That is, there are many different kinds of cells in the body, each having a specific function. The cells are organized into tissues, or groups of cells having similar functions. The tissues are organized into organs. And organs are grouped into systems. All systems are well-developed. As vertebrates, humans have a spinal column and an internal skeletal structure, or endoskeleton, that grows with the body.

The tissues, organs and systems develop from three embryonic germ layers, the **ectoderm** (EK-toe-derm), or outside skin, the **mesoderm** (MESS-o-derm), or middle skin, and the **endoderm** (EN-do-derm), or inside skin. The epidermis, hair, and nervous system begin in the ectoderm. The dermis, connective tissues, and the vascular system begin in the mesoderm. And the liver, the thyroid gland, and much of the gastrointestinal lining begin in the endoderm.

THE CELL

The **cell** is the basic unit of living organisms. The human body consists of trillions of individual cells of varying sizes and shapes, each having a specific function in the body. Cells determine the structure of the person, since they are the basic structural unit of the body. They determine the biological functioning of the person, since each cell carries out the same biochemical processes as the body does on a larger scale. They determine the heredity of the person, since the cells carry the genetic coding materials. And they determine the development of the person, since they multiply to form new tissues and organs.

In the human organism, the cells are highly specialized, each type having a particular function and contributing to the well-being of the body as a whole. Thus, for example, epithelial cells form the

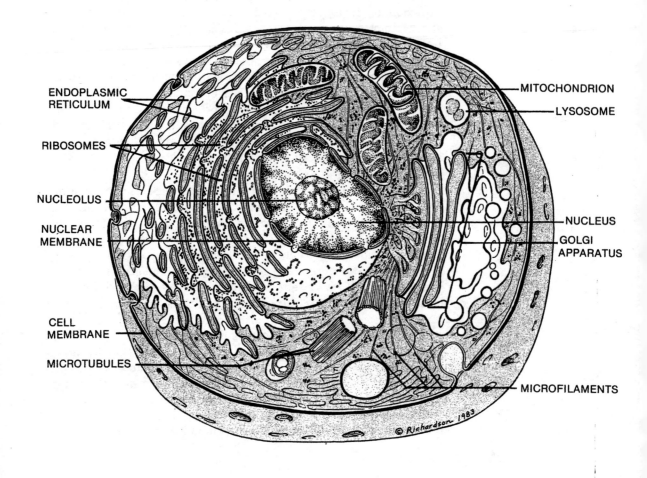

ENDOPLASMIC
RETICULUM

RIBOSOMES

NUCLEOLUS

NUCLEAR
MEMBRANE

CELL
MEMBRANE

MICROTUBULES

MITOCHONDRION

LYSOSOME

NUCLEUS

GOLGI
APPARATUS

MICROFILAMENTS

© Richardson 1983

5.1—Typical human cell

tissues that cover the body surfaces; hair cells form the hair; blood cells form the blood.

All cells, however, despite their degree of specialization, have the same basic structure. They are a mass of **protoplasm** (PRO-tuh-plazm), or living matter, with a nucleus surrounded by cytoplasm, which is, in turn, surrounded by a membrane. The cell consists of a number of parts, called **organelles** (or-gan-ELS), which function within the cell in much the same way organs do within the body (Fig. 5.1).

The cell is surrounded by a semi-permeable membrane made of a combination of protein and lipids. The membrane holds the cell together, much the same as the skin holds the body together. It also acts as a selective filter, letting nutrients, oxygen, and hormones in, while letting waste products out.

The **nucleus** (NOO-klee-us) is the largest organelle of the cell and is responsible for metabolic functions and for reproduction. It holds the RNA and DNA, as well as the genetic materials of the organism. It is surrounded by a nuclear membrane, which separates it from the cytoplasm. The nucleus contains one or more **nucleoli** (NOO-klee-o-lee), which are responsible for the synthesis of RNA, and **chromatin** (KRO-ma-tin), the building bodies that form **chromosomes** (KRO-mo-zom).

The cell is filled with **cytoplasm** (SY-toh-plaz-em), the living matter that surrounds the nucleus and holds the other organelles in suspension. There are two types of organelles, those with membranes, which are responsible for metabolic functions, and those without membranes, which have special purposes. The membraneous organelles include the Golgi apparatus, lysosomes, the endoplasmic reticulum, and mitochondria. The nonmembraneous organelles include ribosomes, filaments, centrioles, and microtubules.

The **Golgi apparatus** (GOL-gee ap-ar-AT-us) consists of a series of fluid filled membraneous pouches that store and transport materials used by the other parts of the cell. It also helps in the formation of lysosomes. **Lysosomes** (LY-so-sohmz) are **vacuoles** (vac-U-ol), little sacs filled with digestive enzymes, which let the cell absorb food. They are surrounded by especially heavy membranes that keep the enzymes from destroying the cell itself.

The **endoplasmic reticulum** (en-do-PLAS-mik re-TIK-u-lum) is a network of membraneous channels and tubes that allow the movement of materials throughout the cytoplasm. The **mitochrondria** (my-toh-KON-dre-ah) are large cylindrical organelles surrounded by a double membrane. These organelles contain enzymes that convert nutrients into the energy needed for the cell processes. They are the largest and most numerous of the membraneous organelles.

Ribosomes (RY-bo-sohmz), the most numerous of the nonmembraneous organelles, may be attached to the endoplasmic reticulum or may float freely in the cytoplasm. These small organelles are responsible for the synthesis of proteins both for use throughout the body and for cellular respiration.

The cell contains a number of filaments arranged in bundles called **fibrils** (FY-brils). These fibrils act much like an internal skeletal structure to support the cell. The **centrioles** (SEN-tree-ohls) are a pair of small, cylindrical organelles, located near the nucleus. They play an important role during cell division. Cells also contain a number of **microtubules** (my-kro-TOO-buhls), tiny tubes that help in cell movement and in the transport of materials throughout the cell.

In addition to the organelles, cells also contain a number of materials that are not part of the cell. These materials, which include stored food particles and pigments, are called **inclusions** (in-KLU-shuns). The stored foods consist of glycogen or fat. The pigments include carotene, melanin, and hemoglobin.

Cells reproduce by **mitosis** (MY-toh-sis), or cell division. When it grows large enough, the parent cell splits into two identical cells called daughter cells. At the beginning of the process, the **prophase** (PRO-faze), the centrioles separate and start to move apart. A series of microtubules, called a **spindle** (SPIN-del), start to form between the two centrioles. Granules of chromatin condense to form chromosomes, which split into pairs of **chromatids** (KRO-mah-tids), which arrange themselves along the spindle.

During the **metaphase** (MET-ah-faze), the next step in the process, the nuclear membrane and nucleoli have disappeared and the centrioles have settled at opposite poles, with the chromatid pairs at the equator. With the onset of the **anaphase** (AN-ah-faze), the third stage, the chromatid pairs split, with one member of each pair moving toward one of the centrioles at the poles.

In the last phase of the process, the **telaphase** (TEL-ah-faze), nuclei form around each polar centriole, and the chromosomes break back down into strands of chromatin. The cytoplasm of the cell pinches inward at its center and separates into two new cells, each with the genetic materials of the old cell.

Cellular reproduction occurs constantly during the life of the body as old cells are constantly being replaced by new cells. The process is ended only by death.

TISSUES

The cells group themselves according to their specialization to form **tissues** (TISH-yu), which are the structural materials of the body. There are five different kinds of tissue, differentiated by the types of cells they contain and their function. These are epithelial tissue, muscular tissue, connective tissue, nerve tissue, and liquid tissue.

Epithelial tissue (ep-ih-THEL-e-ahl TISH-yu) makes up the outer body covering as well as the lining for the hollow internal organs, the digestive and respiratory tract, and the glands. The cells are usually packed closely together, leaving little room for intracellular fluid. There are no blood vessels in epithelial tissue, but there are large numbers of nerve endings.

This sheet-like tissue takes a number of forms, depending on the shape of the cells. **Squamous** (SWKA-mus) epithelial tissue is found in body cavity linings and blood vessel linings as well as in the epidermis, the mouth, esophagus, and the corneas. It consists of thin, flat cells shaped like overlapping tiles. On dry surfaces, such as the outer skin, the tissue is highly keratinized.

The cells in **cuboidal** (ku-BOYD-ahl) epithelial tissue are cube-shaped. This type of tissue is found in gland tissue and kidney linings. **Columnar** epithelial tissue consists of tall, column-like cells and is found in the linings of the stomach and intestines. The columnar epithelial tissue lining the respiratory ducts has cilia, fine hairs, to keep dust away from the lungs. **Goblet cells** (GOB-let SELS), so named because of their wine-glass-like shape, make up a specialized type of columnar epithelium found in secretory organs and glands.

Muscle tissue (MUS-el TISH-yu) has the ability to contract, thus allowing movement in the body. There are three different types of muscle tissue. **Striated** (STREYE-a-ted) muscle tissue is attached to the skeletal system and controls conscious movements. Arm and leg muscles, for example, are striated. **Smooth** muscle, or involuntary muscle tissue, is found mostly in hollow cavity walls and controls movement not under the conscious control of the individual. The small intestine, for example, consists of smooth muscle tissue. **Cardiac** (KAR-dee-ak), or heart, muscle tissue is striated yet is involuntary. This type of muscle tissue is found only in the heart.

Connective tissue ties other tissues together. It also helps protect other tissues and helps support the other tissues. This type of tissue contains relatively few cells with rather loose spacing. There is a good deal of intercellular material, however. This nonliving material is called the **matrix** (MAY-trix), or **ground substance** (GROUND SUB-stanz). Connective tissue contains large numbers of blood vessels. The typical cell in connective tissue is a **fibroblast** (FEYE-bro-blast), a long, irregularly shaped cell that synthesizes protein for tissue growth.

The connective tissue is found under the epidermis and around internal organs and blood vessels. It is the main packing material of the body and contains fat tissue. In addition to the ground substance, the connective tissue contains fibrous materials, including **collagen** (KOL-uh-jin), bundles of white fibers that are inelastic yet flexible; elastic fibers, which contain **elastin** (ee-LAS-tin); and **reticular fibers** (reh-TIK-u-lar FEYE-bers), which are found in lymphatic tissue.

Cartilage (KAR-ti-lij) is a specialized form of connective tissue that helps support the body. It is found in the nose, ears, in the spinal discs, and at the ends of bones. Cartilage gradually changes into bone as calcium and other minerals from bone cells fill in the intercellular spaces.

Nerve tissue consists of neurons, or nerve cells, which are found in the brain, the spinal cord, nerves, and sensory organs. They transmit electrical impulses to and from the brain and coordinate all bodily activities.

The major body fluids, **blood** and **lymph,** may be considered as tissues even though they are liquid. They are composed of specialized cells, like the other tissues, and they have large quantities of intercellular fluids. Blood, important to many body functions, consists of red cells, white cells, plasma, and platelets, each of which has a specialized task. Lymph is similar to plasma. It contains large numbers of white cells, but no red cells.

ORGANS

Just as tissues are composed of groups of cells, **organs** are composed of groups of tissues. And as with tissues, the body contains several types of specialized organs that are vital to its proper functioning. The major organs are the brain, the heart, the lungs, the liver, the kidneys, the glands, the stomach, the intestines, and the skin.

The **brain,** the most complex organ in the body, controls the nervous system. The **heart** pumps blood through the circulatory system. The **lungs** supply oxygen to the blood through the respiratory system. The **liver** and the **kidneys** process and excrete toxic wastes through the excretory system. The **glands** secrete hormones and other substances needed for growth or regulation through the endocrine system. The **stomach** and **intestines** (in-TES-tinz) process nutrients from food through the digestive system. The **skin** forms the tough, outer covering of the body.

SYSTEMS

The body consists of nine **systems** (SIS-tems), groups of organs working together to perform specific functions. These systems are:

The Systems for Support and Movement

1. The **skeletal** (SKEL-e-tahl) **system**—the bones, cartilage and ligaments, which form the supporting structure of the body.
2. The **muscular** (MUS-kyoo-lahr) **system**—the muscles, which allow the body to move and to work.

The Systems for Control and Regulation

3. The **nervous** (NUR-vus) **system**—the brain, spinal cord and nerves, which transmit electrical impulses to process information and direct responses to control the body's functions.
4. The **endocrine** (EN-doh-krin) **system**—the ductless glands, which regulate body processes.

The Systems for the Production of Energy

5. The **circulatory** (SUR-kyoo-lahr-tohr-ee) **system**—the heart, blood, lymph, and the vessels that transport them throughout the body.
6. The **respiratory** (RES-pi-rah-tohr-ee) **system**—the lungs, which bring in oxygen and take out waste gases.
7. The **digestive** (deye-GES-tiv) **system**—the stomach and intestines, which digest food so the nutrients can be converted into energy.
8. The **excretory** (EK-skre-tohr-ee) **system**—the kidneys, bladder, and other organs that remove waste materials from the body.

The Systems for Procreation

9. The **reproductive** (ree-proh-DUK-tiv) **system**—the reproductive organs, which allow for the continuation of the species.

THE SKELETAL SYSTEM

The skeletal system consists of the bones, cartilage, and ligaments. The 206 bones in the body form the structural framework. Cartilage forms part of the supporting structure as well. The ligaments tie the bones together and hold organs in place. The main functions of the skeletal system are to provide the supporting structure for the body and to serve as attachment points for the muscles. In addition, the skeleton encloses and protects vital organs. Bones also store calcium and contain the mechanism for the production of blood cells.

Bone is composed of about one-third living, or organic, matter and about two-thirds nonliving, or inorganic, matter. Bone cells and marrow comprise the living component; minerals, mostly calcium and phosphorus, comprise the nonliving component. Blood vessels run through the bone to provide nourishment to the cells and to remove wastes. **Marrow** (MAHR-oh), found in the spongy areas of the bone, produces red blood cells.

The skeletal structure is divided into two parts—the **axial** skeleton, which consists of the skull, the thorax, and the vertebral column, and the **appendicular** (ap-en-DIK-u-lar) skeleton, which consists of the pectoral girdle and the arm and hand bones, and the pelvic girdle, and the leg and foot bones. The esthetician is most concerned with the bones of the skull, the bones of the arm and hand, and the bones of the foot.

THE AXIAL SKELETON

The Skull   The skull contains twenty-nine bones divided into four sections. The eight cranial bones form a protective shell around the brain (Fig. 5.2). The bones are:

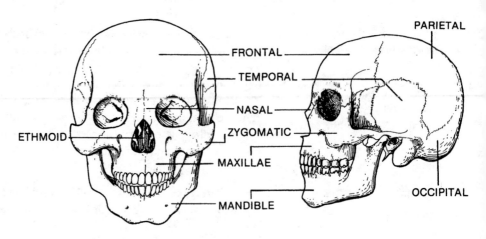

5.2—Human skull bones

1. The **frontal** (FRUNT-al) bone, which forms the forehead.
2. Two **parietal** (pa-RY-e-tal) bones, which form the roof and sides of the skull.
3. Two **temporal** (TEM-po-rahl) bones, which form the lower sides of the skull.
4. The **occipital** (ok-SIP-i-tal) bone, which forms the back of the skull.
5. The **ethmoid** (ETH-moid) bone, which supports the nasal cavity.
6. The **sphenoid** (SFEEN-oid) bone, which forms part of the eye-sockets and ties the rest of the skull together.

There are fourteen facial bones:

1. Two **maxillae** (mak-SIL-ee), which form the upper jaw and the roof of the mouth.
2. Two **zygomatic** (zy-goh-MAT-ik) bones, which form the prominences of the cheeks. These are also called **malar** bones.
3. Two **lacrimal** bones, which form part of the eyesockets and also have grooves for the tear ducts.
4. The **mandible** (MAN-di-bel), which forms the lower jawbone.
5. The **vomer** (VOH-mer), which forms part of the nasal septum.
6. Two **nasal** (NAY-zal) bones, which form the bridge of the nose.
7. Two **nasal conchae** (KONG-kee), which form part of the nasal cavity.
8. Two **palatine** (PAL-i-tyn) bones, which form part of the roof of the mouth and part of the nasal cavity.

The facial bones contain **sinuses** (SY-nuses), air spaces that reduce the weight of the bones without reducing their strength.

The remaining seven bones of the skull are:

1. The **hyoid** (HEYE-oid) bone, or "Adam's apple," which is a horseshoe shaped bone found at the front of the throat.
2. The six **auditory ossicles** (AW-dit-ohr-ee OSS-i-kles), found in the middle ear. These serve as organs of balance and transmit vibrations to the ear drums. There are two **malleus** (MAY-le-us) bones, two **incus** (INK-us) bones, and two **stapes** (STA-pez). These are the smallest bones in the human body.

The Vertebral Column

The **vertebral column** (VER-te-brahl KOHL-um), the main axis of the body, protects the spinal cord and the spinal nerves. It consists of twenty-six bones—twenty-four individual vertebrae, the sacrum, and the coccyx (Fig 5.3).

The twenty-four individual **vertebrae** (VER-te-bray) are divided into three groups. The seven **cervical** (SUR-vi-kal) vertebrae form the neck bones. The first cervical vertebra, at the top, is called the **atlas**; the seventh, at the bottom of the cervix, is called the **axis** (AX-is). The twelve **thoracic** vertebrae extend from the neck through the chest area. The five lumbar vertebrae extend down through the loin area. These twenty-four individual vertebrae are separated by discs of cartilage that allow the column to bend and absorb shock to the system.

The **sacrum** (SAY-krum), which extends down from the lumbar vertebrae, consists of five vertebrae that are fused together into a single bone. The sacrum forms the back of the pelvis. The **coccyx** (KOK-siks) consists of three to five fused rudimentary vertebrae at the bottom of the vertebral column and forms the **caudal appendage** (KAUD-ahl ah-PEN-daj), or the remnants of what may once have been a tail before human beings evolved from lower forms of primate.

The Thorax

The **thorax** (THO-racks) consists of the **sternum** (STIR-num), or breastbone, and twenty-four ribs. The twelve pairs of ribs are connected loosely to the vertebral column. The first ten pairs of ribs are attached to the sternum by flexible strips of cartilage. The thorax forms a protective cage around the lungs, the heart, and other important internal organs. The loose connections and the flexible cartilage let the ribs move when the lungs expand and contract while breathing (Fig. 5.4).

THE APPENDICULAR SKELETON

The **appendicular** (a-pen-DIK-yoo-lar) **skeleton** consists of the bones of the upper extremities and the lower extremities. There are 126 bones in the appendages of the skeletal system.

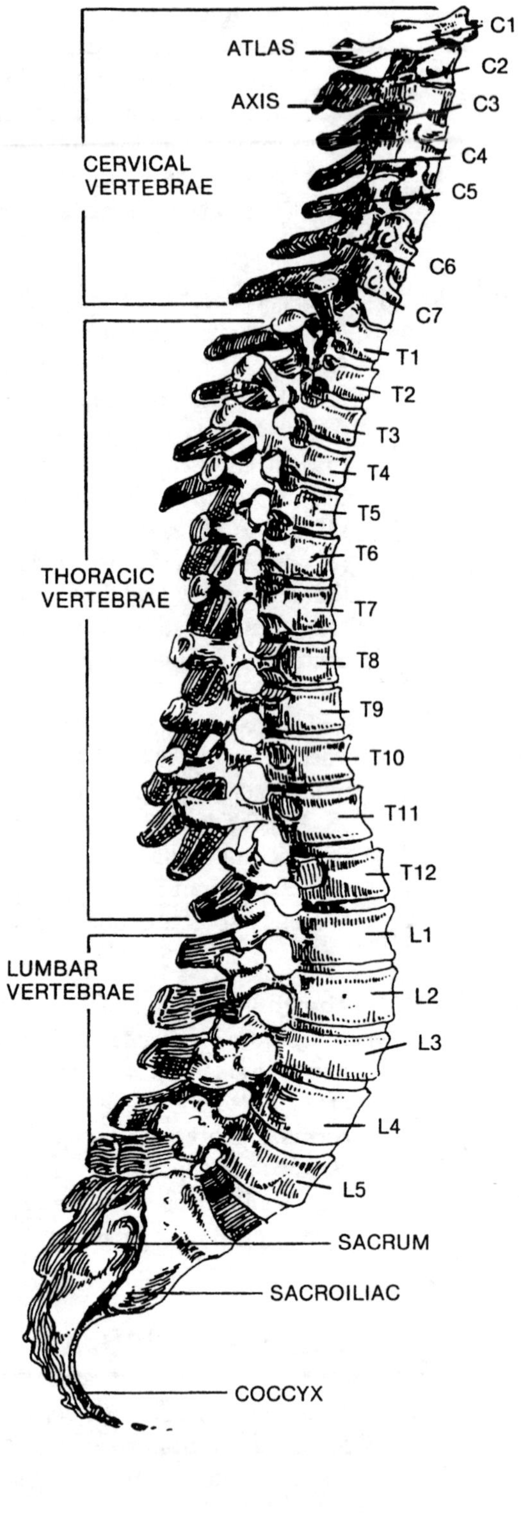

ATLAS — C1
AXIS — C2
C3
C4
C5
C6
C7

CERVICAL
VERTEBRAE

T1
T2
T3
T4
T5
T6
T7
T8
T9
T10
T11
T12

THORACIC
VERTEBRAE

L1
L2
L3
L4
L5

LUMBAR
VERTEBRAE

SACRUM
SACROILIAC
COCCYX

5.3—Vertebral column

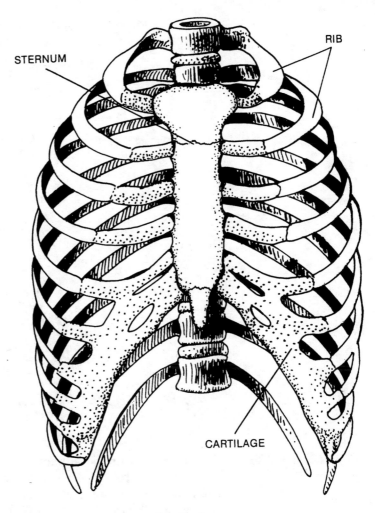

STERNUM

RIB

CARTILAGE

5.4—The thorax

The Upper Extremities

The upper part of the appendicular skeleton consists of the four bones of the **pectoral girdle** (pek-TOR-ahl GIR-del) and the sixty bones of the arms and hands. The pectoral girdle consists of two **scapulae**, or shoulder blades, and two **clavicles** (KLAV-i-kel), or collarbones. The upper arm has one long bone, the **humerus** (HYOO-mo-rus). The forearm has two bones, the **ulna** (UL-nah), the larger of the two, which is on the little finger side of the arm, and the **radius** (RAY-dee-us), on the thumb side of the arm (Fig. 5.5).

The hand is more complex, consisting of eight **carpals** (KAHR-pal), or wrist bones, five **metacarpals** (met-a-KAHR-palz), which form the palm, and fourteen **phalanges** (fa-LAN-jeez), three in each finger except the thumb, which has two.

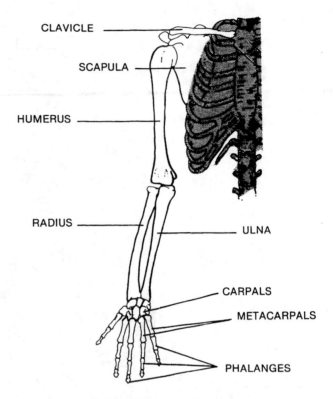

CLAVICLE

SCAPULA

HUMERUS

RADIUS

ULNA

CARPALS

METACARPALS

PHALANGES

5.5—Shoulder, arm and hand bones

The Lower Extremities

The lower part of the appendicular skeleton consists of the two bones of the **pelvic girdle** and the sixty bones of the legs and feet. The bones of the pelvic girdle are the **hipbone,** which consists of three bones, the **ilium** (IL-ee-um), the **ischium** (ISH-ee-um) and the **pubis** (PYOO-bis), fused into a single bone, and the **pelvis** (PEL-vis). The pubis and the pelvis are the only bones that have somewhat different shapes for males and females.

The thigh has one long bone, the **femur** (FEE-mur). The leg has two long bones, the **tibia** (TIB-ee-ah), or shinbone, and the **fibula** (FIB-u-la). The **patella** (pa-TEL-a), or kneecap, is located at the front of the knee.

The foot has twenty-six bones—seven **tarsals** (TAR-sals), including the **talus** (TAY-lus), or ankle bone, five **metatarsals** (met-a-TAR-sals), and fourteen **phalanges** (fa-LAN-jeez), three in each toe except the big toe, which has two. The hands and feet are similar structurally.

Joints, or **articulations** (ar-tik-yoo-LAY-shuns), occur at the junction of two or more bones. Some joints are immovable; others have a limited range of motion; and still others have a full range of motions. The immovable articulations may be joined by interlocking edges, as the cranial bones, or they may be joined by cartilage, as the first ribs are to the breastbone. The articulations of limited motion are joined by a spongy, fibrous cartilage, as the discs between the vertebrae.

The freely movable articulations take a number of forms, varying from a simple hinge, as the elbow; along a plane, as in the wrist or ankle; a pivot, as in the neck or forearm; and a ball and socket, as in the hip bone. The moveable joints contain a liquid, called **synovial** (SY-no-vee-ahl) **fluid,** that lubricates the joint. The bones are held together by muscles and ligaments.

THE MUSCULAR SYSTEM

Muscles account for forty percent of the body's weight. These fibrous tissues allow the various parts of the body to move as they contract and relax. There are three kinds of muscle, the **striated** (STRY-aye-ted) tissues of the skeletal muscles, which are under voluntary control; the **smooth** tissues of the muscles of the internal organs, which are under involuntary control; and the **cardiac** (KAHR-dee-ak), or heart, muscle, which is also under involuntary control.

The smooth muscles perform a number of functions under the direction of the autonomic nervous system. They move food through the digestive tract; expel waste materials from the gallbladder, the urinary bladder and the rectum; regulate the change of size in various openings in the body, such as the pupil of the eye; and they constrict or dilate the blood vessels. The cardiac muscle pumps blood through the circulatory system.

The skeletal muscles control the movement of the body. They allow walking, bending, scratching, etc., over a wide range of motions. The eighty muscles in the face, for example, allow the formation of more than seven thousand different expressions. The esthetician is most concerned with the skeletal muscles, especially of the head, face, neck, arms, and hands, since these are the muscles most often worked on. If full body massage or reflexology treatments are offered in the salon, the esthetician will also be concerned with the muscles of the torso, legs, and feet.

The esthetician can stimulate or soothe the muscles in a number of ways. These include massage, either by hand or with a mechanical vibrator or rotating brush; by the application of chemical solutions; by the use of electrical current, either with the high frequency machine or the iontophoresis machine; or by the application of moist or dry heat.

Skeletal muscles are attached to bones or to other muscle tissue. One end of the muscle, the **origin,** is fixed. The other end, the **insertion,** is moveable. Almost all of the more than 650 muscles in

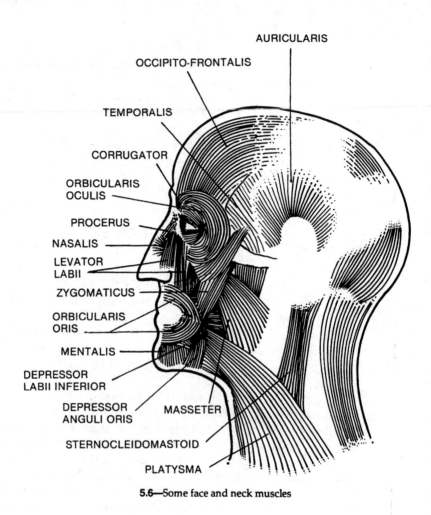

AURICULARIS

OCCIPITO-FRONTALIS

TEMPORALIS

CORRUGATOR

ORBICULARIS
OCULIS

PROCERUS

NASALIS

LEVATOR
LABII

ZYGOMATICUS

ORBICULARIS
ORIS

MENTALIS

DEPRESSOR
LABII INFERIOR

DEPRESSOR
ANGULI ORIS   MASSETER

STERNOCLEIDOMASTOID

PLATYSMA

5.6—Some face and neck muscles

the body are found in pairs. One contracts as the other relaxes, allowing a joint to bend. When the first relaxes and the other contracts, the joint straightens.

Muscles of the Head

The muscles of the head can be grouped according to their function. The muscles of expression allow the physical manifestation of emotional responses, such as laughter, smiling, anger, fear, or grief. The muscles of mastication allow chewing. The muscles of the tongue let the tongue move. The muscles of the pharynx and the muscles of the soft palate allow swallowing. However, the esthetician is concerned only with the muscles of expression and the muscles of mastication (Fig. 5.6). The major muscles of interest to the esthetician include:

1. The **epicranius** (ep-i-KRAY-ne-us), which covers the top of the skull. The front part, called the **frontalis** (front-TAY-lis), elevates the eyebrows and wrinkles the brow. The back part, called the **occipitalis** (ok-SIP-i-ta-lis), pulls the scalp backward. The two parts are connected by a tendon called the epicranial **aponeurosis** (ap-o-noo-ROH-sis).
2. The **corrugator** (KOR-oo-gay-tohr) **supercillii,** which are located under the frontalis on the sides of the eyebrows, pull the eyebrows down and in.
3. The **orbis oculi** (OR-bis OK-yoo-leye), which encircles the eyesocket, lets the eye close, and tightens the skin on the forehead.
4. The **orbicularis oris** (or-bik-yoo-LAY-ris OH-ris), which surrounds the upper and lower lips, lets the lips close or pucker.
5. The **zygomaticus** (zeye-goh-MAT-i-kus), which extends from the zygomatic bone to the corner of the mouth, pulls the corner of the mouth up.
6. The **triangularis** (treye-an-gyoo-LAY-ris), which extends along the side of the chin, pulls the corner of the mouth down.
7. The **risorius** (ri-ZOHR-ee-us), which runs across the cheek, draws the corner of the mouth out.
8. The **quadratus labii inferioris** (kwah-DRAY-tus LAY-bee-eye in-FEER-ee-or-ihs), which encircles the lower lip, draws the lower lip down.
9. The **quadratus labii superioris** (suu-PEER-ee-or-ihs), which encircles the upper lip, draws the upper lip up.
10. The **buccinator** (BUK-si-nay-tor), which lies in the cheek, allows the cheek to compress.
11. The **procerus** (proh-SEE-rus), which covers the bridge of the nose, wrinkles the skin at the top of the nose.
12. The **caninus** (kay-NIGH-nus), which is located under the quadratus labii superioris, raises the angle of the mouth.
13. The **mentalis** (men-TAL-is), which extends from the mandible to the chin, lets the lower lip protrude.
14. The **platysma** (pla-TIZ-mah), which covers the lower jaw and side of the neck, depresses the lower jaw and lower lip.
15. The **masseter** (ma-SEE-tur), which covers the side of the lower mandible and cheek, closes the mouth and clenches the teeth.
16. The **temporalis** (tem-po-RAY-lis), which covers the temporalis bone, also closes the mouth and clenches the teeth.
17. The **external pterygoid** (ex-TER-nahl TER-i-goid), which extends from the side of the sphenoid bone to the joint of the temporalis bone and the mandible, lets the mouth open and move from side to side.

The Muscles of the Neck

The muscles of the neck allow the head to bend and rotate and move the hyoid bone during the process of swallowing. The esthetician is concerned only with the muscles that move the head. The major neck muscles of interest to the esthetician are:

1. The **sternocleidomastoideus** (STUR-noh-KLE-i-doh-mas-toid-ee-us), which extends across the sides of the neck from the clavicle to the **mastoid** (MAS-toid), the area of the temporalis behind the ear.
2. The **splenius capitis** (SPLEE-nee-us KAP-ih-tus), which extends from the cervical vertebrae to the occipital bone.
3. The **rectus capitis** (REK-tus KAP-ih-tus), which extends from the first cervical vertebrae, the atlas, to the occipital bone.

The Muscles of the Upper Extremities

The muscles of the upper extremities—the shoulders, arms, and hands—can be grouped into those that move the scapula, those that move the humerus, those that move the forearm, and those that move the hand (Fig. 5.7). The muscles of most interest to the esthetician are:

1. The **pectoralis minor** (pek-tohr-AL-is MY-nor), which extends from the sternum to the scapula, moves the scapula down and away from the body.
2. The **trapezius** (tra-PEE-zee-us), which covers the upper surface of the back, draws the scapula back and raises the shoulder.
3. The **serratus anterior** (ser-RAT-us an-TEER-ee-or), which extends from the rib cage to the scapula, pulls the scapula forward.
4. The **rhomboid** (ROM-boid), which lies under the trapezius muscle, rotates the scapula to depress the shoulder.

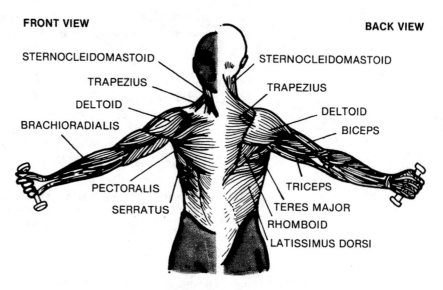

5.7—Shoulder, arm and hand muscles

5. The **latissimus dorsi** (la-TIS-i-mus DOR-see), which covers the lower surface of the back, rotates the humerus and extends the arm.

6. The **pectoralis major** (MAY-jor), which covers the upper portion of the chest, moves the humerus away from the body.

7. The **deltoid** (DEL-toid), which covers the shoulder and gives it its shape, helps flex and extend the arm.

8. The **biceps** (BEYE-seps), which extends along the front of the upper arm, flexes and supinates the forearm.

9. The **triceps** (TREYE-seps), which extends along the back of the upper arm, extends the arm and forearm.

10. The **brachialis** (BRAY-kee-ahl-is), which covers the front of the humerus under the biceps, flexes the forearm.

11. The **brachioradialis** (BRAY-kee-oh-RAY-dee-ah-lis), which extends from the humerus to the front of the radius, flexes the forearm. It also acts as a pronator or supinator, depending on how the forearm is moved.

12. The **supinator** (SUE-pi-nay-tor), which extends from the humerus to the ulna, turns the forearm and hand palm upward.

13. The **pronators** (pro-NAY-tors), **quadratus** (KWOD-rat-us), and **teres** (TEH-rez), which extend from the humerus to the radius, turn the forearm and hand palm downward.

14. The **flexor carpii** (FLEX-or KAHR-py), which are located on the forearm, flex the wrist and forearm.

15. The **flexor pollicis brevis** (pahl-ee-sez BREE-vis), which lies along the top of the carpal bones, flexes the thumb.

16. The **extensor** (ex-TEN-sor) **carpii**, which extend along the top of the ulna, extend the hand.

17. The **extensor digitorum communis** (di-ji-TOR-ee-um ko-MUN-is), which lies along the back of the arm, extends the wrist and fingers.

18. The **extensor pollicis brevis**, which lies under the extensor digitorum communis, extends the thumb.

19. The **opponens** (oh-POH-nens) **pollicis**, which extends from the carpal ligaments to the metacarpal, lets the thumb extend across the palm of the hand.

THE NERVOUS SYSTEM

The **nervous system** is the control center for all of the body's functions. It is essentially a network for information processing and action response. The system receives information from the external environment and from the internal environment, processes that information, and directs the responses to deal with that information.

The nervous system controls all physical and mental functions and coordinates those functions so they work in harmony.

This control system is of importance to the esthetician because of the effects the nerves have on muscles and the skin and the effects the various operations conducted during the facial treatment have on the nerves. Muscles contract or relax as the nerves that control them are stimulated. Nerves, like muscle tissue, may be stimulated in a number of ways: by physical means, such as massage or the application of pressure; by heat, such as steam or infrared radiation; by chemical action, such as various products that are placed on the skin; or by the application of electrical current, such as iontophoresis or high frequency. All of these are involved in the facial process. The esthetician is most concerned with the nerves of the head, face, neck, arms, and hands.

The nervous system consists of the brain, the spinal cord, and the network of nerves that run throughout the body. The brain and the spinal cord form the **central** (SEN-trahl), or **cerebrospinal** (ser-EE-broh-SPY-nahl), nervous system, which is the information processing center. The network of nerve fibers that extend from the brain and spinal cord form the **somatic**, or **peripheral** (pe-RIF-er-al), nervous system and the **autonomic** (aw-toh-NAHM-ik), or **sympathetic** (sim-pah-THET-ik), nervous system, which are the information transmission lines.

The **somatic** (sow-MA-tik) **nervous system** consists of those nerve fibers that are distributed throughout the body. They are of two types, depending on the direction of information flow. The **sensory**, or **afferent** (AF-fer-ent), nerves transmit information from the sensory receptors to the brain. The **motor**, or **efferent** (EF-e-rent), nerves, transmit impulses from the brain to the skeletal muscles. Some nerve fibers may perform both sensory and motor nerve functions. These nerves are responsible for those functions under voluntary, or conscious, control.

The autonomic nervous system consists of those nerve fibers that extend to and from the internal organs and the glands so they can perform their necessary functions. These nerves are responsible for those functions under involuntary, or unconscious, control.

The basic unit of the nervous system is the **neuron** (NOOR-on), which transmits the electrical signals. There are more than 10 billion neurons in the body, most of which are contained in the brain. They vary in size from very small, as the brain cells, to very long, as the neurons running from the spinal cord to the lower extremities (Fig. 5.8).

A neuron consists of a **cell body**, which contains the nucleus, an **axon** (AK-son), a long fiber that transmits electrical signals from the cell body, and a number of **dendrites** (DEN-drytes), short fibers that transmit electrical signals to the cell body. The nerve fibers are pro-

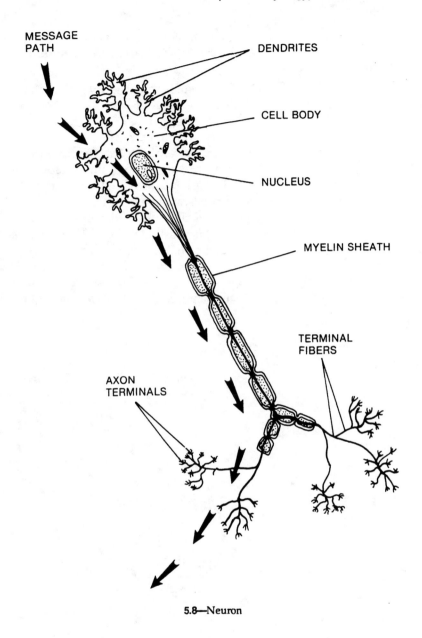

MESSAGE
PATH

DENDRITES

CELL BODY

NUCLEUS

MYELIN SHEATH

TERMINAL
FIBERS

AXON
TERMINALS

5.8—Neuron

tected by a layer of fatty material. This is called the **myelin sheath** (MY-ah-lin SHEETH).

The electrical impulses are transmitted from the axon terminals of one neuron to the dendrites of the next neuron in line. The junction between the two parts is called the **synapse** (SIN-aps). The axon terminals, however, do not touch the dendrites. The electrical impulse is transmitted across a gap, called the **synaptic cleft** (SIN-AP-tik kleft), by chemical particles called **neurotransmitters** (NOOR-o-trans-mit-ers).

The Brain

The brain is the primary information processing facility in the body. It is the most complex and the largest mass of nerve tissue. And, even though it makes up only a small percentage of the weight of the body, weighing from 2.5 to 3.5 pounds, it requires an extraordinarily large percentage of the energy produced by the body for it to function properly. The brain is responsible for all voluntary actions, for all consciousness and awareness, for all emotions, for all mental processes and for all sensations. It is also responsible for the regulation of all bodily processes (Fig. 5.9).

This most vital organ is divided into a number of major areas: the cerebrum, the cerebellum, the diencephalon, the mid-brain, the pons, and the medulla oblongata or brain stem. The **cerebrum** (SER-ee-brum) is the largest area of the brain and is divided into two hemispheres, the left and the right, which are joined by a mass of

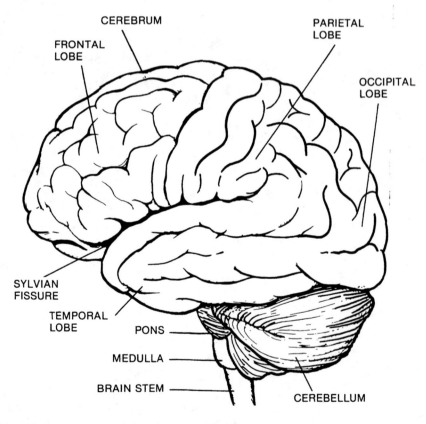

5.9—The brain

nerve fibers, called the **corpus callosum** (KOR-pus kal-O-sum). The outer layer is made up of gray matter, called the **cerebral cortex** (ser-EE-brah KOR-tex). The inner layer is made up of white matter.

The cerebrum controls the voluntary movements of the body and is responsible for receiving all sensory inputs, including sight, hearing, taste, and smell, and for allowing the higher mental processes, such as judgment, learning, memory, and speech. The left hemisphere controls logical processes, analytical reasoning, and speech. The right hemisphere controls spatial relations, artistic ability, and intuitive thought. Right-handed people are controlled predominantly by the left hemisphere; most left-handed people, by the right hemisphere.

The **cerebellum** (ser-ah-BEL-um) is a smaller area of the brain located beneath the rear of the cerebrum and behind the medulla oblongata. This area of the brain is the center of motor coordination, regulating the timing for complex movements. It is also the center for balance and equilibrium.

The **diencephalon** (DY-en-sef-a-lon), the area between the mid-brain and the cerebrum, contains the **thalamus** and the **hypothalamus**. The thalamus is the main relay station for the brain, sorting out and relaying the sensory inputs received from the various sensory nerves. The hypothalamus coordinates the functions of the nervous system and the endocrine system and ties the two systems together. It is the body's temperature control and appetite control center. The hypothalamus controls many emotional responses, as well.

The mid-brain, or **mesencephalon** (mez-en-sef-a-lon), lies above the pons and in front of the cerebellum. This area connects the higher center of the brain with the lower center and assists in maintaining equilibrium. The **pons**, a bulbous area below the mid-brain and in front of the medulla oblongata, connects the medulla with the higher brain centers. The **medulla oblongata**, or **brain stem**, is the lowest portion of the brain, and connects the rest of the brain with the spinal cord. The brain stem regulates the heartbeat, and controls the digestive system, respiratory system, and circulatory system.

The Cranial Nerves

Twelve pairs of cranial nerves extend from the brain to the various parts of the head and neck. These control the head and sense organs and are identified by number and by name. All but the first and second cranial nerves come from the brain stem. Most are sensory-motor nerves although a few are sensory nerves only. All of the nerves have many branches. The twelve pairs are:

1. **Olfactory** (ol-FACK-tur-ee)—the **First Cranial Nerve**, a sensory nerve that controls the sense of smell.
2. **Optic** (OP-tik)—the **Second Cranial Nerve**, a sensory nerve that controls the sense of sight.

3. **Oculomotor** (ock-yoo-lo-MO-tur)—the **Third Cranial Nerve**, a principally motor nerve that controls eye movement.
4. **Trochlear** (TROK-lee-ur)—the **Fourth Cranial Nerve**, a principally motor nerve that also controls eye movement.
5. **Trigeminal** (try-JEM-i-nul)—the **Fifth Cranial Nerve**, a sensory nerve for the face and head and a motor nerve for the muscles used in chewing.
6. **Abducent** (ab-DEW-sunt)—the **Sixth Cranial Nerve**, a principally motor nerve that also controls eye movement.
7. **Facial** (FAY-shul)—the **Seventh Cranial Nerve**, a sensory-motor nerve for the face, head and neck.
8. **Vestibulocochlear** (ves-TIB-u-lo-kok-le-ar) or acoustic—the **Eighth Cranial Nerve**, a principally sensory nerve that controls the sense of hearing.
9. **Glossopharyngeal** (glos-o-fa-RIN-jee-ul)—the **Ninth Cranial Nerve**, a sensory-motor nerve that controls the sense of taste.
10. **Vagus** (VAY-gus)—the **Tenth Cranial Nerve**, a sensory-motor nerve that has the most extensive distribution throughout the body. It controls the movements and sensations of the ear, pharynx, larynx, heart and lungs.
11. **Accessory** (ack-SES-uh-ree)—the **Eleventh Cranial Nerve**, a sensory-motor nerve that controls neck movement.
12. **Hypoglossal** (heye-po-GLOS-ul)—the **Twelfth Cranial Nerve**, a sensory-motor nerve that controls tongue movement.

Of the twelve cranial nerves, the most important to the esthetician are the trigeminal (fifth), the facial (seventh), and the accessory (eleventh) (Fig. 5.10).

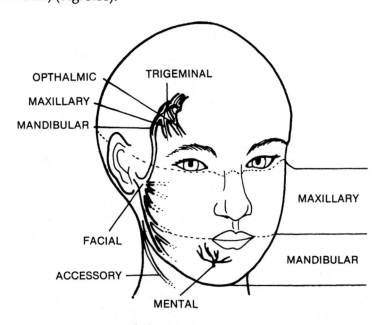

5.10—Major facial nerves

The Spinal Cord   The **spinal cord** is the main pathway for conducting the electrical impulses to and from the brain. It is also a major reflex center, controlling a number of reflex actions. A **reflex** is an automatic response to a stimulus and does not require that the sensation travel from the sensory organ to the brain and back again. The response is triggered directly from the spinal cord.

The spinal cord extends from the brain stem to about two-thirds of the way down the spinal column. Nerve fibers continue to run down the spinal column from the end of the spinal cord. The cord and the brain are wrapped with a protective coating. The three layers of the coating are called **meninges** (men-IN-jes). The meninges are filled with a liquid, the **cerebrospinal fluid**, which cushions the spinal cord and the brain.

Thirty-one pairs of spinal nerves arise from the spinal cord. These include eight pairs of **cervical nerves**, which control the neck and arms; twelve pairs of **thoracic nerves**, which control the chest cavity; five pairs of **lumbar nerves**, which control the legs and feet; and six pairs of nerves from the sacrum and coccyx, which control the pelvic organs and buttocks.

THE ENDOCRINE SYSTEM

The **endocrine system** works along with the nervous system to control and regulate the bodily functions. While the nervous system is the electrical control system of the body, however, the endocrine system is the chemical control system (Fig. 5.11).

Although the esthetician does not work directly with the glands or glandular secretions, an understanding of the endocrine system is important because many of the skin-care products contain hormone derivatives. The essential oils used in aromatherapy contain **phytohormones** (FEYE-tow-hor-monz), plant hormones, which are compatible with human hormones.

There are two types of **glands** in the body, the **exocrine** (EX-oh-krin), or **ducted** glands, so named because their secretions travel through ducts, and the **endocrine**, or **ductless** glands, which inject their secretions directly into the bloodstream. The exocrine glands include the **sebaceous** (see-BA-shus) glands, which secrete sebum; the **sudoriferous** (su-dor-IF-er-us), or sweat glands; and the **salivary** glands.

The endocrine system, however, includes only the ductless glands, which secrete hormones. Most of these specialized glands secrete only hormones. A few, however, have other functions besides the production of **hormones**. A hormone (HOR-mown) is a chemical substance that retards or stimulates the function of another organ. Hormones are responsible for the control of most of the basic life functions, including growth, development, reproduction, even personality.

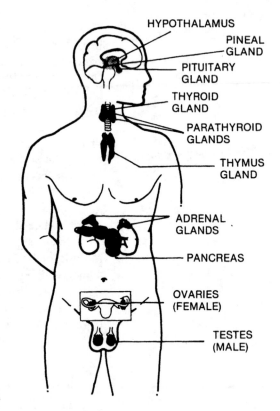

HYPOTHALAMUS

PINEAL
GLAND

PITUITARY
GLAND

THYROID
GLAND

PARATHYROID
GLANDS

THYMUS
GLAND

ADRENAL
GLANDS

PANCREAS

OVARIES
(FEMALE)

TESTES
(MALE)

5.11—Endocrine system

The most important endocrine glands are the hypothalamus, pituitary, pineal, thyroid, parathyroid, thymus, adrenal, and gonads. In addition, the gastrointestinal tract and the pancreas also secrete hormones as well as carrying out other functions.

The **hypothalamus** ties the nervous system and the endocrine system together. As discussed earlier, this gland controls the appetite, body temperature, and a number of emotional responses. It also regulates the pituitary gland.

The **pituitary** gland, located at the base of the brain, is the master gland of the body and regulates the hormone production of many of the other glands. In addition, the pituitary gland produces growth hormone, which regulates the normal growth of the body.

The **pineal** gland, at the rear of the diencephalon, is a small gland that produces hormones that help regulate the gonads, or reproductive glands.

The **thyroid** gland, in the middle of the neck below the larynx, produces hormones that control the metabolic rate of the body and help regulate the growth processes. The thyroid gland also contains four **parathyroid** glands, which produce a hormone that regulates calcium and phosphorus levels in the blood and bones.

The **thymus** gland, located just above the heart, produces hormones important to the maintenance of the immune responses. In addition, the thymus also produces **lymphocytes**, which enter the lymphatic system.

The two **adrenal** glands, located at each kidney, produce a number of hormones important to life maintenance, including salt and water balance and metabolic processes. They also produce hormones that affect the body's response to strong emotions.

The **gonads** are the reproductive glands. They are the **testes** in males and the **ovaries** in females. These glands produce **testosterone** (tes-TOS-tur-ohn) and **estrogen** (ES-tro-jin), hormones that stimulate the development of male and female sex characteristics.

The gastrointestinal tract produces a number of hormones that are important to the proper functioning of the stomach, liver, kidneys, and gallbladder. The pancreas has both exocrine and endocrine functions. Its exocrine secretions are inserted into the duodenum. The endocrine hormones, which include insulin, regulate blood sugar balance and carbohydrate metabolism.

The skin may be considered as part of the endocrine system, since it produces vitamin D, of which one form, cholecalciferol, or vitamin D_3, is considered to be a hormone rather than a nutrient.

THE CIRCULATORY SYSTEM

The circulatory system consists of two parts, the cardiovascular system and the lymphatic system. The cardiovascular system—which consists of the heart, veins, arteries, and capillaries—transports blood throughout the body. The lymphatic system—which consists of the lymph vessels, lymph nodes, thymus gland, and spleen—manufactures and distributes antibodies that help protect the body from disease (Fig. 5.12).

The esthetician is concerned with the cardiovascular system because of the importance of proper circulation to the overall health of the body and the effects of poor circulation on the skin. An understanding of the lymph system is important because of its role in waste removal and the immune system. The esthetician is directly involved with the lymphatic network when lymphatic drainage massage is performed.

The Cardiovascular System

The **cardiovascular system** represents a closed loop in which the heart pumps blood from the right side of the heart to the lungs, where it picks up oxygen, then returns to the left side of the heart. This is known as **pulmonary** (PULL-mo-ner-ee) **circulation**.

The oxygen enriched blood is then pumped through the arteries throughout the body where it provides oxygen, nutrients, and hor-

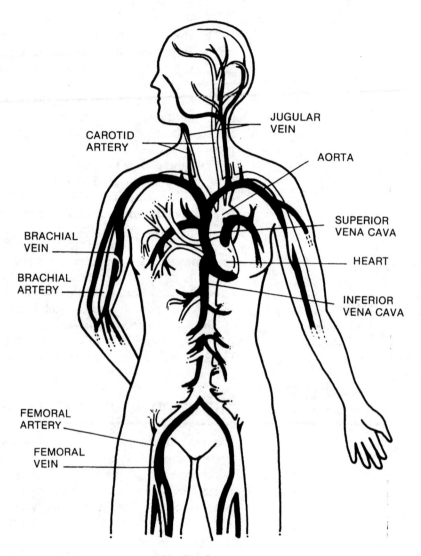

5.12—Circulatory system

mones to the tissues and organs as it filters through capillaries. The oxygen-depleted blood and waste materials are then pumped through the veins back to the right side of the heart. The process is repeated over and over. This is known as **systemic circulation**.

The Heart. The human heart is a fist-sized organ composed of cardiac muscle. It lies in the chest cavity where it is protected by the rib cage. This three-quarter-pound living pump beats an average of

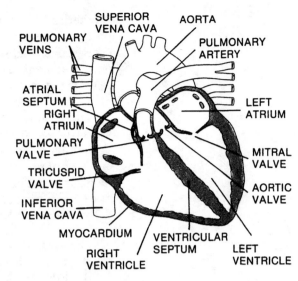

SUPERIOR VENA CAVA

AORTA

PULMONARY VEINS

PULMONARY ARTERY

ATRIAL SEPTUM

RIGHT ATRIUM

LEFT ATRIUM

PULMONARY VALVE

MITRAL VALVE

TRICUSPID VALVE

AORTIC VALVE

INFERIOR VENA CAVA

MYOCARDIUM

VENTRICULAR SEPTUM

LEFT VENTRICLE

RIGHT VENTRICLE

5.13—The heart

seventy to eighty times a minute from the moment of birth until the moment of death (Fig. 5.13).

The **heart** is encased in a double-walled membrane, called the **pericardium** (per-i-KAHR-dee-um). This membrane provides a casing for the heart and contains a lubricating fluid between the walls of the membrane. This fluid minimizes friction and rubbing as the heart expands and contracts.

The heart is divided into four chambers, the left and right atria and the left and right ventricles. The **atria** are the upper chambers; the **ventricles** (VEN-tri-kel) are the lower chambers. Veins carry blood from all parts of the body to the superior and inferior vena cavae, the main veins into the heart, where it enters at the right atrium. Blood then passes into the right ventricle. It is pumped from the right ventricle to the lungs through the pulmonary artery. After picking up oxygen, blood travels through the pulmonary vein back to the heart and is pumped into the left atrium. The blood then enters the left ventricle, where it is pumped into the aorta (the main artery) and through the arteries to the rest of the body. At each stage of its journey into, through, or out of the heart, the blood passes through a one-way valve that keeps it from reversing the flow and backing up.

The Blood Vessels. The **arteries** (AR-ter-eez) carry blood from the heart to the body tissues. **Veins** carry blood from the tissues back to the heart. **Capillaries** (CAP-i-ler-eez) transfer the blood from the arteries to the veins, depleting the blood of oxygen and nutrients in the process. In structure, arteries and veins are similar, except arteries are thicker and more elastic. Veins also contain one-way valves to prevent backflow.

Arteries branch out from the aorta, the large artery at the heart, which is about an inch in diameter, through successively smaller arteries, culminating in **arterioles**, tiny arteries about one-tenth of an inch in diameter. The capillaries are minute vessels, less than one-tenth of the thickness of a hair, through which blood passes slowly on its way to the veins. Tiny veins, called **venules**, take the blood from the capillaries and transfer it through succeedingly larger veins on its trip back to the heart.

The major blood vessels of the pulmonary system are the right and left pulmonary arteries, which take oxygen-depleted blood from the heart to the lungs, and the right and left pulmonary veins, which take oxygen-rich blood from the lungs back to the heart.

The major system arteries in the body are:

1. The **aorta** (AY-or-ta), the largest artery, which extends upward from the heart and arches over and extends downward. All of the other major arteries branch out of the aorta in pairs that supply the left and right sides of the body.
2. The right and left **common carotid** (kah-ROT-id) arteries, which extend up from the arch of the aorta and supply blood to the head.
3. The **external carotid** arteries and the **internal carotid** arteries, which branch from the common carotids. The external carotids supply blood to the outer parts of the neck and face. The internal carotids supply blood to the cranial cavity, the brain, and the eyesockets.
4. The **superficial temporal** arteries, which branch from the external carotids and supply blood to the scalp, top, and sides of the head.
5. The **transverse facial** arteries, which branch from the external carotids and supply blood to the lower part of the face, nose, and mouth.
6. The **occipital** arteries, which branch from the external carotids and supply blood to the back of the head.
7. The right and left **subclavian** arteries, which extend from the arch of the aorta and carry blood to the arms.
8. The **axillary** arteries, which continue from the subclavian arteries and supply blood to the arms.
9. The **brachial** arteries, which continue from the axillary arteries and supply blood to the upper arms.
10. The **ulnar** and **radial** arteries, which branch from the brachial arteries and supply blood to the forearms and hands.
11. The **thoracic aorta**, which extends downward from the arch of the aorta and is the main channel for arteries that supply blood to the internal organs in the chest area.
12. The **abdominal aorta**, which is a continuation of the thoracic aorta and is the main channel that supplies blood to the internal organs in the lower areas of the trunk.

13. The **common iliac** arteries, which branch from the end of the abdominal aorta and channel blood to the pelvic area and the lower extremities.
14. The **internal** and **external iliac** arteries, which branch from the common iliac arteries. The internal iliac arteries, also called the **hypogastric** arteries, supply blood to the pelvis and the reproductive organs. The external iliac arteries extend to the legs.
15. The **femoral** arteries, which extend from the external iliac arteries and supply blood to the thighs.
16. The **posterior** and **anterior tibial** arteries, which branch from the femoral arteries and supply blood to the lower legs and feet.

The veins run roughly parallel to the arteries and, in general, share their nomenclature. So, for example, the femoral artery is paralleled by the femoral vein. The brachial artery is paralleled by the brachial vein, and so on. Arteries are usually located deeper within the body than the veins, which are located closer to the surface of the body.

The major systemic veins in the body that do not share nomenclature with arteries are:

1. The **internal** and **external jugular** veins lie on the left and right sides of the head and neck. The external jugular vein drains blood from the outer portions of the face and scalp. The internal jugular vein is the principal vein draining blood from the head and neck.
2. The **superior vena cava** is the main channel returning blood to the heart from the upper part of the body.
3. The **inferior vena cava** is the largest vein in the body and is the main channel returning blood to the heart from the lower part of the body.
4. The **portal** vein drains blood from the stomach, intestines, gallbladder, spleen, and pancreas into the liver, where toxic wastes are removed. The blood then passes from the liver into the inferior vena cava.

Blood. **Blood** is the most important of the body fluids. It delivers oxygen, hormones and nutrients to the organs and tissues in the body. It carries antibodies to defend the body against disease. It carries toxic waste materials from the organs and tissues. And it regulates the temperature of the body.

Blood consists of **plasma**, the liquid component, which contains **red** and **white blood cells**, or **corpuscles**, and **platelets**. The red cells pick up and transport oxygen to the tissues. The white cells attack invasive organisms such as bacteria and viruses to protect the body from disease. The platelets allow the blood to coagulate to stop leaks when the system is punctured.

The average adult has about six quarts of blood, or about seven percent of body weight. The plasma makes up about fifty-five percent of the blood and consists of about ninety percent water, eight percent protein and two percent inorganic salts. The red and white cells and the platelets make up the remaining forty-five percent of the blood. Red cells are smaller than the white cells, but outnumber them by a ratio of more than 600 to 1. In the systemic arteries, when the blood is oxygen-rich, it is bright red in color. In the systemic veins, when it is oxygen-poor, it is dark brownish-red.

The Lymphatic System

The **lymphatic system** is a separate circulatory system that carries **lymphocytes** that attack disease-causing organisms and that drains tissue fluids back into the bloodstream. It is the body's main sewer system (Fig. 5.14).

The system consists of the lymph, the lymphatic organs, the lymph nodes, and the lymph capillaries and vessels. Unlike the cardiovascular system, the lymphatic system has no mechanism for pumping the fluid through the vessels. Lymph movement relies, instead, on pressure differentials and on muscular activity. The lymph vessels do have valves, however, to prevent backflow.

The **thymus** gland and the **spleen** manufacture lymphocytes for the body's immune system. In addition, the spleen filters out foreign substances. The **lymph** (LIMF) **nodes** are located at intervals along the lymph vessels and act as filters. The lymph vessels collect the lymph from the lymph capillaries. They generally follow a course parallel to the arteries and veins and empty into the main lymph ducts.

THE RESPIRATORY SYSTEM

The nutrients carried throughout the body must be burned to be converted to energy. The respiratory system brings oxygen into the body so the nutrients can be burned. Oxygen, from the atmosphere, passes through the nose and the nasal passages, through the trachea and into the lungs. As discussed previously, the heart pumps oxygen-poor blood through the pulmonary arteries into the lungs, where the oxygen is transferred to the blood and pumped back into the heart through the pulmonary veins (Fig. 5.15).

As the blood picks up oxygen from the lungs, it gives up carbon dioxide as a waste product. The carbon dioxide is then exhaled back into the atmosphere, completing the exchange of gases.

Oxygen is even more important to the body than food or water. Although survival without food or water is possible for days or weeks, oxygen deprivation will cause death in a matter of minutes.

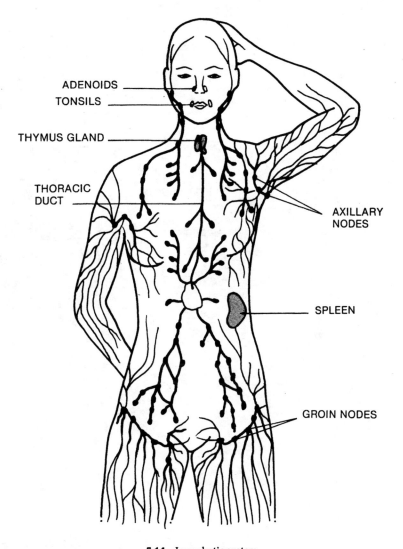

ADENOIDS

TONSILS

THYMUS GLAND

THORACIC
DUCT

AXILLARY
NODES

SPLEEN

GROIN NODES

5.14—Lymphatic system

Brain cells, for example, will start to die if they are deprived of oxygen for as little as four minutes.

The respiratory system consists of the nasal cavity, the pharynx, the larynx, the trachea, the bronchial tree, and the lungs. The **nasal cavity** begins in the nose, which is divided into two **nostrils**. The rear of each nostril, the **vestibule**, contains long hairs and a mucous membrane. The nasal cavity serves as the primary inlet for atmospheric air and warms and moistens the air and filters out dust and dirt before it passes into the throat. This area also contains the **olfactory nerves**, which control the sense of smell.

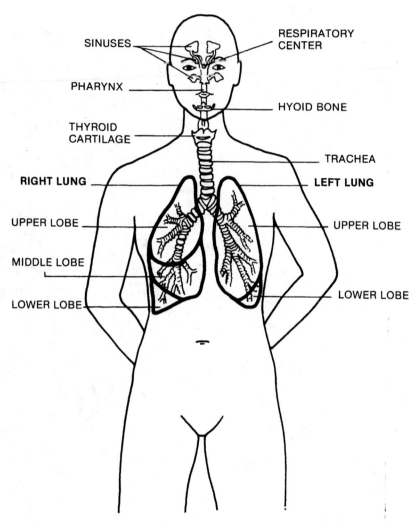

SINUSES

RESPIRATORY
CENTER

PHARYNX

HYOID BONE

THYROID
CARTILAGE

TRACHEA

RIGHT LUNG

LEFT LUNG

UPPER LOBE

UPPER LOBE

MIDDLE LOBE

LOWER LOBE

LOWER LOBE

5.15—Respiratory system

Air may also be brought into the lungs through the mouth. Mouth breathing, however, does not warm, moisten, or filter the air. Prolonged mouth breathing may be harmful, especially under cold, dry or dusty conditions.

The **sinuses** (SY-nus-es), air spaces in the bones around the nasal cavity, supply mucus to the nasal cavity. In addition, the sinuses reduce the weight of the bones and act as resonance chambers for sound waves generated during speech.

The **pharynx** (FAR-inks), or throat, is the first air passageway behind the nasal cavity. Both food and air pass through the pharynx as it branches into the esophagus, or food passageway, and the trachea, or air passageway. A flap, the **epiglottis**, closes off the trachea when food or liquid are swallowed.

The **larynx** (LAR-inks), or voice box, lies at the top of the trachea and contains the **vocal cords**, which vibrate as air from the lungs passes by them, causing the sound waves, which become speech. The larynx is attached to the hyoid bone by a membrane and is protected by the **thyroid cartilage**.

The **trachea** (TRAY-kee-uh), or windpipe, extends from the larynx to the thorax, where it branches off into the left and right bronchi. The trachea is a tubular structure supported by a series of ring-like cartilages, open at the back. The cartilages keep the windpipe from collapsing.

The **bronchial** (BRONK-ee-ul) **tree** carries air from the trachea into the lungs. It consists of two **bronchi**, which branch from the trachea and enter the lungs. As they enter the lungs, they divide and subdivide into smaller and smaller tubes, ending as tiny tubules called **bronchioles**. The bronchioles lead to the **alveolar ducts**, which branch into **alveolar sacs**. Each alveolar sac contains a number of **alveoli** (al-VEE-il-eye).

The **lungs**, the major respiratory organs, are an asymmetrical pair of spongy tissues filled with millions of alveoli, through which the oxygen and carbon dioxide gases are exchanged in the respiratory process. They rest on the **diaphragm** (DY-a-fram), which forces them to expand and contract as it moves. The right lung is shorter and wider than the left lung to allow room for the liver. The left lung is longer and more narrow to allow room for the heart. The right lung has three lobes; the left, only two.

The millions of alveoli in the lungs provide a large surface area for the efficient exchange of gases. As air is inhaled, the diaphragm contracts and moves down. This lowers the air pressure in the lungs and lets the lungs expand. As carbon dioxide is exhaled, the diaphragm relaxes and moves up. This increases air pressure in the lungs, letting the lungs contract and forcing the air outside. Breathing is controlled by the respiratory center in the brain stem. It occurs unconsciously, although an individual can exercise some conscious control over the breathing rate. Coughing and sneezing are protective reflex actions to eliminate foreign bodies from the system.

THE DIGESTIVE SYSTEM

The organs and tissues of the digestive system process and distribute the nutrients derived from food throughout the body. Food is ingested. It is broken down mechanically, then digested chemically. Nutrients are absorbed and distributed for use, and the waste products of digestion are eliminated.

The digestive system consists of the alimentary canal, a twenty-seven-foot long tube that extends from the mouth to the anus, through which food is processed, and the accessory glands that produce the enzymes needed for digestion (Fig. 5.16).

The Alimentary Canal

Food starts its journey through the body at the mouth. As the food is chewed, the teeth cut and grind the food into smaller particles. The **salivary glands** produce **saliva**, which moistens and softens the food and contains enzymes that begin the conversion process, breaking down the carbohydrates in the food into simple sugars. The lining of the mouth cools or warms the food to body temperature, and the tongue manipulates the food in the mouth, moving it to the back of the mouth where it is swallowed. The tongue also contains the taste buds, sensory organs that give the sensations of flavor.

The food moves into the **pharynx**. The **soft palate** raises and closes the nasal passage while the **epiglottis** lowers and closes the trachea so food can't enter the respiratory passages. The autonomic nervous system controls this action so it does not require conscious effort.

The food mass enters the **esophagus** (e-SOF-a-gus), a tube that lies behind the trachea and extends from the pharynx to the stomach. The food moves along the esophagus by **peristaltic** (pair-i-STAL-sik) **action**, a rippling, wave-like motion of the muscles of the esophagus.

The **stomach**, the mixing bowl of the system, lies on the left side of the abdominal cavity under the diaphragm. It is connected to the esophagus by the **cardiac sphincter** muscle, which controls its opening and closing. The food mass is mixed with digestive juices by alternate contractions and relaxation of the stomach muscles to convert it into a thick, semi-liquid mass, called **chyme** (KEYEM). The **gastric juices** are secreted by glands in the stomach wall. They consist of hydrochloric acid and two enzymes, **rennin** and **pepsin**, which digest protein.

The **pyloric sphincter** muscle connects the stomach with the upper part of the **small intestine** and allows the chyme to pass into the small intestine a little at a time. The small intestine is a coiled tube about 21 feet long, which extends from the stomach to the large intestine and which carries on most of the digestive process.

There are three parts to the small intestine. The **duodenum** is the shortest part, about a foot long, and lies just outside the stomach. The **jejunum** is about nine feet long and the **ileum** is about 11 feet long. Bile, from the liver, and hormones and enzymes from the pancreas, feed into the small intestine and complete the process of digestion. The nutrients released by digestion are absorbed from the

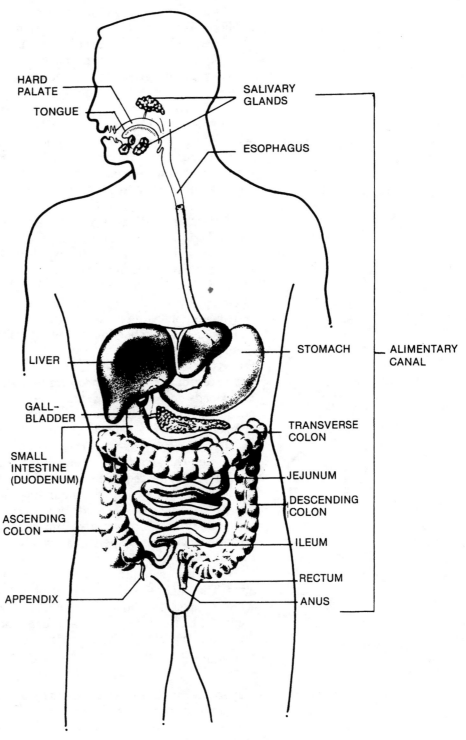

5.16—Digestive system

small intestine into the bloodstream to be transported throughout the body. The small intestine contains millions of **villi**, tiny projections that increase the surface area of the intestine to make the absorption of nutrients more efficient.

Water passes from the stomach through the intestines almost immediately. Foods take from three to five hours to pass through, with carbohydrates being passed first, followed next by proteins and then by fats. The chyme moves through the small intestine by peristaltic action, taking two to four hours to make the journey.

The **ileocecal sphincter muscle** connects the small intestine with the large intestine. It controls the movement of undigested food into the large intestine and prevents waste material from flowing back into the ileum.

Undigested food passes into the large intestine where the water is reabsorbed into the bloodstream and the solid waste materials are processed into **fecal matter** for expulsion from the body. The waste materials travel through the large intestine by peristaltic action. Many of the intestinal bacteria responsible for the synthesis of some vitamins breed in the large intestine.

The large intestine is shorter than the small intestine, about five feet long, but much wider, varying from one to three inches in diameter. It is divided into three parts—the cecum, the colon, and the rectum.

The **cecum** is located at the lower right side of the torso. The **appendix** extends downward from the end of the cecum. The appendix has no known function, but there is speculation that it may be the remnants of an organ that once enabled pre-humans to digest cellulose.

The **colon**, the longest part of the large intestine, is divided into four parts. The **ascending colon** rises vertically on the right side of the body from the cecum to the area of the liver. From there, it turns to the left and crosses the body horizontally as the **transverse colon**. The **descending colon** extends downward vertically on the left side of the body to the pelvic area and ends as the **sigmoid colon**, an S-shaped section in the pelvic cavity. Waste matter is carried through the colon by peristaltic action.

The **rectum** extends from the end of the colon and ends at the anus. The **anus** is under the control of the anal sphincter muscle, which relaxes to allow the expulsion of fecal matter. The **anal sphincter** consists of two parts—the internal anal sphincter, which is under the control of the autonomic nervous system, and the external anal sphincter, which may be controlled consciously.

The Accessory Glands

The accessory glands include the salivary glands, the liver, the gallbladder, and the pancreas. The **salivary glands** are all located in the area of the mouth. These glands produce up to a quart and a half of saliva per day. The saliva contains enzymes that convert carbohydrates into simple sugars as the beginning of the digestive process. In addition, saliva moistens the food, making it easier to swallow and also dissolves some food particles. Saliva also contains chemicals that cleanse the mouth and fight tooth decay.

The **liver**, located just below the diaphragm in the upper right part of the abdominal cavity, produces **bile**, a yellowish-brown liquid that enters the duodenum through the bile ducts. The bile emulsifies fats, letting them mix with water, so they may be digested. Excess bile is stored in the **gallbladder**, where it is concentrated and kept until it is needed. In addition, the liver processes and stores some nutrients and vitamins. The liver also performs a number of metabolic functions and helps remove toxic materials from the blood.

The pancreas, located beneath the liver and the stomach, is both an endocrine gland and an exocrine gland. Its endocrine functions were discussed earlier. As an exocrine gland, it produces pancreatic fluids that are passed into the duodenum through pancreatic ducts. The enzymes contained in the fluids are important to the digestion of all food elements.

THE EXCRETORY SYSTEM

The excretory system removes waste materials from the body to keep the body from being poisoned by the toxic wastes and to maintain a constant internal environment. Excretory functions are carried out by a number of different systems and organs. The lungs, for example, carry out carbon dioxide. The skin carries off wastes through perspiration. Solid food waste is eliminated through the large intestines. Internally, waste materials are carried by the blood and the lymph. And the liver and the spleen both filter out waste products.

The **urinary system**, which consists of the kidneys, the ureters, the bladder, and the urethra, is the major excretory system for removing wastes from the blood. Unfiltered blood enters the kidneys from the aorta. It is filtered in the kidney, then returned to the heart through the inferior vena cava. The wastes filtered from the blood are converted into urine, which flows from the kidneys through the ureters into the bladder, where it is stored until it reaches a sufficient quantity to be excreted through the urethra (Fig. 5.17).

In addition to its excretory function, the system also regulates the water balance of the body. The kidneys eliminate excess salt or excess water from the body to keep the salt content constant.

The **kidneys** are small, bean-shaped organs located on either side of the vertebral column at the back wall of the abdominal cavity. They consist of more than a million **nephrons** (NEFF-ron), the structural units of the kidneys, which perform the filtration function.

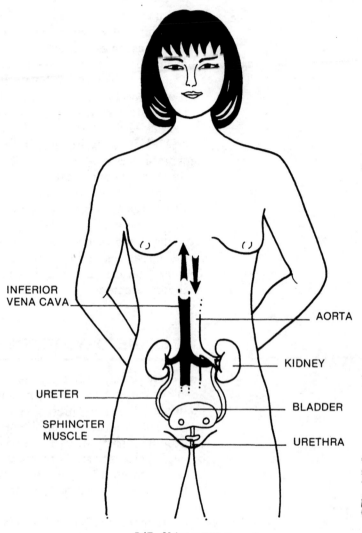

INFERIOR
VENA CAVA

AORTA

KIDNEY

URETER

SPHINCTER
MUSCLE

BLADDER

URETHRA

5.17—Urinary system

Each nephron is a tiny capsule containing a group of capillaries, called a **glomerulus**, and a renal tubule. As the blood passes through the glomerulus, it is filtered and returns to the bloodstream. The filtrate passes through the renal tubules to collecting ducts, which meet at the entrance of the ureters (Fig. 5.18).

In the **renal tubules**, the filtrate is condensed and usable water and minerals are returned to the body. The waste products are converted into **urine**, a liquid consisting of about ninety-five percent water and the rest solid materials, mostly urea and salt.

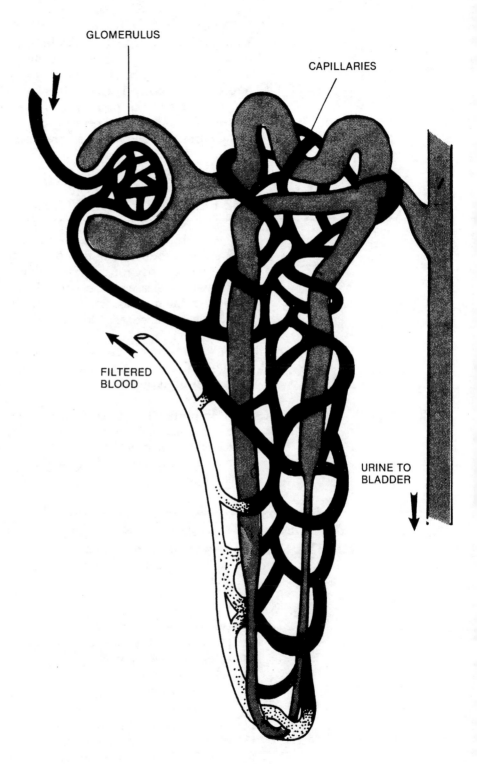

GLOMERULUS

CAPILLARIES

FILTERED
BLOOD

URINE TO
BLADDER

5.18—Nephron

The **ureters** are tubes through which the urine flows from the kidneys to the bladder. The **bladder** is an elastic sack that stores the urine until the quantity stimulates the nerves that signal the need to urinate. The **urethra** is the passageway from the bladder to the outside of the body. There are two sphincter muscles at the end of the bladder and the beginning of the urethra. One is under the control of the autonomic nervous system; the other is under voluntary control. The body normally releases one to two quarts of urine daily.

THE REPRODUCTIVE SYSTEM

The **reproductive system** is designed to perpetuate the species through the production of new human beings. The male reproductive system consists of the **testes**, which produce **sperm**, and the **penis**, which releases the sperm. The female reproductive system consists of the **ovaries**, which produce the egg, and the **uterus**, in which the fertilized egg develops into a **fetus**, which eventually grows into a baby.

Unlike the other systems, the reproductive system has little effect on the skin so far as the esthetician is concerned. A more complete discussion of its structure and function is beyond the scope of this chapter.

It is important to remember that even though the various systems have been discussed as separate entities, in fact, they all work together and their functions are, to a large extent, interrelated. And almost all of the systems have an effect, either directly or indirectly, on the skin.

REVIEW QUESTIONS

1. Define physiology.
2. Why is physiology important to the esthetician?
3. Which organs and systems are important to the health of the skin?
4. What is a cell?
5. How do cells reproduce?
6. What are tissues?
7. How many kinds of tissue are there?
8. What is epithelial tissue?
9. What are organs?
10. Is the skin a tissue or an organ?
11. What are systems?
12. How many systems are there?
13. What is the skeletal system?
14. What bones are of most concern to the esthetician?

15. How many kinds of muscle tissue are there?
16. What is the function of skeletal muscles?
17. How many muscles are there in the face?
18. What factors stimulate or soothe the muscles?
19. What is the nervous system?
20. Why is the nervous system important to the esthetician?
21. What is the difference between afferent and efferent nerves?
22. What are the 12 pairs of cranial nerves?
23. Which cranial nerves are of most importance to the esthetician?
24. What is the endocrine system?
25. What is a hormone?
26. Why is the circulatory system important to the esthetician?
27. What are the four chambers of the heart?
28. What is the function of the respiratory system?
29. What is the function of the digestive system?
30. What organs make up the digestive system?
31. Why is the excretory system important to the body?
32. What is it important to remember about systems?

6 Skin Structure and Function

OBJECTIVES   *After completing this chapter, you should be able to:*

❶ Describe the layers of the skin and the structure and workings of the different types of cells in the skin.

❷ Discuss the cutaneous appendages of the skin, including the hair, nails, sweat glands, and sebaceous glands.

❸ Outline in detail the various functions of the skin, its physiological and chemical functions as well as its psychological functions.

❹ Analyze the skin and determine clients' skin type.

❺ Discuss differences in male and female skin and in ethnic differences in skin.

INTRODUCTION   The human skin is a marvelous fabric. Soft, flexible, and elastic, the skin is at the same time tough, waterproof, and durable. It is the first line of protection against germs and pollution. Virtually impenetrable, the skin keeps out harmful elements, yet it is porous enough to let the body breathe and to excrete waste products. The skin has the ability to let the body move, yet it is firm enough to let the body hold its shape. Along with its appendages—which include the hair, nails, sweat and oil glands, nerve endings, some muscles and the mucous membranes of the mouth and the anal canal—the skin forms the entire **integument** (in-TEG-u-ment), or outer covering, of the human being. One might say that the skin is the wrapping that contains the substance of life.

A multilayered sheet of **epithelial tissue**, the skin is the largest organ of the body. Stretched out flat, the skin of the average adult male would form a blanket six feet long by three feet wide. Yet, this organ is so complex that a piece of skin the size of a postage stamp contains millions of cells; thousands of sensory receptors for pain, touch, heat, and cold; and hundreds of sweat and sebaceous glands. The skin varies in thickness from one-tenth of a millimeter to four millimeters, depending on the location. It is thickest on the palms and soles; thinnest on the eyelids.

One cannot underestimate the importance of the skin to human life. It has physiological functions, as a protective barrier, a temperature regulator, a metabolic organ, and a sensory organ. It also has chemical functions, for producing glucose, lipids and sweat, and for maintaining the acid mantle. But, equally important are the skin's psychological functions, those involved in touching, feeling, communication with the environment, and with esthetics.

A complete understanding of the skin is vital to the professional esthetician, since the skin is the basic working material. Like the canvas on which the artist paints, the skin is the medium on which the esthetician applies lotions, masks, oils—and the personal touch. To be able to treat clients properly, to be able to determine skin types, to recognize skin disorders, and to develop a course of treatment, the esthetician must know the skin. It is important to know what the skin is, its structure, its functions, how it works, and what problems it can experience. Without a thorough understanding of the skin and its mechanisms, it is impossible to give care the client needs and deserves.

STRUCTURE OF THE SKIN

The skin is a complex structure. It consists of a number of disparate elements working together to perform their many functions as a singular unit. For purposes of this discussion, the various elements are considered separately. It is important to keep in mind, however, that they interact with each other to perform their vital work in keeping the body healthy.

The skin is made up of two distinct layers that are structurally dissimilar and arise from different biological origins. The **epidermis** (ep-i-DUR-mis), or outermost layer, stems from the **ectoderm**, the outermost embryonic layer, while the **dermis**, the innermost layer, stems from the **mesoderm**, or middle embryonic layer. The two layers come together unevenly and vary in thickness depending on the location on the body and on the type of skin. They rest on a third layer, the **subcutaneous** layer, which is not usually considered to be part of the skin. In addition, there are a number of cutaneous appendages, embedded in or growing out of the skin. These include the hair and hair follicles, nails, sweat and oil glands, blood and lymph vessels, nerve endings, and muscles (Fig. 6.1).

6.1—Skin structure

The Epidermis   The epidermis, also called the **cuticle** or **scarf-skin,** is the thinner of the two layers of skin. It consists of epithelial tissue made up of several different kinds of cells arranged in five layers. The layers, from outermost to innermost, are:

1. The **stratum corneum** (STRAT-um KOHR-nee-um), or horny layer.
2. The **stratum lucidum** (LOO-si-dum), or barrier layer.
3. The **stratum granulosum** (gran-yoo-LOH-sum), or granular layer.
4. The **stratum spinosum** (spy-NO-sum), or spiny or prickle cell layer.

5. The **stratum germinativum** (jur-mi-nah-TIV-um), or basal cell layer.

The stratum spinosum and stratum germinativum are known collectively as the **Malpighian** (mal-PIG-ee-un) layer.

Most of the biochemical changes that occur in the skin take place in the epidermis. It is here, starting in the Malpighian layer, that cells undergo mitosis and start their migration upwards to the stratum corneum, where they die and slough off, carrying out the skin's constant process of regeneration. There are no blood vessels or sensory receptors in the epidermis, although there are a number of nerve endings present.

Stratum Germinativum. The stratum germinativum, or basal cell layer, is the deepest layer of the epidermis. It is in this very thin layer, only one cell deep, that the cells divide and begin their trek to the surface, a journey that will take approximately twenty-eight days.

The cells in this layer are cube shaped or columnar and are regularly outlined. Melanin, the pigment that gives the skin its color, is also present here. The basal layer has a fat content of up to 14 percent and a moisture content of up to 70 percent.

The basal cell layer functions as the center of reproduction for the epidermis, as the cells constantly undergo mitosis.

Stratum Spinosum. As the cells undergo mitosis, they are pushed upward into the stratum spinosum, or prickle cell layer, which is the upper part of the Malpighian layer. This layer is several cells thick. The cells are polyhedral in shape in the lower part of the layer and progressively flatten as they rise, becoming almost tile-like. The cells are characterized by tiny fibrils that connect the cells together. These fibrils give the layer its name. Like the basal cell layer, the prickle cell layer is also a center for reproduction.

Stratum Granulosum. The stratum granulosum, or granular layer, is a transitional layer. It is the outermost of the living layers of the epidermis. As the cells continue traveling upward, they gradually undergo a transformation. They become larger and their nuclei shrink. The cells change to a polygonal shape and become coarsely granular. These granules contain a substance called **keratohyalin** (KER-a-toe-HY-a-lin), which is a precursor of **keratin** (KER-a-tin).

In the granular layer, the cells begin to die and become keratinized, starting their transformation into a hard, horny substance. At this stage, they have lost a considerable amount of fat content and moisture.

Stratum Lucidum. The stratum lucidum, or barrier layer, is a thin, indistinct, poorly defined layer that varies from as little as one cell thick to a readily discernable thickness in the soles of the feet and the palms of the hand. The cells vary from a flat, dry, indistinct shape to a clear, perfectly outlined shape. They are highly keratinized and have no nuclei. This is the innermost of the two layers of dead cells.

The function of the barrier layer is not well understood, although current thought is that it acts as a barrier in some manner.

Stratum Corneum. The stratum corneum, or horny layer, is the outermost layer of the epidermis. It is here that the cells end their journey begun in the basal cell layer some four weeks earlier. This is the part of the skin actually exposed to the environment. It is a tough, insensitive covering consisting of dead, hard cells, arranged much like shingles on a roof.

This layer is unbroken except where hair follicles or sweat pores penetrate. It is the thickest of the epidermal layers, varying from 0.6 to 0.8 millimeters on the soles of the feet, where it is the thickest, to less than 0.1 millimeter on the eyelids.

The cells in the stratum corneum are flat and have no nuclei. They are composed entirely of keratin, a nonliving substance, and are constantly being shed as they are replaced by cells moving upward from the lower layers of the epidermis. In this layer, the cornified cells have only a seven percent fat content and about ten to twenty-five percent water content remaining.

The stratum corneum, because of its toughness and durability, provides protection for the rest of the skin. Its ability to thicken in response to injury, forming calluses, adds to its protective function, as does its thin coating of sebum and sweat.

The Dermis

The **dermis** (DUR-mis), also called the **corium** (KOH-ree-um), **cutis** (KYOO-tis), or **true skin,** is the thicker of the two layers and is composed mostly of fibrous materials with only a few cells of varying types. The dermis is divided into two layers, the **papillary** (pa-PIL-ah-ry) and the **reticular** (re-TIK-yoo-lar), which are different from each other more in degree than in kind.

Papillary Layer. The papillary layer is the thinner of the dermal layers and lies just below the epidermis, forming at its surface a negative image of the bottom of the stratum germanitivum. This layer derives its name from the cone-shaped projections, or **papillae** (pah-PIL-e), that extend upwards into the epidermis to form the irregular peaks and valleys. The fibrous component of the papillary layer is less dense than the reticular layer and the fibers are thinner. However, it contains more cells than the reticular layer.

A network of capillaries runs through the papillae. The nutrients from the blood diffuse through the papillae to provide nourishment to the living layers of the epidermis.

Reticular Layer. The reticular layer is thicker and more densely packed with fibers than the papillary layer. Unlike the fiber bundles in the papillary layer, which are oriented vertically, perpendicular to the surface, the fiber bundles in the reticular layer are oriented horizontally, parallel to the surface.

Some cutaneous appendages, i.e., follicles, sweat, and sebum glands, are found in the reticular layer, as are most of the sensory receptors and nerve endings.

Both layers, however, contain the same kinds of fibers and the same kinds of cells. The fibrous materials, **collagen** (KOL-uh-jin), **elastin** (ee-LAS-tin), and **reticulin** (reh-TIK-u-lin), are proteins that are formed into bundles to give the dermis its elasticity, resilience, and strength.

Collagen is the supportive component of the skin and is present in the largest amount, providing almost three-quarters of the fibrous bulk. It gives the skin most of its strength. Elastin is a component of the elastic fibers and gives the skin its extensibility. Reticulin is present in the smallest amount and is the least understood of the three fibrous materials. It is possible that the reticulin helps the collagen fibrils form correctly, although its exact function is not yet known.

The fibers are supported in an amorphous gel-like material called the **ground substance**. This material has no structure and is composed mostly of **mucopolysaccharides**, particularly **hyaluronic**

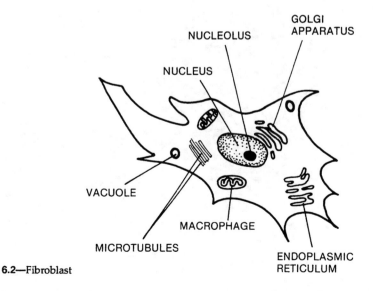

6.2—Fibroblast

acid, which helps retain water and hold cells together. The ground substance resists compression and acts as a shock absorber to help the skin resist pressure.

The cellular components of the dermis consist of fibroblasts, mast cells, and macrophages. **Fibroblasts** are spindle shaped cells present in the largest amount in connective tissue. They are the cells from which the collagen and elastic fibers and ground substance are formed (Fig. 6.2).

Mast cells are large oval cells that contain **histamine,** a vasodilator, and **heparin,** an anticoagulant, and are found mostly around the small blood vessels in the dermis. They help heal injury to the skin and may have some role in the regulation of lipids, the basic component of sebum (Fig. 6.3).

Macrophages are large cells that are important to the immune responses of the body. They attack and degrade foreign bodies and protect against viral infections. Like the mast cells, macrophages are also involved in the production of lipids (Fig. 6.4).

Dermal-Epidermal Junction   The area in which the epidermis and dermis meet is called the **dermal-epidermal junction.** This area is highly irregular in cross-section and has many cones and ridges that extend down from the epidermis into the dermis. The two layers are separated by a submicroscopic membrane, called the **basal lamina.** The function of this

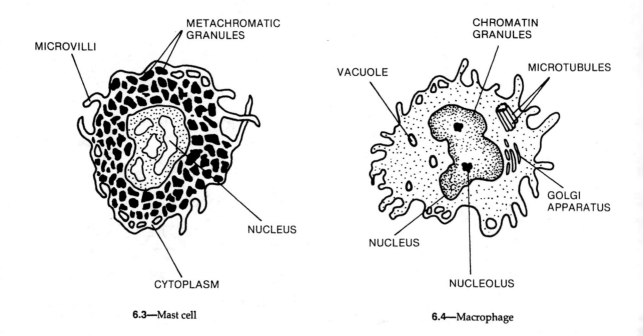

MICROVILLI

METACHROMATIC GRANULES

NUCLEUS

CYTOPLASM

6.3—Mast cell

CHROMATIN GRANULES

VACUOLE

MICROTUBULES

GOLGI APPARATUS

NUCLEUS

NUCLEOLUS

6.4—Macrophage

membrane is not fully understood but it is probable that it has something to do with the attachment of the epidermis to the dermis.

Subcutaneous Layer

The dermis rests on a bed of loose fatty tissue of varying thickness. This tissue is called the **subcutaneous** (sub-kyoo-TAY-nee-us) **layer** or **panniculus adiposus**. It contains a network of arteries from which capillaries branch up into the dermis. The subcutaneous layer helps cushion the skin and gives the body its shape.

CUTANEOUS APPENDAGES

The skin has a number of appendages—the hair and hair follicles, muscles, nails, sebaceous glands, sweat glands, blood vessels, lymph vessels, and nerves.

Hair and Hair Follicles

The **pilary system** consists of the hair and the hair follicles. Hair covers virtually the entire body, whether coarse and thick, as on the head or in the axillary and pubic areas, or very fine and virtually invisible, as on the rest of the body. Hair structure and function is discussed fully in Chapter 10.

Muscles

The skin contains no muscle tissue except for the **arrector pili** muscles attached to each hair follicle. These small muscles are activated by the sympathetic nervous system in response to cold or emotion and cause the hair to stand erect.

Nails

The **nails** are hard, highly keratinized structures located at the ends of the fingers and toes. These protective plates grow outward from the Malpighian layer of the epidermis. The translucent, cornified nail plates lie on the **nail bed**, formed of modified dermal tissue. The nail bed contains a large blood supply. The skin resting on the back edge of the nail plate is called the **eponychium** or **cuticle**. The crescent shaped area just under the cuticle is called the **lunula** (Fig. 6.5).

Sebaceous Glands

The **sebaceous glands** are sac-like structures attached to the hair follicles. They are found over most of the body, except for the palms and soles, and are especially prevalent on the scalp, face, back and chest, where they number from 400 to 900 per square centimeter. The glands have a well-developed blood supply (Fig. 6.6).

The sebaceous glands produce **sebum** (SEE-bum), an oily, waxy substance composed of various kinds of **lipids** (LIP-ids). The sebum is secreted onto the surface of the skin through a duct that leads

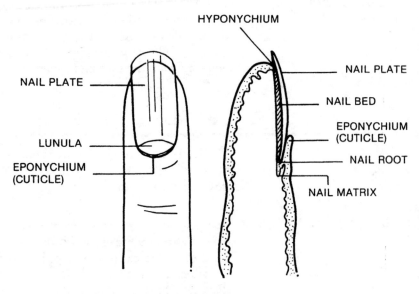

6.5—Nail structure

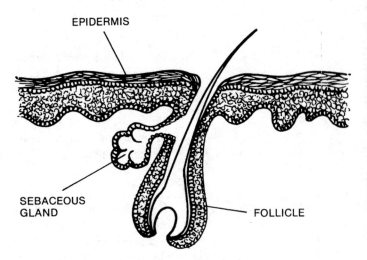

6.6—Sebaceous gland

directly into the follicle. Although the function of sebum is not completely understood, it is generally believed that it acts as a lubricant and emollient for the skin, and has some anti-bacterial function as well. Some researchers feel that the prime function of sebum may be as a **pheromone**, or sex attractant, since it gives the clean body its characteristic odor.

Sweat Glands

There are two types of **sweat** or **sudoriferous** glands—**apocrine glands** and **eccrine glands**. The two types are separate and have different functions (Fig. 6.7 and Fig. 6.8).

Apocrine glands are the larger of the two. These glands are found in the **axillae** (armpits), pubic areas, and in the outside canals of the ears. They are tightly coiled and tubular in shape. Most are contained in the dermis, although some of the larger apocrine glands extend down into the subcutaneous layer. The upper part of the coil narrows to about a third of the diameter of the lower part, then narrows even further into a duct that runs roughly parallel to a follicle. The duct empties into the pilary canal of the follicle at a point above the sebaceous duct.

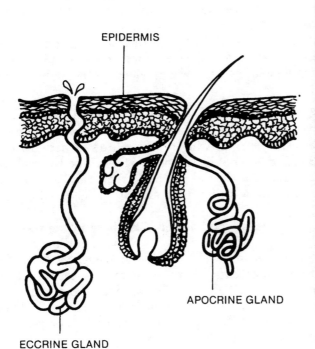

EPIDERMIS

APOCRINE GLAND

ECCRINE GLAND

6.7—Sweat glands

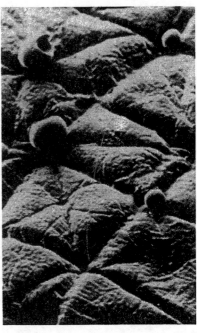

6.8—Electron microphotograph of perspiration on aged skin *(Reprinted with permission from* Les Nouvelles Esthetiques—*American Edition)*

The apocrine glands secrete small quantities of a shiny, viscous substance that can vary in color from clear to yellowish, reddish, or brownish hues. The apocrine secretion mixes with the sebum in the pilary canal. The secretion is odorless, but the decomposition of bacteria on the skin gives it its characteristic odor, especially in the armpit area.

The function of the apocrine secretion is not clear. Modern social customs governing control of body odors notwithstanding, it may be that the sweat, or more specifically its odor, is meant to be a means of chemical communication.

Eccrine sweat glands are smaller than apocrine glands and are far more numerous, about three to five million distributed over the entire body. They are most numerous on the palms and soles and also on the head. Like the apocrine glands, eccrine glands consist of a tubular secretory coil embedded in the dermis or subcutaneous layer, ending in a more narrow duct. The eccrine ducts, however, open directly onto the surface of the skin.

The eccrine glands secrete large amounts of diluted salt water. An adult male can excrete as much as three gallons of sweat in a day. Eccrine secretion is stimulated by heat and by emotional stress. Apocrine secretion is stimulated only by emotional stress. When stimulated by heat, the forehead and neck start sweating first. The palms and soles sweat least. When stimulated by emotion, however, the palms and soles sweat profusely, as do both the eccrine and apocrine glands in the axillary area.

The eccrine glands function as thermal regulators for the body by cooling the skin through evaporation of the perspiration. They also help regulate the salt and water balance of the body.

Blood Vessels

The skin is well supplied with blood vessels. **Arteries** and **veins** that originate in the subcutaneous layer and below travel upwards into the dermal layer where they branch into a vast network of **arterioles** and **capillaries**. The distribution of these blood vessels is complex and irregular. The dermal papillae contain capillary loops. The follicles and sudoriferous glands are intertwined with capillary networks.

The cutaneous blood vessels, like those in the rest of the body, supply oxygen and nutrients to the surrounding tissue and help carry off waste products. Since the cutaneous vessels, however, are present in much larger numbers than necessary for these strictly biological needs of the skin, it is obvious that they serve other functions as well. The major functions of the dermal blood supply are the regulation of temperature and blood pressure.

The blood vessels in the skin have a greater ability to contract and dilate than the blood vessels in the rest of the body. This ability lets them adjust the blood flow through the skin to compensate for external fluctuations in temperature and maintain a constant body temperature. They dilate and allow more blood to flow when the temperature rises to carry off excess heat; and they contract and restrict the blood flow when the temperature lowers to conserve heat. Without this ability to regulate heat, the body temperature would vary whenever the outside temperature changed.

The cutaneous blood vessels contain mechanisms called **arteriovenous anastomoses** or **shunts** that allow blood to pass directly from the arteries to veins. They act as valves, opening when the temperature rises to increase blood flow and closing when the added blood flow is not needed. This is part of the temperature regulatory system of the skin.

The other function of the shunts is to regulate blood pressure. As the vessels constrict, the pressure of the blood rises. The shunts, working almost like safety valves, open to increase the blood flow and keep the pressure in balance.

The blood supply in the skin also contributes to the skin's color, especially in Caucasians. The amount of blood and the location and density of the capillaries running below the surface of the skin play a large part in the overall coloration of the skin. For example, people with many capillaries near the surface will have a characteristically "ruddy" or reddish complexion.

Blood flow to the skin also changes in response to emotional stress, rushing to the skin, for example, with embarrassment, causing the characteristic flushing or "blush." It may also drain away from the skin, for example, with fear, causing the characteristic pallor.

Lymph Vessels

The **lymphatic** (LIMF-a-tik) **system** of the skin is about as extensive as the **vascular** (VAS-kyoo-lahr) **system** and runs parallel with it. Lymphatic capillaries traverse the papillary layer of the dermis and connect with larger lymph vessels in the subcutaneous layer and eventually join the venous system near the heart. Along the way, they filter into lymph nodes.

The lymphatic system is important to maintaining the proper balance of capillary filtration. The lymph vessels remove fluids that leak from the blood vessels into the tissues, thus preventing **edema,** or swelling. They also help remove waste matter from surrounding tissues.

Nerves

As would be expected of the main sensory organ of the body, the skin contains large numbers of **afferent,** or sensory, nerve endings, especially in the fingertips. These nerve endings are of different types and register the sensations of touch, pressure, pain, heat, and cold.

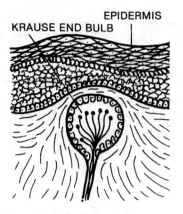

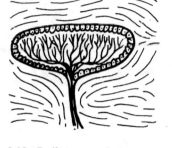

6.10—Ruffini corpuscle (heat receptor)

6.9—Krause end-bulb (cold receptor)

Krause's end-bulbs are round nerve endings that register the sensation of cold. The other thermoreceptors are **Ruffini's corpuscles**, elongated, tubular nerve endings, which register the sensation of heat (Fig. 6.9 and Fig. 6.10).

Meissner's corpuscles are small, oval nerve endings found in the papillary layer of the dermis. These are the tactile endings that register the sensation of light touch. The **Pacinian corpuscles** are the largest nerve endings in the skin. These register the sensation of deep pressure and vibration. The sensation of pain is registered through the multitude of free nerve endings distributed throughout the skin (Fig. 6.11 and Fig. 6.12).

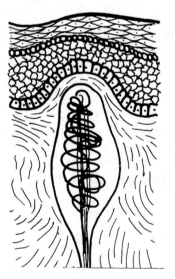

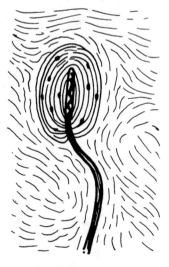

6.11—Meissner's corpuscle (touch receptor)

6.12—Pacinian corpuscle (pressure receptor)

In addition to the afferent, or sensory, nerves, the skin also contains **efferent,** or motor, nerves under the control of the autonomic, or sympathetic, nervous system. These nerves operate the arrector pili muscles, the glands, and the blood vessels.

FUNCTIONS OF THE SKIN

The skin has a number of physiological and chemical functions. Equally important, however, is the psychological functioning of the skin. Physiologically, the skin is a protector, a regulator, and a sensory organ. Chemically, it is a producer of sebum, sweat, glucose, lipids, keratin, and melanin. Psychologically, the skin is a communicator, an arouser, and a comforter. It can be a source of both pleasure and anguish. All of these functions are important—the psychological no less than the physiochemical.

Physiological Functions of the Skin

The primary physical function of the skin is as a protective barrier. The unbroken skin keeps out harmful bacteria, dirt, and pollution. It protects internal organs by absorbing shocks and bumps. It also protects the body from the ultraviolet rays emanating from the sun.

The horny layer of the skin (the outermost layer of the epidermis) is relatively impermeable to most foreign substances. The surface of the skin is covered with a thin layer of sebum. It is the combination of these two factors that gives the skin its protective barrier function. The melanin cells in the stratum germinativum layer of the epidermis and the papillary layer of the dermis help protect the body from ultraviolet radiation by darkening on exposure and absorbing more of the sun's rays. The fat cells in the subcutaneous layer provide a cushion that absorbs the bumps and bruises of daily life, thus protecting the internal organs of the body.

The second function of the skin is as a temperature regulator for the body. It maintains the body temperature at an almost constant level of 98.6°F. (37°C.) through the reactions of the blood vessels and the sweat glands to heat or cold. When the body gets too hot, the blood vessels dilate to provide greater flow of blood. At the same time, the sweat glands produce sweat, which evaporates from the skin's surface to provide cooling. When the body gets too cold, the blood vessels constrict to reduce the flow of blood and conserve heat.

The third function of the skin is as a sensory organ. Large numbers of sensory receptors for touch, pain, pressure, heat, and cold are located throughout the skin in the dermal and subcutaneous layers. These receptors respond to external stimuli and make the skin an active channel of communication—on both the physical and psychological levels. Through touching, the skin communicates much about the environment to the body—cold, heat, damp, physical presence. It also communicates human needs, desires, affection, and personality.

Chemical Functions of the Skin

Chemically, the skin functions as a secretory organ, an excretory organ, and as a chemical factory to produce the materials needed for its own nutrition, protection, maintenance, and growth. The sebaceous glands secrete a lipid substance, called sebum, which is a mixture containing free fatty acids, squalene, waxes, cholesterol, and triglycerides. When the sebum reaches the surface of the skin, it mixes with the epidermal lipids, the water from the sweat glands, and the keratin of the dead cells of the stratum corneum to produce an oily, viscous, slightly acid emulsion that forms a film on the surface of the skin.

Because of its oily characteristic, this film lubricates the skin and helps retain moisture to keep the skin from drying out. Its weakly acid characteristic gives it bacteriostatic and fungistatic properties. This characteristic is called the **acid mantle** of the skin, and is an important concept for the esthetician to remember. The acid mantle is removed from the skin during cleansing, leaving the skin susceptible to attack by germs. Although the acid mantle will gradually reappear, it is necessary to protect the skin with a lotion immediately after finishing a facial.

The pH of the skin varies from about 3 to 9, depending on the location and the type of skin. Male skin tends to be slightly more **acidic** than female skin, which conversely, is more **alkaline.** Skin pH can be affected by environmental conditions, especially temperature.

The skin is an important organ of excretion for the elimination of waste products from the body. Perspiration, in addition to its importance in cooling, also carries off waste materials and toxins. Sweating also helps maintain the water and salt balance of the body metabolism.

The skin is also an organ of respiration. Oxygen is absorbed through the skin. Although the amount is small compared with the amount taken in through the lungs, it is, nevertheless, important to skin metabolism. Much of the oxygen taken in through the skin is absorbed into the bloodstream. Carbon dioxide is removed from the blood and eliminated through the skin as well.

The chemical functions of the skin serve to provide the energy the skin needs for its regeneration and growth. Most of the energy is supplied through respiration. A significant portion of it, however, comes from **glucose** (GLEU-kos) entering the epidermis from the blood. The glucose is metabolized into **lactic acid,** which is converted to energy for growth. It is interesting to note that the amount of glucose present in the skin increases in the presence of a wound to the skin, thus hastening its recovery.

One of the most important products of skin metabolism is keratin, a sulfur-containing protein which, as discussed previously, is the major component of the epidermis, hair, and nails. There are two types of keratin—high sulfur content and low sulfur content. Epidermal keratin is of the low sulfur type, containing 2 to 4 percent **cystine** (SIS-teen). Hair and nails are composed of the high sulfur type of keratin, containing up to 18 percent cystine. Cystine is an amino acid that contains sulfur.

The other important product of skin metabolism is **melanin** (MEL-ah-nin), the brown pigment that gives the skin, hair, and eyes their coloration. Melanin is necessary to human life, since it protects the body from exposure to sunlight. The epidermis absorbs most of the radiation in the ultraviolet end of the spectrum. It is these rays that cause sunburn. The melanin in the skin acts as a filter by darkening on exposure. This is the phenomenon called **tanning,** which is nothing more than the protective response of the skin to exposure to ultraviolet light.

Sunlight isn't all bad, however. It stimulates the production of vitamin D in the skin, and this is necessary for proper calcium metabolism.

Psychological Functions of the Skin

From the psychological point of view, the skin can be considered the body's most important sensory organ. Tactile responses are the earliest formed and the most numerous sensory responses, and are vital to the development of the person. As Ashley Montagu points out in *Touching: The Human Significance of the Skin,* "It appears probable that for human beings tactile stimulation is of fundamental significance for the development of healthy emotional or affectional relationships."

Because of its ability to receive tactile stimuli, the skin is an active channel of communication. It communicates much about the environment to the body—cold, heat, damp, physical presence. Beyond mere physical sensation, however, touching communicates much about the quality of the sensation—comfort, discomfort, affection, dislike, pleasure, pain. Pure silk cloth, for example, which feels smooth, cool, and soft, is a pleasure to hold. Steel wool, on the other hand, which feels rough and hard, is displeasing to hold. A caress is pleasant; a slap is not.

Affection, care, concern, anxiety, fear—almost any emotion—can be transmitted through touching. Thus, the esthetician must be alert to the psychological implications of touch when working on a client, especially during the facial massage. Carelessness or roughness on the part of the esthetician will be evident to the client and will make the facial treatment less pleasurable than it should be.

SKIN TYPES

For purposes of analysis, skin can be classified according to type. The types vary according to appearance, texture, pore size, coloration, and how well or poorly the glands function. The client's skin type is the key to the treatment that will be followed and the products that will be used. Skin can be classified into six basic types—normal, oily, dry, couperose, blemished, and mature. There are variations of both characteristics and degree within each type. Note that there is no separate category for sensitive skin. All skin types may be sensitive to one degree or another at any given time. Some skin types are more sensitive than others, as well.

Normal Skin   The skin is in proper balance. The glands produce just the right amount of sebum and sweat, so the skin is properly lubricated and moistened. It has a soft, smooth texture and is clear. Pores are small to medium sized, but are not evident. There are very few, if any, blemishes. Color is even and translucent. The client probably has very few skin problems, except for an occasional pimple caused by stress or minor break-out during the menstrual cycle. Normal skin fluoresces blue-white under the Wood's lamp. This type of skin does not usually show any unusual sensitivity (Fig. 6.13).

Normal skin is an ideal condition. However, very few people have normal skin.

Oily Skin   The skin is out of balance. The sebaceous glands produce more oil than is necessary for proper skin function. The skin has a rougher, thicker texture than normal skin and tends to be shiny and have a greasy feel. The pores are medium size to enlarged and may be quite evident, especially if the skin is extremely oily. The pores will probably be clogged, and there may be a considerable number of blackheads. There may be relatively few blemishes or there may be many (Fig. 6.14).

It is important to note, however, that the presence of blackheads is not, of itself, a positive indication of oily skin. The blackheads could be formed by the oxidation of cosmetic products trapped inside the pores and not by sebum deposits. And, as discussed earlier, pore size alone is not a positive indication of skin type.

Also, skin can be oily yet be dehydrated. This condition occurs when the pores become clogged and sebum can't get to the surface

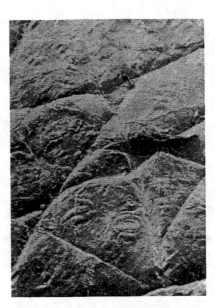

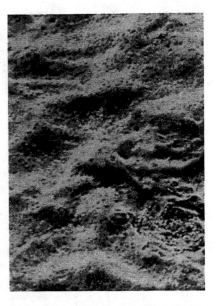

6.13—Electron microphotograph of normal skin around age 40 *(Reprinted with permission from* Les Nouvelles Esthetiques—*American Edition)*

6.14—Electron microphotograph of oily skin *(Reprinted with permission from* Les Nouvelles Esthetiques—*American Edition)*

to lubricate the skin. The skin may be erroneously classified as dry in this case. And oily skin can lack moisture, either because it has been overscrubbed or alcohol-based products have dried it out.

Skin tones can range from ruddy to sallow, depending on the amount of irritation or the amount of sebum on the skin. Oil deposits and clogged pores fluoresce orange under the Wood's lamp. Oily skin tends to be less sensitive than other types of skin, although under some circumstances it may show considerable sensitivity.

Dry Skin

Dry skin may be oil-dry, where the sebaceous glands don't produce enough sebum, or it may be water-dry, or dehydrated, with insufficient moisture in the surface layers. These two conditions should not be confused with oily skin that has clogged pores or that has had the oils stripped by harsh cleansing, as discussed in the section on oily skin (Fig. 6.15 and Fig. 6.16).

Dry skin has a dull appearance without a sheen to it. It has a fine texture but feels dry and rough. Pore size is small. Pores are almost invisible in extreme cases. The skin is thin. Skin is pale to white in coloration and appears almost transparent. Dead cells are usually quite evident and there may be considerable flaking. The skin may

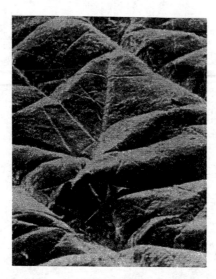

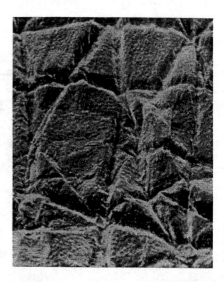

6.15—Electron microphotograph of dry skin with tiny wrinkles *(Reprinted with permission from* Les Nouvelles Esthetiques—*American Edition)*

6.16—Electron microphotograph of dehydrated skin *(Reprinted with permission from* Les Nouvelles Esthetiques—*American Edition)*

feel tight to the client. Dry skin fluoresces light to deep purple, depending on the degree of dryness. Dead cells fluoresce white. Dry skin may show some degree of sensitivity.

Couperose Skin

Couperose skin contains broken capillaries near the surface. These broken capillaries give the skin a "spidery" appearance. This type of skin is thin and very fragile. It also will tend to be dry. Apart from the fine red lines, the overall color tends to be pale, although it may be quite red at times from irritation. Care must be taken when treating this type of skin. Couperose skin is usually quite sensitive.

Blemished Skin

Blemished, or acneform, skin is the most obvious of the skin types. The skin is generally extremely oily. It shows inflammation and redness, and has relatively large numbers of pimples, pustules, and blackheads. Because of the inflammation, the skin is usually quite sensitive. Pores will probably be enlarged and will be clogged with excess sebum.

In many cases, the client's face will be sore because of overwashing in an attempt to clear the excess oil.

Mature Skin

Mature, or aging, skin is generally both oil and moisture dry. Character lines and wrinkles have formed. In some cases, these lines may be quite deep. The skin has lost elasticity and tends to sag, especially

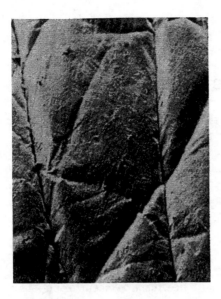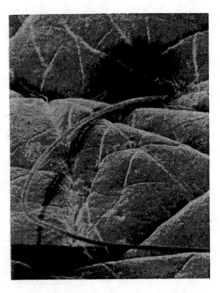

6.17—Electron microphotograph of first wrinkles *(Reprinted with permission from* Les Nouvelles Esthetiques—*American Edition)*

6.18—Electron microphotograph of aged skin *(Reprinted with permission from* Les Nouvelles Esthetiques—*American Edition)*

around the eyes, cheeks, and throat. The skin tends to be fragile and may be quite sensitive. There will probably be an abundance of dead surface cells, as well. There may also be changes in pigmentation, such as age spots (Fig. 6.17 and Fig. 6.18).

Aging skin may be oily instead of dry. In this case, the onset of some of the other signs of aging, such as wrinkles, will be retarded. Seborrheic keratoses may be present.

The esthetician should be alert for signs of skin cancer. If there are suspected carcinomas or melanomas present, however, the esthetician should not alarm the client but should merely suggest a consultation with a physician.

It is important to remember that aging skin is not limited to the elderly. Young people can have old skin, too, especially if they have abused it by improper care or by baking it in the sun.

Combination Skin

A client will rarely have skin of just one type. Most often the esthetician will see combination skin—oily in some areas; dry in others. Blemishes may be confined to one or two small areas. The most common combination skin is oily in the "T-zone"—the forehead, nose and chin—and dry everywhere else. As with any type of skin, the degree of oiliness or dryness varies.

Combination skin is more complicated to treat because it requires that techniques for oily skin be used on the oily areas and techniques for dry skin be used on dry areas.

Determining the skin type of the client lets the esthetician map out a strategy for the facial treatment so that the client derives the full benefit.

ETHNIC AND GENDER DIFFERENCES IN SKIN

Human skin is essentially the same in basic structure and function regardless of sex or ethnic origin. There are some slight differences, but these exist more as tendencies than as structural or functional changes. Skin is skin. It works the same, and is treated the same, whether it is on a woman or man, a caucasian, black, Asian, hispanic, or Indian.

Gender Differences

Men and women are different—structurally as well as psychologically. The external physical differences are obvious. The differences that affect the skin are less so. In part, these differences stem from the predominant hormone concentration—testosterone in men; estrogen in women.

Generally, men have high testosterone levels, have larger, more dense bones, and up to twenty percent more muscle mass. As a result, men tend to be bigger, stronger, and faster, with more endurance than women. Women, on the other hand, have high estrogen levels and tend to have more fatty tissue than men.

The distribution of fat deposits also differs between the sexes. In men, fat tends to be distributed evenly, and excessive fat tends to concentrate in the stomach area. In women, fat tends to concentrate around the breasts, hips, buttocks, and thighs. The rough, "orange-peel" fat deposits around the thighs that some members of the beauty industry call "cellulite" occur only in women.

Hormonal differences also account for differences in hair growth and distribution between the sexes. Men have thicker, coarser, more evenly distributed hair on their bodies and faces and are more prone to genetic baldness than women.

When it comes to skin, however, the differences are slight and subtle indeed. A woman's skin tends to have smaller sebaceous glands than a man's skin. In addition, a woman's sebum production is influenced by her estrogen level. Once a woman reaches menopause and her estrogen level drops, her skin's production of sebum also diminishes. Men, on the other hand, produce sebum in larger amounts with no corresponding decrease in sebum production with age. This makes men more prone to acne than women. In addition, female skin tends to be thinner, finer, and more alkaline than male skin. And women tend to perspire less than men.

From the point of view of the esthetician, there are few differences in treatment for male or female skin. Analysis remains an important step. Male skin will tend towards oiliness, be more prone to acne, and be affected more by environmental dirt and pollution. Also, men will tend to have fewer wrinkles than women and will tend to have fewer concentrations of dead cells on the skin surface, simply because daily shaving removes them constantly. However, beard stubble may interfere with some steps during a facial. By and large, the esthetician will be able to use the same techniques and products used on female skin.

Ethnic Differences

All human beings belong to a single species, **homo sapiens**. However, humans can be classified, somewhat loosely, by racial characteristics. The U. S. Census Bureau recognizes four categories of race:

- black
- white
- Indian and Eskimo
- Asian.

Although genetic differences result in a number of specific physical characteristics within racial groups, such as high cheekbones, hair texture and color, eye shape, etc., the most prominent difference is in skin coloration. Thus, whites tend to have pink skin; blacks, brown skin; Asians, yellow skin; and Indians and Eskimos, red skin. Within groups, however, there is a wide range in skin tones, which tend to overlap from group to group. So, for example, white skin may range from almost alabaster white to deep olive tones; black skin from light tan to almost ebony black; Asian skin from light yellow to deep tan; and Indian and Eskimo skin, various tones of reddish brown. These differences are caused by the melanin content of the skin. In terms of the important characteristics that make up the human condition, there are no differences from one racial group to another. We are all, literally, "brothers and sisters under the skin."

Sebaceous glands tend to be more numerous and large in black skin, and follicles tend to be larger, so black skin tends toward oiliness, although it is less acne-prone. It also tends to be thicker and, of course, has a higher concentration of melanin. The greater pigmentation, however, gives black skin better protection from ultraviolet radiation, which means it resists the effects of sun exposure better and stays younger looking longer. And, because of its coloration, heavy concentrations of dead cells on the surface tend to give it an ashen appearance.

Black skin is more prone to developing **keloids** (KEE-loyd), thick scars caused by fibrous growth resulting from healing of abrasions and cuts. Black males are especially prone to keloid formation because of shaving irritation. Unevenness in pigmentation is also more evident in darker skin.

Except for melanin content, there are few differences in skin structure and function among the racial groups, and, in general, the esthetician may use the same treatments and products for all. The esthetician should be aware, however, that analysis of the skin will be somewhat more difficult as the skin tone gets darker, simply because the darker the skin, the harder it will be to see blemishes and imperfections on the skin's surface.

REVIEW QUESTIONS

1. How many layers does the skin have?
2. What are the cutaneous appendages?
3. How many layers does the epidermis have?
4. What is the Malpighian layer?
5. How long does it take cells to migrate from the innermost to the outermost layer of the epidermis?
6. Which is the thickest layer of the epidermis?
7. Why is the stratum corneum important?
8. How many layers does the dermis have?
9. Where are most sensory receptors found?
10. What is collagen?
11. What is the function of mast cells?
12. What is the subcutaneous layer?
13. What muscles are found in the skin?
14. What is sebum?
15. What are the two types of sweat glands?
16. What is the difference between apocrine and eccrine glands with respect to sweating?
17. What is the purpose of the eccrine glands?
18. Match the sensory receptor with its function.

    1. Krause end-bulbs   a. light touch
    2. Ruffini corpuscles   b. cold
    3. Meissner's corpuscles   c. pain
    4. Pacinian corpuscles   d. heat
    5. free nerve endings   e. deep pressure

19. What are the physiological functions of the skin?
20. What are the chemical functions of the skin?
21. What are the psychological functions of the skin?
22. What factors determine a skin's type?
23. Why is it important for the esthetician to determine the client's skin type?
24. What are the six basic skin types?
25. Match the Wood's lamp indication with the skin type.

    1. blue-white   a. oily
    2. orange   b. dead cells
    3. purple   c. normal
    4. white   d. dry

7 Skin Disorders

OBJECTIVES   *After completing this chapter, you should be able to:*

❶ Describe the factors that are harmful to the skin.

❷ List various types of skin disorders, such as sebaceous gland disorders; papulosquamous disorders; eczematous disorders; fungal, bacterial, and viral disorders; skin tumors; and pigmentation disorders.

❸ Understand various cosmetic surgery options.

INTRODUCTION

The skin, as shown in the previous chapter, is a marvelous protective organ. When unbroken, it shields the inner body from attack by pollutants, dirt, and germs, yet it allows oxygen and nutrients in and waste products out. It produces an oily, slightly acidic chemical barrier that acts as a germicide and as a lubricant. Through the production of sweat, the skin helps control body temperature. Yet, in spite of its toughness, the skin remains flexible and elastic.

It is evident, then, that the proper functioning of the skin is vital to the overall health of the body. Without a healthy skin, the body suffers. Conversely, many physical abnormalities in the inner body are mirrored in the appearance of the skin. To the trained eye, a change in the way the skin looks can signal the onset of a disease.

Estheticians are concerned with wellness, with the holistic aspects of health. We are not physicians. We do not cure disease. But we can work to normalize skin functions and help alleviate certain skin disorders by the proper use of skin-care products and techniques.

And we are educators, teaching clients how to care for their own skin, for both health and appearance.

To work effectively on the skin, the esthetician must be able to recognize various skin disorders and diseases. To choose the proper course of action, he or she must be able to assess the condition of the skin. It is important to remember, however, that the esthetician is *not* a medical doctor and can neither treat diseases nor prescribe medication. Nor should the esthetician attempt to diagnose a skin ailment. If a client has a skin condition beyond the scope of the esthetician's responsibility, the esthetician should suggest that the client see a dermatologist. Under no circumstances should the esthetician try to characterize the condition for the client.

There are many risks involved in trying to diagnose diseases. Many conditions closely resemble other conditions and require extensive testing to diagnose properly. Estheticians are *not* qualified to do this.

FACTORS HARMFUL TO THE SKIN

Many factors, external as well as internal, can affect the health of the skin. Among these are sunlight, smoking, drugs, alcohol consumption, poor nutrition, chemicals, and time. By understanding how these factors can damage the skin, the esthetician can counsel the client on how to avoid them or minimize their effect.

Sunlight "Give me the splendid silent sun with all his beams full-dazzling," was how Walt Whitman characterized the sun. This splendid silent sun is vital to the continued existence of all life on this planet. It gives us light and heat; it provides energy. Yet, this beneficent giver of life can also do great damage to the skin.

The sun generates ultraviolet radiation. These rays penetrate both layers of the skin and cause damage to the structure. The ultraviolet radiation dries out the skin and destroys its elasticity, resulting in wrinkling and premature aging. These adverse reactions take place over long periods of time. So overexposure to the sun in youth, as in sunbathing, is likely to cause wrinkling and other signs of aging starting in the late thirties to early forties, much sooner than would be expected through the natural aging processes alone.

The ultraviolet spectrum extends from 400 **nanometers** (nm) to 200 nanometers and is divided into three bands. The **UV-A** band, from 400 to 320 nanometers, is the tanning region. The **UV-B** band, from 320 to 290 nanometers, is the erythemal, or burning, region. And the **UV-C** band, from 290 to 200 nanometers, is the germicidal band. Most of the radiation in the UV-C band is absorbed by the earth's ozone layer.

Over the short term, overexposure to the sun causes the skin to burn. Even mild cases of sunburn lead to redness, soreness, and discomfort; more severe cases result in pain and nausea. If not properly treated, sunburn can become infected. There is also considerable evidence that long-term exposure to the sun can lead to certain forms of skin cancer.

Tanning, in vogue by modern standards of fashion, is nothing more than the attempt of the skin to protect itself from the ravages of the sun. As the ultraviolet rays penetrate the skin, the dermis produces more melanin, the pigment that gives the skin its color, and darkens. The melanin acts as a barrier to the ultraviolet radiation. So, that heavily tanned body—a symbol of beauty—is in reality a sign of overexposure to the sun and damage to the skin. The phrase "healthy tan" is a contradiction in terms.

Artificial tanning devices, popular in some salons, are only marginally safer than natural sunlight. The body's tanning mechanism is the same, regardless of the source of ultraviolet energy. The claim to safety for these devices is that they screen out the UV-B "burning" rays and admit only the UV-A "tanning" rays. While this is true to some extent, current research shows that the UV-A rays penetrate the skin more deeply than UV-B rays and can also cause harmful effects, including blood vessel damage, adverse reactions to certain medications, and premature aging.

The FDA has established standards for the use of artificial tanning devices. They must have warning labels and instructions for proper use. They must have automatic timers to limit the exposure. The tubes must be shielded from direct contact by the customer, and protective goggles must be worn during use.

To avoid problems, both now and in the future, the client should limit exposure to the sun. If the clients must sunbathe, they should avoid exposure between eleven in the morning and four in the afternoon when the sun's rays are at their strongest. In addition, they should use a good quality sunblock, the higher the Sun Protection Factor (SPF) number the better. The manufacturer's instructions for proper use should be followed. Keep in mind, however, that a sunblocker will not eliminate the risk of sunburn; it only extends the time the client may expose skin to the sun before burning begins.

The SPF number on sunscreen products indicates the relative degree of protection provided. Thus, products with an SPF rating of 2 to 4 give minimal protection from sunburn while allowing considerable tanning, whereas products with an SPF rating of 8 to 15 allow virtually no tanning but give considerably more protection. Products rated above SPF 15 provide maximum protection.

Smoking

Short of becoming addicted to narcotics, smoking is about the single most self-destructive act one can indulge in. Smoking causes emphysema and cancer and is a major factor in the onset of heart attacks. The effect of smoking on the skin is also devastating.

The nicotine in tobacco contracts the small blood vessels and capillaries. As a result, blood circulation decreases, preventing the skin from receiving oxygen and nutrients. This dries the skin and makes it prone to wrinkling and premature aging.

The smoke particles serve as nuclei for airborne dust and dirt, allowing the residue to settle on the skin and clog the pores. And nicotine can stain the skin or give it a yellowish hue.

In addition, constant exposure to smoke causes smokers to squint their eyes in reaction to the irritation of the smoke. The long-term effect of squinting is premature wrinkling.

The remedy for this harmful factor is simple—stop smoking. Clients should be counseled to quit smoking, and not only for the health of their skin. Their bodies will love them for it.

Drugs and Alcohol

Like smoking, the habitual use of narcotics and other illicit drugs can have severe effects on the skin. They also rob the skin of oxygen and essential nutrients and can leave the skin dry or cause acne-like symptoms.

Many medications, both over-the-counter and prescription drugs, can produce side effects that manifest themselves in various skin disorders such as hives, rashes, eczema-like eruptions, and pigment changes. In the initial consultation with the client, it is necessary to ask questions about the use of medicines. A client who shows symptoms of drug side effects should be referred to a physician.

Light to moderate use of alcohol is not generally harmful to the skin. Heavy use, however, can deprive the skin of moisture, leading to dull, dry skin. It can also cause broken capillaries, which show as red blotches under the skin. Chronic overindulgence is also linked to the development of the skin condition rosacea.

Nutrition

There is an old adage that says we are what we eat. And to a large extent, this is true. The skin is, in many ways, a mirror of what we eat and drink. As a working organ of the body, the skin takes nourishment from the food that is ingested. Like the other organs of the body, the amount of nourishment the skin receives is largely dependent on the quality of the food. As discussed in Chapter 8, proper nutrition, therefore, is important to the health of the skin.

While poor nutrition may not affect the skin directly, its effects may lead to conditions that show up as skin disorders. Severe vitamin deficiencies, for example, can lead to a number of different kinds of skin conditions. Most estheticians probably will never see clients suffering from that degree of nutritional deficiency. It is more likely that the esthetician will see clients who have poor nutritional habits and whose skin is dehydrated and looks dull and lifeless.

During the initial consultation, the esthetician should question the clients on their dietary practices. What kinds of food do they eat? Are they overweight or underweight? Are they on any kind of diet? Do they drink enough water?

By getting a picture of the way the client eats and drinks, the esthetician can, in many cases, gain insights into the internal conditions that affect the client's skin. The esthetician can then suggest changes in the client's diet that will help the skin function more efficiently.

Chemicals

Chemicals, both synthetic and those found in nature, can have harmful effects on the skin, causing conditions that vary from dryness and redness to blistering and burning. Many common household chemicals, such as laundry detergents, bleaches, and drain cleaners, can cause contact dermatitis. Alcohols can dry the skin. The plasticizers in synthetic fabrics can cause rashes and itching. Cosmetics, hair dyes, nail polish, even some skin-care products, can cause allergic reactions in people who are sensitive to those substances.

Even natural chemicals can cause severe skin eruptions in some people. Bee stings and poison ivy are examples.

Smog, dirt particles in the air, exhaust fumes, sulfur compounds from industrial wastes, etc., are all potentially damaging to the skin. These sulfur-containing pollutants convert to a sulfuric acid solution on contact with the skin, the same chemical process that forms acid rain. This dehydrates the skin. Similarly, airborne dirt and impurities lodge in the pores and provide breeding grounds for harmful bacteria.

Most soaps are harshly alkaline and dry the skin. The chemical reaction also strips the skin of its protective acid mantle, leaving it open to germicidal attack.

Time

All of the factors discussed so far have one thing in common. Their effects can be eliminated by moderation, avoidance, or change of habits. No one, however, can eliminate the effects of aging. Everyone ages. It is a natural process that occurs in the body.

As the body ages, physical and chemical changes in the internal structure of the skin occur, and these changes alter both the functioning of the skin and its appearance. The tissues in the dermal and subcutaneous layers become thinner. Collagen and elastin content diminish and the amount of ground substance is reduced. As the skin loses its elasticity, lines and wrinkles begin to form.

At the same time, the walls of the capillaries tend to harden, causing a decrease in blood circulation. The sweat glands become less active. The skin loses some of its ability to regulate temperature, and so becomes less sensitive to changes in heat and cold. The reduced circulation also diminishes the supply of oxygen and nutrients to the skin.

With advancing age, the sebaceous glands secrete less sebum. As the production of the sebum diminishes, the horny layer of the epidermis dries out and tends to crack and become rough. Changes in pigmentation also occur as the skin ages. Freckles and age spots start to appear. Growths, such as skin tags, keratoses, corns, and calluses develop.

These effects of aging start to appear in the forties. If the skin has been damaged by long-term exposure to the sun, however, they may appear much earlier and will be much worse. The epidermis thickens and becomes rough and leathery, lines and wrinkles are deeper, and keratoses develop. Some of these may become malignant.

Wrinkles, lines, cracking, dryness, poor circulation, roughness, itching—these are the legacy age leaves to the skin. Proper care by a trained esthetician can retard the effects of aging on the skin. While they cannot be eliminated, the effects of aging can be slowed.

SKIN DISORDERS

Perfect skin is a joy to behold. It is firm, moist, and has good elasticity. It is free of blemishes. There are no blackheads, pimples or other blemishes to mar its surface. The pores are small and virtually unnoticeable. The pigmentation is even and there are no discolorations. The glands produce just the right amount of sweat and sebum. Such a skin represents an ideal. And like most ideals, it seldom exists in real life.

Few people have such perfect skin. The glands produce either too much or too little sebum. The skin is either too dry or too oily. Pigmentation is uneven and blotchy. Pores are too big or too small. Or there are blemishes, lesions of the skin.

A **lesion** (LE-shun) is an unnatural change in the structure or function of tissue and may take a number of forms. Among the lesions caused by injury are:

- **Abrasion**—a scraping away of the skin, as in a superficial scratch. An abrasion is also known as an **excoriation** (ek-skohr-i-AY-shun).
- **Bruise**—a **hematoma**, i.e., a mass of blood located outside of the blood vessels, without a cut being present. Bruises are generally superficial lesions. They are also known as **contusions**.
- **Hicky**—a hematoma caused by a bite or pinch, generally given during play.
- **Laceration**—a wound or tear in the tissue.

- **Scab**—a hard covering formed on the outer surface of a lesion, usually composed of dried pus and blood.
- **Scar**—the tissue formed as a wound heals. A scar is also known as a **cicatrix**.
- **Welt**—a linear wheal, or ridgelike swelling, caused by a blow.

Other lesions include:

- **Blister**—a circumscribed elevation on the skin filled with pus. A blister less than one centimeter in diameter is called a **vesicle**. If it is larger than one centimeter in diameter, it is called a **bulla**.
- **Boil**—a painful, pus-filled infection of a hair follicle. Boils are also known as **furuncles**.
- **Carbuncle**—a cluster of furuncles, also painful. A carbuncle is more severe than a single boil.
- **Corn**—a circumscribed thickening of the skin.
- **Cyst**—an air or fluid filled sac beneath the surface of the skin. Cysts vary from small to large and appear as smooth, firm, dome-shaped lumps in the skin.
- **Macule** (MAK-yool)—a flat, discolored spot on the skin.
- **Pimple**—an infected elevation on the skin, generally one centimeter in diameter or less. If the pimple is filled with pus, it is called a **pustule**. If it is solid, it is called a **papule**.
- **Scale**—a dry, flaky piece of the epidermis left on the surface of the skin. An example is dandruff.
- **Stain**—a discoloration of the skin. An example is a port-wine **hemangioma**.
- **Tubercle** (TOO-ber-kel)—a solid nodule on the skin, similar to a papule, but larger.
- **Ulcer**—an open sore below the level of the skin surface.
- **Urticaria**—an eruption of wheals caused by the release of histamines from the cells, usually in reaction to certain drugs, foods, or psychological stresses. Urticaria is also known as **hives**.
- **Wen**—a sebaceous cyst.
- **Wheal**—a linear or round swelling of short duration.

Other terms used in the description of skin disorders are:

- **Acute**—a condition that develops suddenly and lasts a relatively short time. There is no pattern of recurrence. An acute condition is usually more severe than a chronic condition.
- **Chronic**—a condition that often recurs and lasts for a relatively long time, but is generally less severe than an acute condition.

- **Edema** (e-DEE-muh)—the medical term for swelling caused by fluid gathering in the tissues.
- **Erythema**—the medical term for reddening of the skin.
- **Pruritus** (proo-RYE-tus)—the medical term for itching.
- **Purpura** (PUR-pyoo-ra)—the medical term for purple colored patches on the skin as a result of bleeding in the subcutaneous tissues.
- **Purulent** (PUR-yoo-lent)—the medical term for something containing or producing pus.

There are many different skin disorders. While the esthetician will be concerned with only a few of them, it is necessary to have some understanding of the different types of disorders. It is important to remember that the esthetician is *not* a medical doctor and may work only with skin disorders that are not contagious and that can be helped without medication.

Skin disorders can be classified by type. The more important of these are:

Sebaceous Gland Disorders

Blackheads, or **open comedones** (KOM-e-donz), are plugs of accumulated sebum and other matter that collect in the opening of follicles and turn black on exposure to air as the melanin oxidizes. They may occur on anyone at any age, but are most prevalent on adolescents and on adults with oily skin. They occur mostly in areas in which the oil glands are most numerous and active, such as the nose, forehead, and chin. Blackheads are also found often on the chest and back (Fig. 7.1).

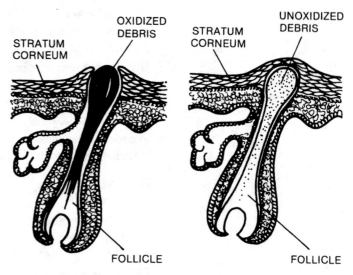

7.1—Blackhead   7.2—Whitehead

Removal of blackheads is an important aspect of skin cleansing and may be done by properly trained estheticians.

Whiteheads, also called **milia** (MIL-ee-uh) or **closed comedones,** are plugs of sebum and other matter trapped just below the surface of the skin. Since they are not at a surface opening on the skin, they do not oxidize, therefore they remain white. Like blackheads, these should also be removed by the esthetician (Fig. 7.2).

Acne is a common disorder of the sebaceous system. When blackheads and whiteheads are present on the skin, the condition is called **noninflammatory** acne. When the comedones become infected and pimples form, the condition is called **inflammatory** acne (Fig. 7.3).

The causes of acne are not fully understood, but it is generally believed that it is connected to the production of male hormones called androgens. Acne typically begins at puberty, when the glands start producing androgens, which stimulate the sebaceous glands. Both males and females may be afflicted with acne, but since females do not produce as much androgen as males, they are not usually afflicted as severely. The fact that **eunuchs** (YOO-nuk), castrated males, never develop acne lends credence to this theory. There is also some evidence that predisposition to acne is a genetic trait.

It is known, however, that acne is not caused by chocolate, greasy foods, lack of sufficient washing, or by either too much or too little sexual activity. Nor is acne caused by bacteria or viruses. Acne may become infected by bacteria, however, forming the characteristic pimples of inflammatory acne.

In many cases, acne will stop as the person reaches adulthood, although the disorder may occur in later years as well. Anxiety or tension can result in acne flare-ups. Acne may also develop from wearing tight clothing, such as headbands or turtleneck sweaters, or

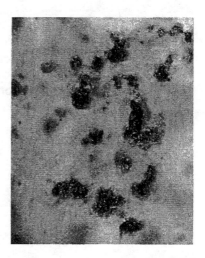

7.3—Acne *(Courtesy of Allergan Laboratories)*

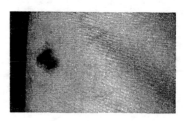

7.4—Rosacea *(Courtesy of Allergan Laboratories)*

from the use of greasy cosmetics. Acne-like lesions may be caused by exposure to chemicals or by some drugs.

Although the condition cannot be cured, acne can be controlled with proper care by a qualified esthetician. Control, however, does require time and effort on the part of the client. Severe cases of acne that do not respond to salon treatment should be referred to a dermatologist.

Rosacea (ro-ZA-se-a) is a chronic inflammation of the sebaceous glands, generally appearing in the middle third of the face. It occurs in middle-aged adults, both male and female. Typical lesions include redness, papules, pustules, and dilated capillaries. In severe cases, the nose becomes bulbous, greasy, and enlarged (Fig. 7.4).

The causes of rosacea are unknown, but its onset is influenced by inherited traits such as oily skin and brunette hair. The condition can be aggravated by climatic extremes or excessive consumption of alcoholic beverages or spicy foods.

Since it is a condition involving excessive oiliness of the skin, rosacea may be helped with proper cleansing and normalization of skin functions.

Papulosquamous Disorders

Papulosquamous disorders are the result of the accumulation of excessive keratin on the surface of the skin and are characterized by scaling. The most important of these disorders to the esthetician are seborrheic dermatitis and psoriasis.

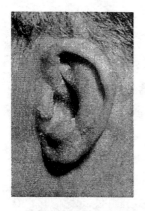

Seborrheic (seb-o-REE-ik) **dermatitis** is a chronic condition found commonly in middle-aged adults. It varies in severity from mild itching and small, loose, greasy scales to red patches of skin with large greasy scales. It occurs mostly on the scalp or face. When this condition occurs on the scalp, it is called **dandruff**. Its cause is unknown, but it is found most often in persons who have oily skin. This condition may respond to proper cleansing and normalization of skin functions (Fig. 7.5).

Psoriasis is a chronic disorder of the skin that affects about two percent of the population. Like seborrheic dermatitis, psoriasis is characterized by scaling. It differs, however, in that the scales are larger, less greasy and are silvery in color. The skin may or may not itch (Fig. 7.6).

The cause of psoriasis is not known but it may be hereditary, since there is often a family history of psoriasis. It may occur at almost any

7.5—Seborrheic dermatitis *(Courtesy of Allergan Laboratories)*

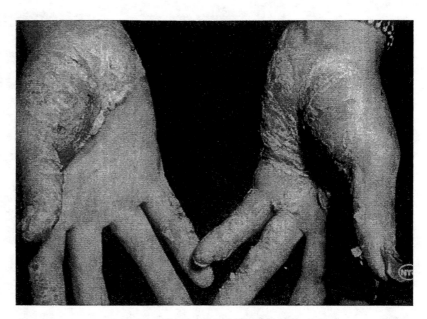

7.6—Psoriasis *(Courtesy of Allergan Laboratories)*

age, from the teens to late middle age. It generally appears on the elbows, knees, scalp, and trunk. About half of the cases of psoriasis also involve the fingernails. There is no cure for psoriasis, but it can be controlled to some extent. Clients with psoriasis should be referred to a physician. Since psoriasis is not contagious, however, estheticians may give facial treatments to clients afflicted with this disorder.

Eczematous Disorders

Eczema (EK-se-mah), or **dermatitis**, covers a number of chronic and acute disorders of the skin. Chronic cases of dermatitis are less severe and may be characterized by scaling and the formation of papules. Acute cases, on the other hand, show redness, oozing, and the formation of vesicles and bullae. Both are accompanied by burning and itching sensations. Clients showing signs of dermatitis should be referred to a physician (Fig. 7.7).

Contact dermatitis is an inflammation of the skin caused by exposure to an irritating substance or an **allergen** (AL-er-jen), a substance that triggers an allergic reaction. Poison ivy is one example of contact dermatitis.

Atopic eczema is a chronic form of dermatitis occurring in persons who have an inherited predisposition to hay fever, asthma or similar allergies. The condition is characterized by severe itching and burning of the skin, along with blisters, oozing, excoriations and thickening of the skin. The skin also becomes excessively dry. It is

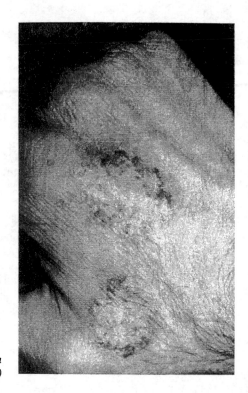

7.7—Eczema *(Courtesy of Allergan Laboratories)*

usually necessary to lubricate and protect the skin and to avoid cleansing with soap.

Miliaria rubra (mil-ee-AY-reé-ah ROOB-rah), or **prickly heat,** is an acute condition caused by the blocking of the sweat ducts in the dermis. It is characterized by severe itching and multiple small, red papules and vesicles. This condition is most common in hot, humid climates.

Fungal Disorders

Fungi are parasitic and saprophytic organisms belonging to the biological kingdom fungi. They differ from green plants in that they do not contain chlorophyll and, therefore, can't obtain food through photosynthesis, but must absorb it from either dead or living organic matter. A few species of parasitic fungi are pathogenic, or disease causing. **Dermatophytes** are fungi that attack and digest keratin. **Tinia,** also called **ringworm,** is the term given to skin, hair, or nail infections caused by dermatophytes. Tinia is characterized by redness, itching, and scaly patches.

Yeasts, unicellular species of fungi, also cause infections. These infections, however, have deeper, systemic roots. These disorders are also characterized by itchy, red patches.

The fungal infections are long lasting and respond very slowly to treatment. They are contagious and should not be handled. Clients should be referred immediately to a physician.

Bacterial Disorders

Pathogenic skin bacteria are responsible for a number of skin disorders other than the infection of comedones. The bacterial disorder of most interest to the esthetician is **folliculitis,** an infection of the hair follicles caused by **staphylococci.** This disorder is characterized by itching and redness in mild cases to the formation of furuncles and boils in severe cases. The condition is not contagious. Mild cases may be treated by thoroughly cleansing the skin. Severe cases should be referred to a physician.

Viral Disorders

Herpes simplex (HUR-peez SIM-pleks), the common **fever blister,** is a chronic viral infection caused by a herpes virus. The disorder is characterized by groups of vesicles on a red base and is found usually around the mouth and lips. The lesions usually heal themselves within two weeks of their appearance. Recurrence of the disorder is likely (Fig. 7.8).

Herpes zoster, also called **shingles,** is an acute viral infection caused by the same herpes virus that causes chicken pox. Like herpes simplex, this disorder is characterized by groups of vesicles. These vesicles are usually found along **dermatomes,** sensory fibers from the spinal cord. The disorder is quite painful. The lesions heal themselves in two to three weeks. Recurrence is rare.

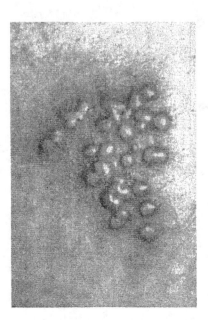

7.8—Herpes simplex *(Courtesy of Allergan Laboratories)*

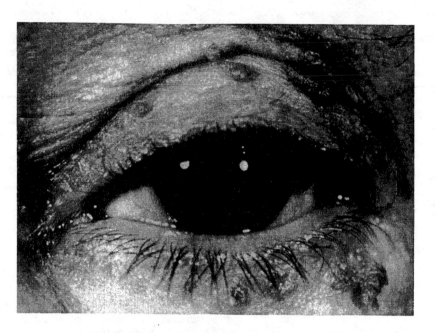

7.9—Verrucae *(Courtesy of Allergan Laboratories)*

Although the herpes viruses are not contagious, they can be transmitted by contact. Clients with these disorders should not be handled in the salon, but should be referred to a physician.

Verrucae, the scientific name for **warts,** are common viral infections characterized by round, rough surfaced lumps on the skin. They vary in size up to one centimeter. They can be removed surgically or chemically, but most often disappear spontaneously. Since they sometimes respond to suggestion, it is possible that they have psychosomatic origins (Fig. 7.9).

Skin Tumors

Tumors are abnormal growths of tissue. They vary in size, shape, and color and can be either benign or malignant.

Seborrheic keratoses are common skin tumors occurring in elderly people, particularly if their skin tends to oiliness. These normally benign growths range up to three centimeters in size and vary in color from flesh-toned to almost black. They have a greasy, wartlike texture, and look as though they were stuck onto the skin. Seborrheic keratoses tend to increase in size and numbers and grow darker with advancing age. Although they can be removed surgically, they have a tendency to recur (Fig. 7.10).

Actinic keratoses are premalignant skin tumors that occur in elderly people, especially those who have light complexions. These keratoses develop in areas that have been damaged by long-term exposure to the sun. Untreated, these tumors can become malignant.

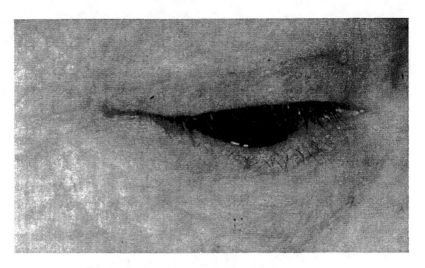

7.10—Seborrheic keratoses *(Courtesy of Allergan Laboratories)*

Actinic keratoses are flat, grainy, scaly lesions that vary in size up to about 1.5 centimeters and are tan to reddish-brown in color. They may cause some burning or stinging sensations. Because of their potential for malignancy, clients with suspected actinic keratoses should be referred to a physician.

Keloids are tumors that form on the skin after an injury. They appear as firm, reddish nodes and may be itchy or painful. Keloids tend to enlarge and radiate outward from the original point of the injury. They occur most often in black people. Surgical removal is possible, but there is a considerable risk involved that they will become more extensive as a result.

Melanocytic nevi, more commonly known as moles or beauty marks, are the most common tumors found on the body. These take many forms. They may be flat or elevated, pigmented or skin colored, and with or without hairs. Hairs in moles should never be plucked. Melanocytic nevi are normally benign, but sudden changes in coloration or size could indicate a potential malignancy.

Ephelides (ef-EE-lee-des), or freckles, are small, flat, brown macules that are very common, especially in red or brown haired people who are genetically predisposed to their formation. They are found mostly in areas of the skin that are exposed to the sun, and are most prevalent in the summer.

Lentigines (len-ti-JEE-neez) are multiple, flat, brown macules that appear as sharply demarcated patches of uniform color. They are differentiated from freckles in that they are not related to sun exposure. The **liver spots** of the elderly are lentigines.

Telangiectases, or **hemangiomas,** are tumors of the blood vessels in which the capillaries in the skin become permanently dilated. The cause is usually unknown, but some telangiectases may be caused by burns or sun exposure. **Birthmarks** are a type of hemangioma present at birth, characterized by a circumscribed discoloration of the skin. The discoloration can vary in size from very small to very large, and can be present on any part of the body.

The **port-wine hemangioma** is a very large, pink to reddish-purple mark usually found on the face. While not life threatening, it is a very disfiguring disorder. There is no effective means of treating port-wine stains, but they can be hidden with corrective makeup.

Acrochordons, or **skin tags**, are stalk-like papules that grow up to about one centimeter long. They can be pigmented or skin colored. Skin tags are very common growths found mostly on the eyelids and neck, especially in obese, middle-aged people. These usually benign tumors can be removed by electrosurgery.

Sebaceous hyperplasia is a condition in which small round papules develop on the face, especially on the forehead and cheeks. These flesh-toned to yellowish lumps are most often found in the elderly. They are benign and require no special treatment.

Basal cell carcinomas (kahr-si-NO-muh) are malignant tumors starting in the basal cell layer of the skin, and are the most common form of skin cancer. They are found in areas most often exposed to the sun, especially in people with fair complexions. The lesions are generally small and smooth surfaced with raised borders. They may be slightly pigmented or skin-colored. They also tend to bleed easily (Fig. 7.11).

Basal cell carcinomas are the least malignant form of skin cancer in that they tend to spread over the skin rather than invade the body tissues. And treatment is almost totally effective, if started early enough. The lesions may be removed surgically or treated by X-ray therapy.

Squamous (SKWAY-mus) **cell carcinomas** are malignant tumors that begin in the epidermal layers that form keratin. These tumors

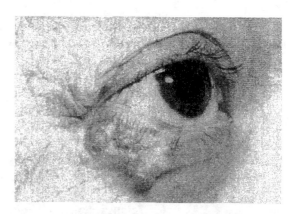

7.11—Basal cell carcinoma *(Courtesy of Allergan Laboratories)*

are found on any part of the body but are most common on the face, especially the lower lip and ears. In many cases, they develop from actinic keratoses, although they may also develop from burn scars or from occupational injury or chemical exposure. The lesions are reddish, round nodules that resemble scaly warts.

These skin cancers are more malignant than basal cell carcinomas and should be treated as soon as possible. Treatment is similar to that for basal cell carcinomas.

Malignant melanomas are the most dangerous form of skin cancer. Although more rare than the other two forms, the mortality rate for this type is much higher. The deeper the invasion, the worse the chances for survival.

The lesions, which may vary from pink to black in color and may be flat or raised, are found most often on areas of the body that have suffered from chronic overexposure to the sun. Early treatment of malignant melanomas is generally effective. The longer the delay, however, the worse the prognosis.

Pigmentation Disorders

Pigmentation disorders may travel in either of two directions. The skin may become more deeply colored, **hyperpigmentation**, or lose coloration, **hypopigmentation**.

Chloasma (kloh-AZ-mah) is a hyperpigmentation of the skin, occurring as irregular brown patches on the face and neck. The cause of this condition is unknown, although it often develops during pregnancy. When it appears in pregnant women, it is called the **mask of pregnancy**, and usually fades after delivery. The skin may respond to treatment with bleaching agents, but the best course of

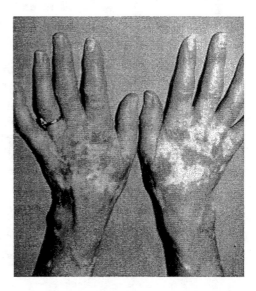

7.12—Vitiligo *(Courtesy of Allergan Laboratories)*

action is probably to cover the spots with a concealing makeup.

Certain drugs can also induce hyperpigmentation. Oral contraceptives, for example, can cause discolorations resembling chloasma.

Vitiligo (vit-i-LY-goh) is a condition of hypopigmentation in which large patches of the skin lose their coloration completely and become milky-white. This condition appears most often on the face and hands, but may occur anywhere on the body. The cause is unknown, but it may be an inherited trait. Vitiligo has been treated with some success with a combination of medication and ultraviolet exposure (Fig. 7.12).

Albinism (AL-bi-niz-em) is an inherited condition of hypopigmentation in which some or all of the pigment is lost in the skin, hair, and irises. Albinos have milky-white skin, gray or white hair and pink eyes. People suffering from this condition generally have shorter life spans than those with normal coloration. There is no known treatment for this disorder.

COSMETIC SURGERY TREATMENTS

During the course of a professional career, the esthetician will encounter clients who have undergone cosmetic surgery. Because of this, the esthetician should have some understanding of the different types of cosmetic surgery available, as well as some idea of what these procedures will and won't do.

The esthetician should remember that these are all medical techniques and may be practiced only by a qualified plastic surgeon. Under no circumstances should the esthetician recommend that a client undergo any specific type of cosmetic surgery. If asked, the esthetician may refer clients to plastic surgeons who have been recommended by other clients or who are personally known.

If the client has had recent cosmetic surgery, it may be harmful to give a standard facial treatment. During the consultation, the esthetician should ascertain if the client has undergone any cosmetic surgery within a year. If so, the esthetician should call the surgeon and find out if it is safe to give the facial.

In general, cosmetic surgery will alleviate problems pertaining to appearance. These include such items as nose and chin reshaping; removal of some wrinkles, scars, and excess fatty tissue; and smoothing the skin. The problems addressed by cosmetic surgery are seldom life-threatening. Correcting these problems, however, often enhances the quality of the patients' lives.

Cosmetic surgery may be performed on virtually every part of the face and neck. Some procedures are invasive; that is, they require cutting the skin to work under the surface or require injecting substances under the skin. Some are noninvasive, that is, they are limited to the outer layers of the skin.

The most common noninvasive procedures include skin pigmentation, chemical peels, dermabrasion, and dermaplaning. Since they are limited to the skin surface, these procedures generally may be performed in the surgeon's office on an out-patient basis and recovery times are shorter.

Skin pigmentation (pig-men-TA-shun) procedures, like tatooing, involve injecting dye into the skin with tiny needles. The technique is most commonly used to darken the lash lines along the upper and lower eyelids as a permanent eyeliner. The effect is permanent.

Chemical peels (PEELS) are used to smooth skin and remove fine wrinkles. The procedure will not remove deep scars or furrows in the skin. A strong caustic, usually phenol, is applied to the skin along the wrinkle lines and covered with tape. The caustic chemically burns off the outer layers of skin, leaving the skin somewhat smoother. The technique is most effective on fair-skinned people. Darker skins may experience discoloration or mottling.

Dermabrasion (dur-muh-BRAY-zhun) and **dermaplaning** (dur-muh-PLAY-ning) are also skin smoothing procedures for removing scars and wrinkles. The outer layers of the skin are removed by sanding with a rotary metal brush or file (dermabrasion) or by shaving them off with a razor-sharp surgical instrument called a **dermatome** (dur-muh-TOHM). Neither procedure will remove deep scars.

Invasive procedures include injecting substances, such as collagen or silicone, into the tissues under the skin, and cutting through the skin and underlying tissues. The injection procedures can usually be performed in the doctor's office on an out-patient basis. The other procedures, however, generally require at least an overnight stay in the hospital and have longer recovery periods.

Collagen (KOL-a-jen) and **silicone injections** are used to remove or minimize light scars, age lines, and wrinkles. The material is injected under the skin in the area to be treated, where it puffs out the underlying tissue and smooths out the surface of the skin. The collagen used in this procedure comes from cattle and is similar to human body tissue. The body tends to absorb the collagen after a few years, so the procedure is not permanent. Silicone, on the other hand, is a nonorganic material and is not absorbed into the body. Although permanent, the silicone may harden and shift its position over time.

There are specific cosmetic surgery procedures for each part of the face and neck. Starting from the top of the head and working down, these include brow lifts, blepharoplasty, rhinoplasty, malar implants, otoplasty, mentoplasty, and rhytidectomy. Each of these can improve the appearance of that part of the face by minimizing wrinkling, or correcting defects of shape or size. None of the procedures, however, will substantially alter the structure of the face or eliminate the effects of aging.

Brow lifts smooth out furrows and lines in the forehead. In addition, they raise the eyebrows and upper lids. In this operation, the skin is cut behind the front hairline. Part of the frontalis muscle is cut away and the skin is stretched back until the brow has been tightened. The skin is sewn in place, leaving a scar behind the front of the hairline.

Blepharoplasty (blef-ah-row-PLAS-tee) can be performed on either the upper or lower lids. Performed on the upper eyelid, the operation makes the eyes larger and tightens the skin. Performed on the lower eyelid, the operation removes bags under the eyes. The procedure will not remove crow's feet at the corners of the eyes or laugh lines and wrinkles. The skin is cut either above the eyebrows or under the lashes on the lower lid. Excess tissue is removed and the skin is pulled tight and sewn. The procedure leaves slight scars in the folds of the eyes.

Rhinoplasty (RY-no-plas-tee) removes humps and straightens out the nose. When performed on the tip, the operation can improve the shape. The procedure, however, cannot make major changes in the shape of the nose. Since rhinoplasty is done from the inside of the nose, there is no external scarring. The surgery removes excess bone and cartilage. In some cases, the nose can be lengthened by implanting a piece of bone from another part of the body in the tip.

Malar (MAY-lur) **implants** add shape to the face by raising the cheekline. In this operation, a groove is cut between the upper lip and gum line and an implant is inserted. As with rhinoplasty, there is no external scarring.

Otoplasty (oh-tow-PLAS-tee) improves the appearance by flattening ears that protrude. The back of the ear is cut and excess cartilage is removed. This lets the ear lie closer to the head. The operation leaves only a small scar in the crease of the ear.

Mentoplasty changes the shape of the chin to improve the profile. This is accomplished either by removing excess bone to reshape the chin or by adding a silicone implant to enlarge it.

Rhytidectomy (rit-i-DECK-tuh-mee), or face and neck lift, is the most extensive of the cosmetic surgical procedures and is often performed in conjunction with one or more of the others. This procedure tightens loose skin in the face and neck. It will not eliminate wrinkles or alter the appearance, however. The skin is cut from the hair line to behind the ear. The skin is separated and loose tissue is removed, then the skin is stretched back and sewn.

REVIEW QUESTIONS

1. How can an esthetician work with skin?
2. What are the factors harmful to the skin?
3. Why is sun a problem to skin?
4. What are the three bands of the ultraviolet spectrum?
5. What is the difference among the three bands?
6. What is tanning?
7. Why is smoking bad for the skin?
8. How do medications affect the skin?
9. What kinds of chemicals can cause dermatitis?
10. What are some of the effects of age on the skin?
11. What can the esthetician do about aging?
12. Match the type of lesion with its description.

1. Abrasion	a.	hard covering over a wound
2. Bruise	b.	flat, discolored spot
3. Scab	c.	discoloration
4. Blister	d.	scrape of the skin
5. Corn	e.	infected elevation of the skin
6. Cyst	f.	contusion
7. Macule	g.	thickening of the skin
8. Stain	h.	sebaceous cyst
9. Pimple	i.	sac beneath the skin
10. Wen	j.	pus filled elevation on the skin

13. Define pruritus.
14. What are blackheads?
15. What are whiteheads?
16. Why are males more prone to acne than females?
17. How can rosacea be helped?
18. What are papulosquamous disorders and why are they important to the esthetician?
19. How should the esthetician handle cases of dermatitis?
20. What are warts?
21. What are actinic keratoses?
22. What are the most common tumors found on the body?
23. What are basal cell carcinomas?
24. What is the most dangerous form of skin cancer?
25. What are the two types of pigment disorders?
26. Why should the esthetician have some knowledge about cosmetic surgery procedures?
27. What should the esthetician do before giving a facial to a client who has had cosmetic surgery?
28. What is dermabrasion?
29. What is rhinoplasty?
30. What is mentoplasty?
31. What is a rhytidectomy?

8 Nutrition

OBJECTIVES *After completing this chapter, you should be able to:*

❶ Understand the importance of a balanced diet to the body and its functions.

❷ Discuss the nutritional process, the various types of nutrients, as well as the value of vitamins and minerals to skin health.

❸ Review the guidelines to good nutrition, as established by the government.

INTRODUCTION

The importance of good food has been recognized since antiquity. And food has always been a preoccupation with human beings. Indeed, it was the development of the ability to cultivate food that allowed for the change from a wandering forager to a village dweller, thus paving the way for civilization.

We are what we eat. The skin, like the other organs of the body, relies on a regular supply of proper nutrients to function properly. When these nutrients are taken in adequate quantities and in balance, the skin is healthy, with good color and vitality, adequate moisture and sebum production, and normal functioning. When some or all of the required nutrients are missing from the diet, the skin may appear dull and lifeless, with poor color and improper functioning. The skin is the second biggest consumer of nutrients in the body. The nervous system is first. When the body is short of nutrients, preference goes to the nervous system, so the skin goes hungry.

Poor nutrition has a direct effect on the health of the skin. It also has an indirect effect. As other organs in the body malfunction, the symptoms are often mirrored in the skin. For this reason, it is impossible to separate the effects of nutrition on the skin from its effects on the rest of the body.

It is important that the esthetician understand the principles of nutrition and diet and how they affect the skin. Knowing how the various nutrients work, what they do, and what happens when they are deficient, can help the esthetician reach the root causes of the client's skin problems.

An understanding of the client's eating habits can let the knowledgeable esthetician suggest changes in diet that will help meet the client's skin-care needs.

THE NUTRITIONAL PROCESS

Think of the body as a chemical factory. Like a manufacturing plant, raw materials are taken in; products are manufactured; and waste materials are thrown away. In the case of the body, the raw materials are the nutrients that come from food, water, and air. The food and water are ingested and pass through the digestive system; the air comes in through the lungs. The products manufactured are energy and tissue, resulting from the complex chemical process called metabolism. The waste products—carbon dioxide, feces, and urine— are eliminated through the excretory system. And, like the manufacturing plant, the quality of the products is only as good as the raw materials that go into making them.

Thus, the nutritional process forms, in effect, a triad—three points of an equilateral triangle. One point is **ingestion**, the second point is **digestion**, and the third point is **elimination**. All three are equally important and all three work together to fuel the body and keep it healthy.

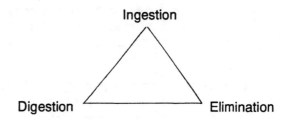

At the first point, ingestion, food is chosen, prepared, and taken into the body. Good nutrition starts with the choice of food. Modern man has an almost infinite variety of foods from which to choose. Some are good, containing the necessary nutrients to fuel the body. Others are poor in nutrients, offering only empty calories. The better one chooses which foods are taken, the better the nutritional process will be.

Preparation is also important. Good foods, improperly prepared, can lose much of their nutritive value. Overuse of pesticides, additives, and preservatives can lower the quality of the food, as can overcooking.

When the food is placed in the mouth, digestion, the second point of the triangle, begins. As the food is chewed, it is broken into smaller pieces that are easier to digest. **Saliva**, the first enzyme encountered in the digestive process, is secreted by the salivary glands in the mouth. These **enzymes**, proteins that act as catalysts to change other substances while retaining their own identity, start the breakdown of the food into a useable form.

After swallowing, the food travels down the esophagus to the stomach where gastric juices consisting of hydrochloric acid and other enzymes continue the breakdown of the food. The food becomes a liquid, called **chyme** (KEYEM). From the stomach, the chyme moves into the small intestine. The pancreas and the liver produce more enzymes that break the food down even further.

The nutrients digested from the food, in the form of glucose, amino acids and fatty acids, are absorbed into the bloodstream and lymphatic system through the walls of the small intestine. From here, they are transported to the various organs where they are converted into energy or tissue by the process of metabolism.

The undigested portion of the food passes from the small intestine to the large intestine, where the third point of the triangle, elimination, starts. The waste products are then expelled from the body in the form of feces and urine.

Proper elimination is just as vital to the health of the skin as the other two legs of the triangle. It is important that the body rid itself of the waste materials before they putrefy and spread toxins throughout the body.

The process by which the nutrients are converted into either tissue or energy is called **metabolism**. There are two phases—**anabolism**, the chemical conversion of nutrients to build up tissue and body chemicals, and **catabolism**, the breakdown of nutrients to supply energy. Both phases occur simultaneously.

Nutrients

Nutrients consist of carbohydrates, proteins, fats, vitamins, minerals, and water. All of these work together synergystically and their effects are interrelated. Each type of nutrient performs a different function for the body, providing fuel for energy, for building tissue or for helping to regulate the processes of the body. The fuel value of a given nutrient is expressed in **calories**, a measure of the amount of heat produced when the nutrient is oxidized. Thus, high calorie foods have more potential for producing energy than low calorie foods.

Carbohydrates. **Carbohydrates** supply most of the body's energy needs, whether for the production of heat, to keep the body temperature constant; for mechanical energy, to enable the muscles to work; or for electrical energy, to allow the nervous system to work.

Sugar, starch, and **cellulose** are the main carbohydrates. Through the action of certain enzymes, sugar, a simple carbohydrate, and starch, a complex carbohydrate, are converted into **glucose**, much of which is either used immediately for energy or is further converted into **glycogen** (GLEYE-ko-jen) and stored in the liver or in muscle tissue. The remainder is converted into fat and stored throughout the body for later use. Cellulose is not digestible, so is not useful for energy conversion.

Protein. **Protein** provides the materials for building tissue and for the production of **hormones** and enzymes. When carbohydrates and fat are deficient, protein is also burned as a source of energy. Excess protein, like excess carbohydrate, is converted into fat and stored in body tissue. The first areas to feel the effects of protein deficiency are the skin, hair, and nails.

Amino acids, the building blocks of the body, are produced by the action of digestion of the proteins. The body needs twenty-two different amino acids. However, the body is capable of producing only fourteen of them. The other eight, called the **essential amino acids**, must come from food. All eight of these must be present in specific proportions for synthesis to take place. Animal products generally contain all eight essential amino acids; therefore, these foods are called **complete proteins**. Fruits and vegetables, **incomplete proteins**, generally lack one or more of these eight, so care must be taken to combine these foods to get the proper mix of the essential amino acids (Table 8.1).

Fats. **Fats** provide a concentrated source of energy, giving up twice as many calories as carbohydrates and proteins as they are oxidized. They also carry the fat soluble vitamins. And they are the slowest of the main nutrients to be digested. Animal fats are **saturated**; that is, they can't accept any more hydrogen atoms in their structural chain and tend to be solid at room temperature. Vegetable fats are **unsaturated**; that is, they can accept more hydrogen atoms and tend to be liquid at room temperature. Vegetable oils, however, can be **hydrogenated** by adding gaseous hydrogen under pressure to convert the oil into solid form.

Fatty acids give fats their characteristic taste and texture. During digestion, the fatty acids are split from the structural chain and pass through the intestinal wall into the bloodstream. Three of the fatty acids—linoleic, arachidonic and linolenic—are collectively known as vitamin F and are discussed in more detail in the section on vitamins.

TABLE 8.1—Amino Acids

AMINO ACID	FORMULA	AMINO ACID	FORMULA
ALANINE	$H_7NC_3O_2$	ISOLEUCINE*	$H_{13}NC_6O_2$**
ARGENINE	$H_{14}N_4C_6O_2$	LEUCINE*	$H_{13}NC_6O_2$**
ASPARAGINE	$H_8N_2C_4O_3$	LYSINE*	$H_{14}N_2C_6O_2$
ASPARTIC ACID	$H_7NC_4O_4$	METHIONINE*	$H_{11}NSC_5O_2$
CYSTINE	$H_{11}N_2S_2C_6O_4$	PHENYLALANINE*	$H_6NC_9O_2$
GLUTAMIC ACID	$H_9NC_5O_4$	PROLINE	$H_{10}NC_5O_2$
GLUTAMINE	$H_{10}N_2C_5O_3$	SERINE	$H_7NC_3O_3$
GLYCINE	$H_5NC_2O_2$	THREONINE*	$H_9NC_4O_3$
HISTIDINE	$H_9N_3C_5O_3$	TRYPTOPHAN*	$H_8N_2C_{11}O_2$
HYDROXYLYSINE	$H_{14}N_2C_6O_3$	TYROSINE	$H_7NC_9O_3$
HYDROXYPROLINE	$H_{10}NC_5O_3$	VALINE*	$H_{11}NC_5O_2$

*Essential Amino Acids.
**Isoleucine and Leucine have the same chemical formula but are different structurally.

Vitamins. **Vitamins,** certain organic substances found in food, are essential to life and health, even though they don't provide energy or build tissue like the three major nutrients. Vitamins are **catalysts** that help manufacture enzymes and regulate the metabolism so the carbohydrates, proteins and fats can do their work. Since the body can form very few of the vitamins on its own, they must be supplied through the diet. There are at least twenty vitamins known at present. Some are water-soluble; others are fat-soluble (Table 8.2).

Vitamin A, a fat-soluble vitamin, is found as preformed vitamin A in fish-liver oil, cream and butter. It is found as **carotene** in green leafy vegetables and carrots. The body converts carotene to vitamin A for use. This vitamin is necessary for proper growth of the bottom layer of skin and is used in the treatment of acne. The **Recommended Dietary Allowance** (RDA) for vitamin A is 5,000 **International Units** (IU) for adults. Vitamin A can be toxic in extremely high doses.

TABLE 8.2—Vitamins

VITAMIN	COMMON NAME	SOURCE	REMARKS
A		Green leafy vegetables, carrots, fish-liver oil, butter, cream	Important for skin, RDA—5,000 IU. Toxic in large doses.
B Complex			
B$_1$	Thiamine	Wheat germ, bran, brewer's yeast	Important for skin.
B$_2$	Riboflavin	Wheat germ, bran, brewer's yeast	Important for skin.
B$_3$	Niacin	Poultry, fish, peanuts, lean meat	Important for skin.
B$_5$	Pantothenic Acid	Organ meats, egg yolks, whole grains	
B$_6$	Pyridoxine	Meat, whole grains	
B$_{12}$	Cobalamin	Organ meats, fish, dairy products	
B$_{13}$	Orotic Acid	Whey, root vegetables	
B$_{15}$	Pangamic Acid	Whole grains, seeds, brown rice	
	Biotin	Organ meats, egg yolks	Also known as Vitamin H.
	Choline	Wheat germ, liver, egg yolk	
	Inositol	Whole grains, liver, citrus fruit	Important for hair growth.
	Folic Acid	Liver, leafy green vegetables	Also known as Vitamin M.
	PABA	Liver, wheat germ, yeast	Important for skin. Sunscreen
C	Ascorbic Acid	Fruits, vegetables	Important for skin. RDA—60 mg.
D		Fish-liver oils.	RDA—400 IU.
E	Tocopherol	Wheat germ oil, seeds, nuts, soybeans	Important for skin. RDA—5–15 IU.
F	Fatty Acids	Vegetable oils, cod-liver oil	
K	Menadione	Kelp, leafy green vegetables	Synthesized in body.
P	Bioflavonoids	Citrus fruit, grapes, cherries	Important for skin.
T		Egg yolk, sesame seeds	
U		Raw cabbage	

Vitamin B complex, a group of water-soluble vitamins, are found in bacteria, yeasts, and molds. These vitamins are necessary for the conversion of carbohydrates to glucose, which is burned to provide the body with energy. They are also necessary for proper metabolism and for the nervous system. All of the members of this group are interrelated in their function and should be taken together. Brewer's yeast and green vegetables are good sources of the B complex vitamins.

Vitamin B$_1$ (thiamine) is needed for the conversion of carbohydrates to glucose and is found in wheat germ and bran. Thiamine is synthesized in the body by the intestinal flora.

Vitamin B$_2$ (riboflavin) is vital to cell respiration and is important to healthy skin. It is found in the same foods that the other B complex vitamins are in. Riboflavin may also be synthesized by the intestinal flora.

Vitamin B$_3$ (niacin) is necessary for healthy skin and as a coenzyme for breaking down the major nutrients. It is found in lean meats, poultry, fish and peanuts. The body also converts the amino acid, tryptophan, into niacin.

Vitamin B$_5$ (pantothenic acid) is needed for healthy skin and is important in cellular metabolism. It also helps retard aging and wrinkling. It is found in organ meats, egg yolks, and whole grains. Pantothenic acid is also synthesized by the intestinal flora.

Vitamin B$_6$ (pyridoxine) aids in the production of hydrochloric acid and helps linoleic acid, one of the essential fatty acids, work better. It is also needed for the synthesis of DNA and RNA. This vitamin is found in meat and whole grains.

Vitamin B$_{12}$ (cobalamin) contains mineral elements and is needed for proper metabolism. It is found in organ meats, fish, and dairy products. Unlike other vitamins, vitamin B$_{12}$ cannot be produced synthetically.

Vitamin B$_{13}$ (orotic acid) helps in cellular restoration and is used in the production of folic acid and vitamin B$_{12}$. It is found in whey and in root vegetables.

Vitamin B$_{15}$ (pangamic acid) helps cell respiration and is needed for the metabolism of protein. It is found in whole grains, seeds, and brown rice.

Biotin, sometimes called **vitamin H,** is a coenzyme that aids the production of fatty acids and is essential for proper nutrition. It is found in organ meats and egg yolks.

Choline is necessary for a healthy liver and kidneys and for the absorption of fat by the body. It is found in lecithin, liver, wheat germ, and egg yolk.

Inositol works with choline in the metabolism of fat. It is also important to hair growth. Inositol is found in lecithin, whole grains, liver, and citrus fruits.

Folic acid, sometimes called **vitamin M**, helps in the formation of red blood cells and in the formation of nucleic acid. It also helps the liver function properly. Folic acid is found in liver and in green leafy vegetables.

Para-aminobenzoic acid (PABA) helps the intestinal flora produce folic acid and is important to the health of the skin. PABA is also effective as a sunscreen. It is found in liver, wheat germ, and yeast.

Vitamin C (ascorbic acid) is a water-soluble vitamin. It is less stable than the other vitamins and is oxidized easily. It is found in most fruits and vegetables, especially in citrus fruits. Vitamin C is important to the maintenance of collagen and the formation of connective tissue. It also helps many of the other nutrients function properly. In addition, vitamin C helps combat stress and acts as a natural antibiotic. Unlike some other vitamins, humans cannot synthesize vitamin C, so the entire requirement for this vitamin must be supplied through the diet.

The RDA for vitamin C is sixty milligrams, although smokers may need additional quantities of this nutrient, since smoking destroys vitamin C. There is no toxicity from excessive intake of vitamin C, although some people may experience some side effects, such as diarrhea or a rash.

Vitamin D, the "sunshine vitamin," is fat-soluble. It is synthesized in the body through the action of sunlight on the skin, and is also present in fish-liver oils. Vitamin D aids normal growth and bone formation, and helps maintain stability in the central nervous system. The RDA for vitamin D is 400 IU. Extremely large doses of vitamin D can be toxic. Milk is generally fortified with synthetic vitamin D.

Vitamin E (tocopherol) is fat-soluble. It is found in wheat germ oil, whole raw seeds, nuts, and soybeans. Vitamin E is an anti-oxidant and helps prevent the breakdown of fatty acids and other vitamins and the formation of free radicals. This nutrient is also important to cellular respiration and helps increase stamina and endurance. It also helps prevent the formation of scars on the skin. The RDA for vitamin E varies from 5 IU for infants to 15 IU for adults. Although vitamin E is generally not toxic, it may be harmful to persons with high blood pressure.

Vitamin F, which consists of the three unsaturated fatty acids, **linoleic, linolenic,** and **arachidonic**, is necessary for normal functioning of the glands and for the regulation of blood coagulation. The unsaturated fatty acids (UFA) also lubricate cells and nourish skin cells. Linoleic acid is an essential fatty acid; that is, it cannot be synthesized by the body and must be supplied in the diet. The other two, linolenic and arachidonic acids, can be synthesized from linoleic acid.

Although there is no RDA established for UFA, it is generally recommended that linoleic acid make up about one percent of the daily caloric intake. Although vitamin F is not toxic, excessive consumption of fatty acids can result in weight gain. Food sources for UFA include natural vegetable oils, cod-liver oil, and wheat germ.

Vitamin K (menadione) is fat-soluble and is manufactured in the body by intestinal flora. It is also found in kelp and leafy green vegetables. Vitamin K is important for proper liver function and for the formation of some of the chemicals required for various body processes. It also helps foster proper blood clotting. Natural vitamin K is not toxic although excessive doses of synthetic vitamin K can produce toxic symptoms. Since it is synthesized by the body, deficiencies are rare, so no RDA has been established. Other sources of vitamin K are yogurt, alfalfa, and fish-liver oils.

Vitamin P (bioflavonoids) consists of a water-soluble group of nutrients that occur with vitamin C in many fruits and vegetables. These nutrients, which consist of rutin, hesperidin, citrin, flavone, and flavonals, are needed to allow vitamin C to be utilized effectively. They also help in the formation of collagen and strengthen capillary walls. No RDA has been established for the bioflavonoids and they are considered to be nontoxic. Food sources include citrus fruits, buckwheat, rose hips, grapes, and cherries.

Vitamin T and **vitamin U** are little known and their use is not yet fully understood. Vitamin T does assist the blood coagulation process and is found in egg yolks and sesame seeds. Vitamin U, found in raw cabbage, helps heal ulcers. Since so little is known about these two vitamins, no RDA has been established for either of them.

Minerals. Like vitamins, **minerals** (MIN-e-rals) are essential to proper body functioning. Minerals are inorganic nutrients that let vitamins work. Without them, vitamins would be unable to function. All of the minerals needed by the body must be supplied in the diet. None can be synthesized by the body. In their pure mineral form, these substances are largely indigestible. Before the body can use them, they must be made digestible through the process of **chelation** (kee-LAY-shun), in which the mineral bonds with an amino acid.

At present, eighteen minerals are known to be important to life. The most important—calcium, iodine, iron, magnesium, phosphorus, and zinc—have had Recommended Daily Allowances established. The other twelve minerals—chlorine, chromium, cobalt, copper, fluorine, manganese, molybdenum, potassium, selenium, sodium, sulfur, and vanadium—though also important, have not had RDA's set (Table 8.3).

More **calcium** is found in the body than any other material. Calcium operates in conjunction with phosphorus for forming bones

TABLE 8.3—Minerals

MINERAL	SOURCE	REMARKS
Calcium	Bone meal, milk, soybeans, salmon	Important to skin, RDA—800–1200 mg
Chlorine	Salt	
Chromium	Eggs, liver, mushrooms, brewer's yeast	
Cobalt	Meat, sea vegetables, milk, shellfish	
Copper	Seafood, liver, whole grains, legumes, leafy green vegetables	Important to skin.
Fluorine	Seafood, cheese, fluoridated water	
Iodine	Fish, sea vegetables	RDA—1 mg/kilo of body weight.
Iron	Organ meats, whole grains, leafy green vegetables	RDA—10–18 mg.
Magnesium	Green vegetables, whole grains, soybeans	RDA—300–350 mg.
Manganese	Whole grains, nuts, green vegetables, eggs	
Molybdenum	Meats, cereals, dark green leafy vegetables	
Phosphorus	Meat, poultry, fish, eggs, whole grains	RDA—800 mg.
Potassium	Leafy green vegetables, bananas, potatoes	Important to skin.
Selenium	Organ meats, fish, brewer's yeast	Important to skin.
Sodium	Salt	
Sulfur	Eggs, meat, fish	Important to skin.
Vanadium	Organ meats, seafood	
Zinc	Meats, eggs, wheat germ	Important to skin.

and teeth. It also helps maintain healthy skin and helps prevent sun damage to the skin. Sources of calcium are milk, dairy products, soybeans, salmon, and bone meal. The RDA for calcium varies from 800 to 1200 milligrams.

Chlorine is generally found combined with sodium or potassium in the form of chloride. Chlorine is needed to regulate the acid/alkali balance of the blood and to help maintain intercellular pressure. Most chlorine is supplied through the ingestion of salt in the diet. Chlorine deficiency may lead to hair loss.

Chromium is essential for the proper enzymatic action in metabolism, and for regulating blood sugar levels. It is needed in very small concentrations. Food sources include eggs, liver, mushrooms, and brewer's yeast.

Cobalt, a component of vitamin B_{12}, is necessary for proper cellular functioning. Meat—especially organ meats, sea vegetables, shellfish, and milk—are food sources for cobalt.

Copper is important to the skin, nerves, and blood. It helps the amino acid, tyrosine, function to pigment the skin and works with vitamin C to form elastin. In addition, it helps form the myelin sheaths around nerve fibers and assists the development of hemoglobin in the blood. Copper is found in seafood, liver, whole grains, legumes, and leafy green vegetables. Copper deficiency may inhibit healing of skin sores.

Fluorine helps strengthen bones and teeth. Although needed in small quantities for good health, fluorine is toxic in high concentration. In the U.S., most fluorine is supplied in fluoridated water. Food sources include seafood and cheese.

Iodine is necessary for the proper functioning of the thyroid gland. This mineral helps regulate energy, control the metabolism, and influence growth and development. The RDA for iodine is about one microgram per kilogram of body weight. Pregnant women should ingest slightly higher amounts. The best food sources for iodine are fish and sea vegetables. Iodine deficiency may lead to dry hair.

Iron is important to the quality of the blood. This mineral combines with copper to help produce hemoglobin, which carries the oxygen in the blood. In addition, iron helps form myoglobin in muscle tissue. The RDA for iron is between ten and eighteen milligrams. Women require more iron than men. Organ meats, whole grains, and leafy green vegetables are the best dietary sources of iron.

Magnesium is essential to metabolism and the maintenance of a suitable acid-alkaline balance. It also helps convert blood sugar into energy. The RDA for magnesium varies from 300 to 350 milligrams, the lower amount for men, the higher amount for women. This mineral is found in most foods, especially in green vegetables, soybeans, whole grains, and apples.

Manganese helps activate a number of enzymes that promote the functioning of vitamins. It also helps feed nerves and brain tissue. Food sources of manganese include whole grains, nuts, green vegetables, and eggs.

Molybdenum helps iron and copper function properly in the body. Meats, cereals, and dark green leafy vegetables are good food sources for this mineral.

Phosphorus is second only to calcium in its presence in the body. Like calcium, phosphorus is necessary to proper growth and healthy bones and teeth. For best functioning, these two minerals should be combined in specific proportions. The RDA for phosphorus is 800 milligrams. All high protein foods contain phosphorus. These include meat, poultry, fish, eggs and whole grains.

Potassium works with sodium to help regulate the balance between intercellular and intracellular fluid. These two minerals also help equalize the acid-alkali balance and are important for muscle functioning. Potassium also helps promote healthy skin. Potassium is found in green leafy vegetables, bananas, potatoes, and whole grains.

Selenium is necessary to maintain elasticity in tissues and for reproduction. An antioxidant, selenium works with vitamin E to help retard aging. Organ meats, fish, brewer's yeast, and whole grains are food sources for this mineral.

Sodium, in addition to working with potassium, helps maintain the solubility of other minerals in the blood. It also helps produce hydrochloric acid in the stomach. Present in most foods, sodium is one of the few nutrients for which there is little chance of deficiency. Table salt is the principle source of sodium in the diet.

Sulfur, a component of keratin, is essential for healthy skin and hair. It also helps in tissue respiration. Eggs, meat, fish, and dairy products are good food sources for sulfur. Sulfur is necessary for a good complexion. It keeps the skin smooth and youthful and it keeps hair glossy and smooth.

Vanadium helps in the proper development of bones and teeth. It also helps iron function in blood formation. Food sources of vanadium include organ meats, seafood, and whole grains.

Zinc is important for the proper functioning of many vitamins and enzymes as well as for normal growth and development. It also assists the body's natural healing processes. Zinc is essential for healthy skin. The RDA for this mineral is fifteen milligrams. Food sources include meats, eggs, wheat germ, and brewer's yeast.

Water. **Water** is probably the most important nutrient of all. It comprises almost two-thirds of the body's weight and is a part of virtually every bodily process from digestion through elimination. Water carries the other nutrients through the body and carries the waste products from the body. It also helps regulate body temperature. The amount of water the body needs daily varies according to how much is lost due to activity and environmental conditions. Generally, however, a minimum of six to eight glasses of water should be ingested daily. Water is contained in all potable liquids and most foods.

GUIDELINES TO GOOD NUTRITION

As part of the overall skin-care regime, the esthetician may counsel the client on good nutritional habits. The U.S. Department of Health and Human Services has published a list of seven dietary guidelines that can serve as a model for this advice (*Nutrition and Your Health: Dietary Guidelines for Americans*).

1. Eat a Variety of Foods

Although most foods contain more than one of the nutrients needed for good health, no one food contains them all. The only way to insure an adequate intake of nutrients is to eat a balanced diet that contains foods from the following groups: fruits and vegetables; cereals, whole grains and grain products; dairy products (i.e. milk, cheese, and yogurt); meats, poultry, fish, and eggs; and legumes, such as beans and peas.

With a balanced diet, there will be little need for taking extra vitamins or food supplements, although some people, notably pregnant women, the elderly, and women of child-bearing age, may need additional nutrients.

Men's nutritional needs differ from those of women. Men need about 2,300 to 2,700 calories per day, while women require only 1,600 to 2,400. In addition, women need food that is richer in nutrients.

2. Maintain an Ideal Weight

Everyone has an ideal weight, at which all the body systems operate most efficiently and at which health is optimized. This weight is based on one's height, build and metabolism. Significant deviation from this ideal weight can lead to a variety of disorders (Table 8.4).

Obesity increases the risk of high blood pressure, high triglyceride levels, increased cholesterol, diabetes, and heart attack and strokes.

To have the best chance for success in the long term, a program for weight loss must be based on reducing the caloric intake and increasing the amount of exercise. Weight loss should be gradual, no more than one to two pounds per week. Unfortunately, there are no quick and easy ways to lose weight permanently. It takes an adjustment of dietary habits.

TABLE 8.4—Suggested Body Weights[1]

Range Of Acceptable Weights		
Height (feet-inches)	Men (pounds)	Women (pounds)
4'10"		92–119
4'11"		94–122
5'0"		96–125
5'1"		99–128
5'2"	112–141	102–131
5'3"	115–144	105–134
5'4"	118–148	108–138
5'5"	121–152	111–142
5'6"	124–156	114–146
5'7"	128–161	118–150
5'8"	132–166	122–154
5'9"	136–170	126–158
5'10"	140–174	130–163
5'11"	144–179	134–168
6'0"	148–184	138–173
6'1"	152–189	
6'2"	156–194	
6'3"	160–199	
6'4"	164–204	

Note: height without shoes; weight without clothes.
[1]*Nutrition and Your Health: Dietary Guidelines for Americans*, U.S. Department of Health and Human Services, February, 1980.

3. Avoid Too Much Fat, Saturated Fat and Cholesterol

High blood **cholesterol** (ko-LES-ter-ol) increases the risk of heart attack. Diets rich in fats and saturated fats tend to increase blood cholesterol levels in most people. To control the cholesterol level, it is wise to limit the intake of foods high in fats. Fat intake should be limited to about thirty percent of the calorie total.

Good low cholesterol protein sources include lean meat, fish, poultry, dry beans, and peas. Organ meats and eggs are high in cholesterol but contain many vitamins, minerals, and other important nutrients, so should be eaten in moderation.

Butter, cream, and most shortenings are high in cholesterol, so their intake should be limited. Foods should be prepared by boiling, baking, or broiling, rather than by frying.

4. Eat Foods With Adequate Starch and Fiber

The energy the body needs is supplied by both carbohydrates and fats. If fat intake is limited, the intake of carbohydrates should be increased to maintain the required caloric level.

In general, a low-fat, high-carbohydrate diet is healthiest. Carbohydrates contain about half as many calories per ounce as fats. In addition, the energy from fats is stored in the stomach and hips where it becomes body fat. The energy from carbohydrates, however, is stored in the muscles and liver.

Complex carbohydrates provide energy along with other vitamins and minerals. They also increase the amount of fiber consumed in the diet. Diets higher in fiber reduce chronic constipation and may help reduce the risk of some forms of cancer.

Whole grain breads, cereals, pasta, fruits and vegetables, beans, peas, and nuts are good sources of starch and fiber.

5. Avoid Too Much Sugar

The average American consumes 130 pounds of sugar per year, either through direct use or through sweeteners added to foods or naturally present in foods. The major dietary problem with added sugar is the risk of tooth decay. It is best to limit the use of white and brown sugar, honey, and syrups and to use moderation in the consumption of foods containing these substances.

6. Avoid Too Much Sodium

The body needs sodium to function properly. The amount needed is about 1,000 milligrams per 1,000 calories consumed. One teaspoon of salt equals three grams. The American diet, however, contains much more sodium than is needed. Most processed foods, many beverages and condiments contain large quantities of salt. In addition, many people add additional table salt to their food.

Excess sodium consumption may lead to high blood pressure, which is a significant health risk. It is best to limit the use of salt to reduce the intake of sodium. Add only small amounts of salt during cooking and don't add salt to the food at the table. Limit the intake of salty foods, especially snack foods such as potato chips and pretzels. Use other herbs and spices for flavoring.

7. If You Drink Alcohol, Do So In Moderation

Alcohol has little or no nutritional value but is high in calories. In addition, alcohol alters the rate of absorption of some nutrients, making them less useful to the body. Heavy drinkers may, therefore, suffer from vitamin and mineral deficiencies. In addition, heavy alcohol consumption may lead to diseases such as cirrhosis of the liver and to some types of cancer, and may cause birth defects. The high caloric content of alcohol makes it difficult to drink while on a diet.

Alcohol consumed in moderation, 1½ ounces of pure alcohol—that is, one or two mixed drinks, eight ounces of wine, or twenty-four ounces of beer—per day, does not seem to be harmful to adults, however. So, drink only in moderation.

REVIEW QUESTIONS

1. Why is nutrition important to the skin?
2. What is the result of poor nutrition on the skin?
3. What are the three points of the nutritional triad?
4. Where does good nutrition start?
5. Why is proper elimination vital to the skin?
6. What are the two phases of metabolism?
7. How is the fuel value of a nutrient expressed?
8. What kind of nutrient supplies most energy needs?
9. What are the main carbohydrates?
10. What kind of nutrient builds tissues?
11. What are essential amino acids?
12. What is the difference between complete and incomplete protein?
13. What are vitamins?
14. What are the two types of vitamins?
15. Why is vitamin A important to the skin?
16. Why is vitamin C important to skin?
17. How is vitamin D synthesized in the body?
18. Why are minerals important?
19. Can minerals be synthesized in the body?
20. Which minerals are most important to life?
21. Which mineral is contained in the body in the largest amount?
22. Why is copper important to the skin?
23. Why is sulfur important to the skin?
24. Why is water an important nutrient?
25. What are the seven guidelines to good nutrition?

9 Massage Theory

OBJECTIVES *After completing this chapter, you should be able to:*

❶ Describe various types of massage and understand the energy flows in the body.

❷ Discuss the physical and psychological benefits of massage.

❸ Describe the various physical manipulations used in massage.

❹ Locate and identify the pressure points of most importance to the esthetician.

❺ Describe a typical facial massage.

INTRODUCTION

The massage may not be the most important step in the facial treatment, but it probably will be the step the client remembers most. Properly done, the massage relaxes the client, stimulates and soothes the skin, and prepares both the client and the skin for the steps to come. It is the most emotional part of the facial and it also forges the links of trust between client and esthetician.

Touch works wonders. From earliest childhood, we've known the value of touch and gentle rubbing to ease the hurt of those everyday bumps and scrapes. The phenomenon of touch is nothing new. Massage, in one form or another, was practiced by the ancient Egyptians, Greeks, and Romans. The use of massage was one of **Hippocrates'** precepts for therapy. **Galen,** the father of anatomy, taught the values of massage, as well.

In the west, massage lost its reputation as a therapy from the time of the fall of Rome through the Dark Ages, as things of the flesh were made subservient to the spiritual. Massage therapy emerged from the Dark Ages gradually through the Renaissance. And in the sixteenth century, the French physician **Ambroise Pare** advocated its use and developed techniques that were adopted by his peers. Early in the nineteenth century, **Henry Peter Ling** developed his technique of Swedish massage, which remains the most widely utilized form of massage in use today.

In the east, however, massage never lost its value as a theraputic tool. Most of the Oriental and Arabic cultures have a tradition of sophisticated massage techniques.

Massage has once more come into its own in western civilization as new techniques, many borrowed from the east, have been developed and are becoming more and more widely practiced.

TYPES OF MASSAGE

There are many types of massage currently being practiced. Some systems are based on body structure; that is, on the manipulation of muscle tissue, bones and connective tissue, to achieve the theraputic goal. Others are based on energy, on the manipulation of the life force of the body to achieve the theraputic goal. Both use physical manipulation of one kind or another. A number of these massage techniques are of considerable interest to the esthetician.

- **Swedish massage** is a structure-based system in which deep muscle tissues are manipulated by a series of kneading, slapping, or rubbing strokes. This type of massage affects both deep and superficial muscles and the joints, and has some effect on the internal organs and nerves. It is used to stimulate circulation, improve muscle tone, and relieve soreness.

- **Shiatsu** (she-AT-su) is an energy-based system of massage that involves pressure on accupressure points along the body's energy meridians, combined with stretching of the spine and limbs. Pressure is applied with the fingers, hands, feet, elbows, and knees, depending on the part of the body being worked on.

  The underlying philosophy of shiatsu is that the vital life force of the body, called **ki** (KEE), flows along twelve **meridians** (mer-ID-ee-enz), each of which is associated with an organ, and which transmits that organ's energy. In addition to the twelve organ meridians, there are two others, the **governor vessel**, which extends along the centerline of the back, and the **conception vessel**, which extends along the centerline of the front. Pressure is applied to specific points, or **tsubos** (SUE-bow), along the meridians. There are 365 major tsubos in the body.

- **Accupressure** is similar to shiatsu and follows the same principles. The only difference between the two is that accupressure relies solely on pressure point manipulation.

9.1—Reflexology points

- **Reflexology** is an energy-based system of theraputic massage that manipulates areas on the hands and the soles of the feet to achieve balance in the inner organs. The principle behind reflexology is that reflex points in the hands and feet correspond to various organs. Manipulation of these reflex points has a beneficial effect on those particular organs (Fig. 9.1).
- **Aromatherapy massage** is a structure-based system that utilizes essential oils along with the body manipulation. During the manipulations, the essential oil penetrates and affects the organ underlying the point of manipulation.

- **Lymphatic drainage massage** is a structure-based system that utilizes gentle strokes and pressure along the lymphatic channels that lie just under the skin. The purpose of lymphatic drainage is to speed the passage of toxic waste materials through the lymphatic system to rid the body of toxins more rapidly.

The esthetician borrows elements from all of these massage techniques to deliver the most effective and beneficial massage to his or her client. Thus, the massage utilized by the esthetician will be part Swedish, part accupressure, part shiatsu, part aromatherapy, part lymphatic drainage. Sometimes, one technique will be more appropriate than another. The techniques will vary from client to client. An effective massage utilizes both body manipulation and energy flow manipulation.

THE BENEFITS OF MASSAGE

Regardless of type, massage has many physical and psychological benefits. Physically, almost every system of the body is affected. Psychologically, it brings relaxation and a tremendous sense of well-being to the client. The massage gives that same sense of well-being to the esthetician, as well.

Ideally, the massage is just as rewarding for both parties. Massage helps the body cope with the stresses of the environment by relieving the tensions of everyday life. And by relieving those tensions, it lets the body utilize its natural energy more productively.

Massage helps the body feed. It improves the circulation of the blood throughout the body. It lets blood return to the heart more easily, thus reducing the effort the heart has to exert. It increases the supply of blood to the muscles. By improving blood flow, massage increases the amount of nutrients and oxygen delivered to the cells, tissues, muscles, bones, and organs.

Massage helps cleanse the body. It helps remove waste products from the body. It increases the efficiency of the liver. It increases lymphatic flow. It helps cleanse the blood. And it helps restore normal breathing patterns.

Massage soothes the body. It sedates the nervous system. It releases **endorphins** (en-DOR-fins), the natural pain-killers of the body. It reduces muscular tension. It relieves fatigue by eliminating lactic acid that builds up in muscles after exertion. It relaxes muscle spasms and breaks down adhesions in the tissues. Massage also lowers blood pressure.

Massage tones the body. Although it can't replace exercise, massage can restore tone to flaccid muscles. It increases the flexibility of joints and increases muscle size. It does not increase muscle strength, however.

Massage revitalizes the body. It balances the nervous system and brings the energy flow of the body into balance. It increases the level of energy and helps the body heal itself. Once the body is healed, massage lets it stay well. It maintains a level of health and vitality in the body.

Massage beautifies the body. It improves the texture and appearance of the skin. It softens the skin. It loosens and helps remove dead surface cells. By toning the facial muscles, it helps reduce wrinkles and prevent sagging. By improving circulation, it brings color to the face.

Massage helps recontour the body. It helps eliminate the fat deposits sometimes known as **cellulite** (SEL-yu-lite). It also helps maintain correct posture and balance. Because a high level of health and vitality are being maintained, all systems are in balance and clients feel good about themselves. This good feeling promotes the body's natural beauty.

There is a link between the physical aspects of massage and the psychological aspects. Emotions are retained in the cells, just as tensions are retained in the muscles. Emotions can be massaged away just as tensions are. Relaxation is a psychological state of mind as well as a physical state of body. In addition, the communicative aspects of touch, the physical contact between two people, adds its own psychological impact to the massage experience. Massage reduces mental fatigue as well as muscle fatigue.

BODY ENERGY

Many massage techniques, especially those with roots in eastern civilization, rely on the manipulation and balancing of the body energy. This energy, which the Japanese call **ki,** is the body's vital force and constantly circulates through its own vessels, called **meridians** (mer-IH-dee-ans). Ki is created by the interplay between two opposite yet complementary forces known in eastern philosophy as **yin** and **yang.** Yin is feminine, passive, dark, moist, soft, and cool. Yang is masculine, active, light, dry, hard, and hot. Yin is the moon; yang is the sun (Fig. 9.2).

This vital energy, or ki, has five different aspects, each associated with one of the **Five Agents**—fire, earth, metal, water, or wood— which are the elements from which, according to eastern philosophy, all material things are made. Humans are a blend of all five elements, each of which controls one solid organ and one hollow organ. The solid organs—the heart, spleen, lungs, kidneys, and liver—are yin. The hollow organs—the small intestine, stomach, large intestine, bladder, and gallbladder—are yang.

According to the **sheng cycle,** the energy flows in a clockwise direction from fire to earth to metal to water to wood and back to fire in a never-ending cycle of creation. Fire burns wood to produce ashes. Ashes become earth. Earth becomes metal. Metal comes from

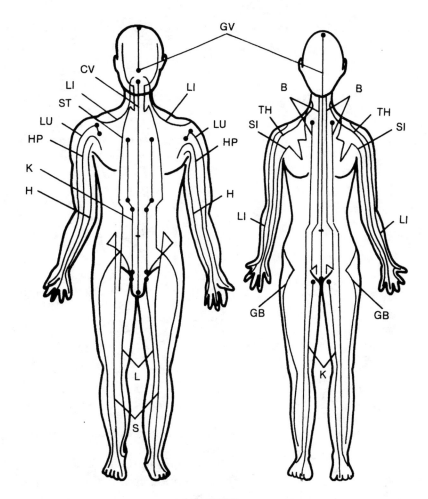

9.2—Meridians

mud, which is a mixture of earth and water. Water makes trees and plants grow to produce wood, which provides fuel for fire.

By the **ki cycle**, the energy is counterbalanced in a star-shaped pattern from fire to metal to wood to earth to water to fire in a never-ending cycle of control. Fire melts metal. Metal cuts wood. Wood tills earth. Earth absorbs water. Water douses fire (Fig. 9.3).

Except for fire, which controls two pairs of meridians, each of the five elements controls a pair of meridians associated with a pair of organs, one solid, or yin; one hollow, or yang. Thus, there are twelve organ meridians. The yin meridians, in which the energy flows upward, are the heart protector and the heart (fire), the spleen (earth), the lungs (metal), the kidneys (water), and the liver (wood).

The yang meridians, in which the energy flows downward, are the triple heater and the small intestine (fire), the stomach (earth),

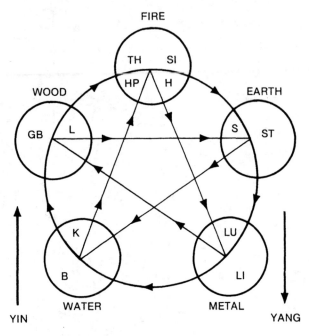

FIRE

TH   SI
HP / H

WOOD

EARTH

GB   L

S   ST

K

LU

B

LI

YIN

WATER

METAL

YANG

9.3—Sheng and ki cycles

the large intestine (metal), the bladder (water), and the gallbladder (wood).

In addition to the twelve organ meridians, there are two others. The conception vessel transmits energy up the centerline of the front of the body and is yin. The governor vessel transmits energy downward along the centerline of the back of the body and is yang.

In Oriental medicine, when yin and yang are in balance and energy flows along the meridians unobstructed, the body is healthy. When the two factors are out of balance, however, because of obstructions along the meridians, illness results. An excess of yin energy causes damp, cool diseases, with symptoms of fatigue, poor circulation, and chilliness. An excess of yang energy causes dry, hot diseases, with symptoms of nervousness, fever, and insomnia. Pressure on the tsubos, points along the meridians that amplify the energy, unblocks the meridian, letting the energy flow freely and balancing yin and yang to restore health.

Western science cannot verify the existence of this vital life force. It can't be seen or measured. The effectiveness of shiatsu, accupressure and accupuncture techniques, however, have been amply demonstrated, whatever the principle involved. Science does know that all matter, including human beings, consists of atoms. These atoms are in constant motion. They vibrate and radiate energy. Each body, therefore, is surrounded by an electromagnetic field.

Just as the body is surrounded by an electromagnetic field generated by the material body, it is surrounded by an emotional field generated by the psyche. This emotional field manifests itself as an invisible **aura,** which has three planes. The **etheric plane** is closest to the body. It extends outward about an inch and matches the electromagnetic field. This plane transmits the ki. The **astral plane** extends outward about twelve inches and transmits moods and emotions. The **mental plane** extends outward to several feet. Strong negative emotions cause eddies in the aura. These eddies disrupt the smooth flow of energy and manifest themselves as physical disease.

The energy field is important to the quality of the massage. During the massage, the energy field of the client and the esthetician mesh. The more the vibrations of both are in tune, the more satisfying the experience will be for both. If the esthetician feels ill or is in a bad mood, this will be transmitted to the client, and the quality of the massage will suffer accordingly.

PHYSICAL MANIPULATIONS

The physical basis of massage is manipulation of both superficial and deep muscle tissue delivered to the client in a series of rhythmic strokes, stretching movements and the application of pressure at selected points on the body.

Effleurage

Effleurage (ef-LOO-rahzh), or **stroking,** is the most basic and the most utilized movement in the massage. The movements are done with only light to moderate pressure. Work over an area of the body begins with gentle stroking, which gradually becomes more firm and finishes up as gentle stroking again. **Feathering,** the lightest touch, is used to break contact with the body, to avoid the unpleasantness of a sudden loss of touch between the client and the esthetician.

Stroking movements induce relaxation and sedate the nervous system. All stroking movements are done slowly and rhythmically. The wrists are loose and flexible and the hands are relaxed. The movements are controlled by the arm and upper body muscles. Gentle stroking is done by gliding the hands over the body in broad, long movements. Friction is kept to a minimum.

Feathering requires an extremely light touch, with the hands just lightly brushing the body. Stroking, regardless of the amount of pressure used, is done in one direction only. The movement does not go back and forth over an area, but moves around it in broad circles.

Stroking movements should be repeated a minimum of three times over any given area.

Friction   **Friction** utilizes heavier pressure than stroking. The hands apply light pressure before starting to move, then they move back and forth over the area being worked on, with pressure gradually building from light to heavy. Friction increases circulation and promotes warmth in the deeper muscle tissues. These movements are soothing.

As with stroking movements, friction movements should be controlled by the arm and upper body muscles with the wrists and hands relaxed and flexible. These movements should be repeated a minimum of three times over an area.

Petrissage   **Petrissage** (PE-tre-sahzh) movements involve kneading, wringing, pulling, and rocking motions and are used to massage the deeper muscle masses of the limbs and fleshy areas of the body. These maneuvers relax deep muscle tissue while stimulating the skin. They also increase circulation and promote waste removal from the tissues and firm and tone weak muscles. Petrissage is very good for oil-dry skin, since it stimulates sebum production. All of the variations of petrissage are accomplished with a rhythmic hand-to-hand alternation of pressure and release.

In **kneading,** the hand grasps a section of muscle and pulls upward and squeezes at the same time. Pressure is released with that hand as the other hand simultaneously grasps another section of muscle, pulls upward and squeezes. This alternating grasping, squeezing, and releasing movement is continued along the bone, moving up the body. The muscle mass should not be twisted during kneading. Contact with the body should not be lost between strokes. The motion is the same as used when kneading dough.

On the fleshy areas of the body, the palms and fingers are used for deep kneading. On bony areas or on the face, the flesh is grasped between the thumb and middle finger as only superficial kneading is done.

Wringing is used mostly on the limbs. The hands are placed on opposite sides of the limb and moved toward each other in slow, twisting movements. The movement is started at the end of the limb and the hands are moved up toward the trunk. The motion is similar to that used in wringing out a wet towel. Care must be taken to move the muscle tissue without sliding the hands across the skin and creating friction.

Pulling is used on the fleshy areas and involves a back and forth rolling movement of the deep muscle tissues over the supporting bone. The movement is done more rapidly than in the other petrissage movements. The hands should be moved along the area in an overlapping manner.

Rocking is a gentle, soothing technique in which the palm and fingers of one hand are placed over the muscle and gently rocked back and forth with a minimum of pressure. The free hand should be placed on the joint directly above the muscle being rocked. Care should be taken not to slide the hand over the muscle.

Tapotement

Tapotement (tah-POT-ment) movements involve various forms of percussion, including hacking, clapping, pummelling, tapping, and pinching. Tapotement movements are stimulating to the body. They tone muscles and the skin and improve circulation. Hacking, cupping, and pummelling are used only on the fleshy areas of the body and are never used on the face. **Hacking** uses the edges of the little fingers and the hands; **clapping** uses the cupped palms; **pummelling** uses the fleshy sides of the clenched fists. The hands and wrists are relaxed. The hands are bounced rapidly in alternating strokes up and down the muscle areas being worked on. The pressure should be heavy enough to stimulate the muscles, but not so heavy that they cause pain.

Tapping is done by rapidly alternating finger strokes over the area being massaged, much like playing a piano. Only the pads of the fingertips are used. This movement is appropriate for use on the face and is stimulating to the skin.

In **pinching,** small bunches of skin and muscle tissue are grasped between the thumb and middle finger, picked up and quickly released. This is also done rapidly. Pinching is suitable for use on the face, although care should be taken not to stretch the skin or cause bruising.

Vibration

Vibration is a rapid shaking movement of muscle tissue and can be either soothing or stimulating. It can be used to stimulate organs directly below the muscle tissue and is suitable for use on the face to stimulate the more fleshy areas. Vibratory motion is accomplished by rapidly contracting and relaxing the muscles of the forearm. For soothing vibrations, the entire relaxed hand is placed on the muscle tissue and vibrated. For stimulating vibrations, only the fingertips are used. This gives motion much like a mechanical vibrator.

Stretching Maneuvers

Gentle stretching maneuvers relieve tightness, improve flexibility in the joints and are soothing and relaxing. The joint should be moved through its full range of motion, first in one direction, then in the other. The joint should be stretched through its full range, but care must be taken not to force the movement. The client should relax while the esthetician does all the work. The esthetician will be mostly concerned with stretching maneuvers of the neck, wrists, and ankles.

Pressure Application

Finger pressure is applied to pressure points, or tsubos, along the meridians to remove energy blockages and to sensitive areas in the muscles to relieve tightness. The amount of pressure applied varies from light to heavy, although it should never be heavy enough to cause pain. The fingers should remain relaxed while applying pressure, with the force coming from the weight of the body.

The pressure may be applied rhythmically by gradually increasing and decreasing the pressure as the fingers remain still. Or it may be applied while moving the fingers in a circular or zig-zag motion over the area, moving the underlying tissues but not sliding over the skin.

MAJOR PRESSURE POINTS

Although there are many pressure points in the body, the esthetician will be concerned with relatively few of these. Most of the pressure points the esthetician will manipulate will be on the head and face, although there are a few points of importance on the hands and legs, as well. All of the points lie along a meridian. Controlled pressure to these points relieves tension, eases fatigue, and removes energy blockages, all of which help clear the skin and improve its functioning (Fig. 9.4).

Bladder Meridian

- B-1 At the inside corner of the eye above the tear duct. Relieves tired eyes.
- B-2 At the inner end of the eyebrow. Relieves bloodshot eyes.
- B-4 At the hairline directly above the inside corner of the eye. Relieves headache and clears sinuses.
- B-10 At the junction of the trapezius muscle with the skull. Relieves headache and eyestrain.

Conception Vessel

- CV-24 In the center of the chin below the lower lip. Helps smooth wrinkles below the lips.

Gallbladder Meridian

- GB-1 At the outside corner of the eye. Helps remove wrinkles around the eyes.
- GB-11 Just behind the flap of the ear. Helps relieve dizziness.
- GB-21 At the top of the shoulder at the base of the neck. Relieves tension in the shoulders.

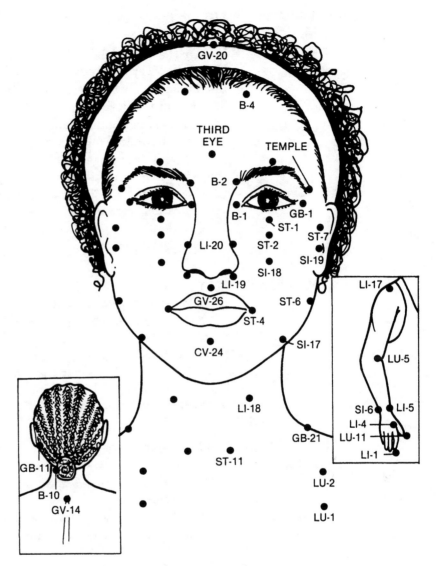

9.4—Major pressure points

Governor Vessel
- GV-14 At the base of the neck on the back. Helps relieve tension in the neck and helps relieve migraine headache. Helps clear blemishes.

- GV-20 On the centerline of the head at the top of the ears. Helps relieve heaviness in the head and relieves headache.
- GV-26 In the hollow between the upper lip and the base of the nose. Helps smooth wrinkles around the nose and lips.

Large Intestine Meridian

- LI-1 On the index finger at the base of the nail. Helps remove blemishes.
- LI-4 On the back of the web between the thumb and index finger. Helps relieve eye fatigue and headache. Helps remove blemishes.
- LI-5 In the hollow area between the two tendons at the base of the thumb. Helps relieve pain in the wrist.
- LI-17 At the apex of the triangle formed by the trapezius and the sternocleidomastoid muscle. Helps improve circulation.
- LI-18 About four finger widths to the side of the hyoid bone. Helps improve respiration.
- LI-19 In the depression between the wings of the nose and the upper lip. Helps remove wrinkles around the nose and lips.
- LI-20 At the sides of the wings of the nose just as they start to flare. Helps open sinuses.

Lung Meridian

- LU-1 About two inches below the outer edges of the clavicles. Helps relieve congestion in the chest.
- LU-2 Just below the clavicles. Helps relieve tension in the shoulders.
- LU-5 Just below the crook of the elbow on the inside of the arm. Helps improve circulation in the arm.
- LU-11 At the base of the thumb nail. Helps relieve fatigue in the throat and vocal cords.

Small Intestine Meridian

- SI-6 In the groove of the bone at the outside of the wrist. Helps relieve facial blemishes and boils.
- SI-17 At the front of the midpoint of the sternocleidomastoid muscle. Helps relieve sore throat.
- SI-18 In the hollow below the cheekbone. Helps remove wrinkles around the cheeks. Helps tone cheek muscles to prevent sagging. Helps ease facial swelling.
- SI-19 Just at the front of the tragus. Helps relieve headache and dizziness.

Stomach Meridian

- ST-1 Below the center of the eye in the hollow of the orbicular bone. Helps remove bags beneath the eyes.
- ST-2 One finger width below ST-1. Helps remove bags beneath the eyes and helps relieve eye fatigue. Helps clear blemishes.
- ST-4 One finger width to the side of the corner of the mouth. Helps remove wrinkles around the nose and lips.
- ST-6 At the pivot point of the jaw. Helps relieve tension in the lower jaw.

- ST-7 In front of the ear at the masseter muscle. Helps tone cheek muscles to avoid sagging cheeks.
- ST-11 At the top of the sternum at the tip of the clavicle. Helps relieve tension in the neck.

In addition to these meridian points, there are a number of other pressure points of importance to the esthetician. These are:

The "third eye," the point between the eyes just at the line of the eyebrows. Helps relieve tension and headache. Helps clear sinuses. Improves circulation and restores color to the complexion.

The temples, about two finger widths from the corners of the eyes and slightly above. Helps relieve headache.

A number of points exist around the perimeter of the eyesockets on the bony protuberances.

FACIAL MASSAGE DEMONSTRATION

Massage has its roots in both science and art. As a science, it relies on knowledge of physiology and manipulation of energy fields. As an art, it relies on empathy, sensitivity, and an almost intuitive feel for the movements. Because of this, there is no one right way to give a good massage. There are almost as many techniques as there are practitioners. What is important is not a mechanical adherance to rote procedures, but working in a logical sequence and working rhythmically.

The esthetician must teach clients how to react to the massage. It is necessary to tell clients what they should do—or not do—during the massage. The clients should be receptive. They should relax and give in to the esthetician's movements. They should concentrate on the massage and the sensations it produces and should try to forget worries. If the client fully relaxes, he or she may fall asleep during the massage. The esthetician should take this as a compliment.

The esthetician must be relaxed as well, concentrating on the massage, paying attention to the client's needs. The esthetician's mood or state of mind will transmit itself to the client. If the esthetician is angry or upset, or is not confident, the client will sense the mood, and the massage will not have its full pleasurable and beneficial effect.

The esthetician should tell the client what will be done before the treatment and should encourage questions. Once the massage has begun, however, talking should be discouraged. Everything should be ready once the massage is started, so the esthetician does not have to fumble around for materials, such as essential oils or massage creams.

The mood should be relaxed. Soothing music or special relaxation tapes should be played. During an aromatherapy massage, the scent from the essential oils will contribute to the mood. The room should be warm.

Before starting, the esthetician's hands should be clean. Fingernails should be short and all jewelry should be removed. The esthetician should pause for a moment, closing eyes, breathing deeply, and aligning the two auras by holding his or her hands over the client.

A small amount of massage cream should be warmed in the hands and gently applied to the client's face, smoothly and evenly. Initial contact with the face should be made firmly, but with light pressure. Pressure should be increased gradually. Once contact with the skin has been made, it should not be broken unnecessarily. If contact must be broken, the hands should be removed slowly, with pressure gradually diminishing until it is feather-light.

Massage should not be given if the skin is infected or there is skin disease. If the client has had cosmetic surgery within a year, the surgeon should be consulted and permission obtained before attempting the massage. Massage should be given carefully and sparingly if the client has high blood pressure, a heart condition, or is pregnant. Stimulating maneuvers should not be used under these conditions.

The following is an example of a basic facial massage. It is to be studied only as a guide. All of the movements listed are not necessarily used in any one given massage. It does illustrate a logical sequence of movements and utilizes virtually every movement discussed in this chapter. Movements, especially those in which moderate pressure is used, should be made in an upward direction to avoid pulling down the skin and promoting sagging. Pressure is usually applied with the middle, ring, and little fingers. The index fingers and thumbs are used only occasionally. The total massage should take approximately twenty minutes.

Phase 1—Relaxation

This phase utilizes stroking and friction movements along with pressure and stretching.

Forehead.

1. Starting at the left temple, stroke across the forehead with three fingers of each hand alternately, until reaching the right temple. One hand should be touching the forehead as the other is withdrawn, to maintain constant contact. Repeat this step four times, using light pressure (Fig. 9.5).
2. Starting at the left temple, stroke across the forehead with the middle fingers in a zig-zag motion until reaching the right tem-

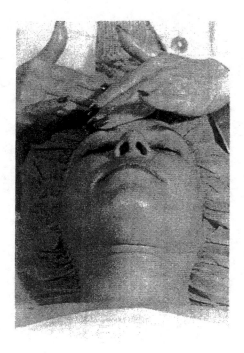

9.5—Massage step 1

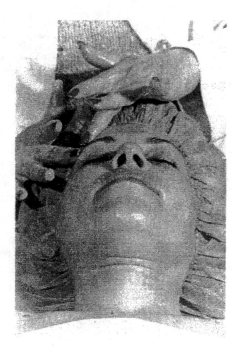

9.6—Massage step 2

ple. Repeat this step four times, using somewhat heavier pressure than in step 1 (Fig. 9.6).

3. Hold the skin on the forehead tight with the thumb and middle finger of one hand. Using the edge of the other middle finger, iron out the horizontal wrinkles in the forehead. Repeat four times. Repeat the motion using zig-zag strokes four times, then repeat four times using circular strokes. Use moderate pressure (Fig. 9.7).

4. Hold the skin between the eyebrows at the bridge of the nose tight with the forefinger and middle finger of one hand. Using an upward stroke, iron out the vertical wrinkles at the bridge of the nose. Repeat four times. Repeat the motion using zig-zag strokes four times and using circular strokes four times. Use moderate pressure (Fig. 9.8).

5. Starting at the left temple, stroke across the forehead with circular motions using two fingers. Repeat four times. Use moderate pressure (Fig. 9.9).

6. Apply moderate pressure to each temple with the middle fingers. Hold the pressure for 10 to 15 seconds (Fig. 9.10).

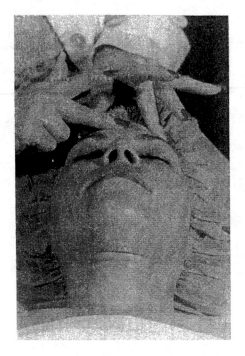

9.7—Massage step 3

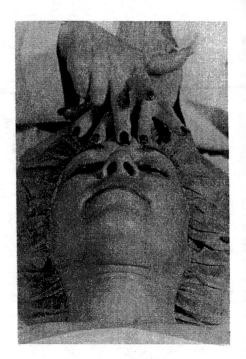

9.8—Massage step 4

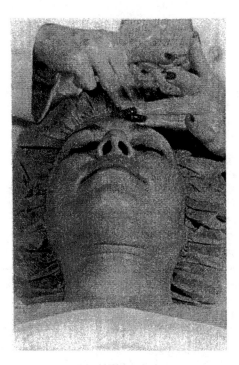

9.9—Massage step 5

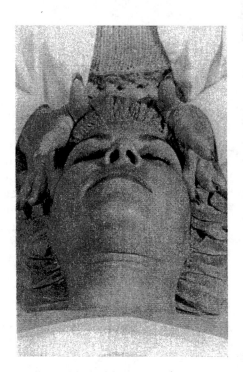

9.10—Massage step 6

Eyes.

7. Maintain pressure on the left temple with the left middle finger. With the right middle finger, apply moderate pressure in a circular motion at the outside corner of the right eye (Point GB-1). Do four circles. Repeat four times using a zig-zag motion (Fig. 9.11).
8. Maintaining pressure on the left temple as above, stroke underneath the right eyebrow with the right middle finger from inside to outside. In the same motion, apply moderate pressure at four pressure points underneath the eye, from outside to inside. Repeat three times (Fig. 9.12).
9. Maintain pressure on the right temple with the right middle finger and repeat steps 7 and 8 on the left eye.
10. Repeat steps 7 and 8 on both eyes simultaneously.
11. Lightly tap around the eyes and the forehead with the fingertips in a piano-like motion (Fig. 9.13).

Nose.

12. Intertwine the fingers loosely together and place the hands under the chin. Using the thumbs, circle the nose and bring off sharply. Repeat three times using moderate pressure (Fig. 9.14).

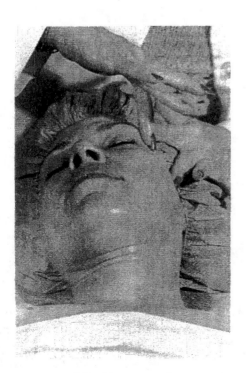

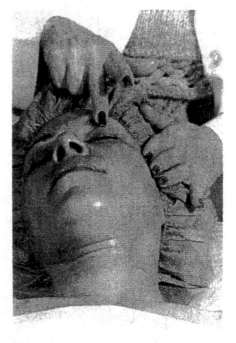

9.11—Massage step 7   **9.12**—Massage step 8

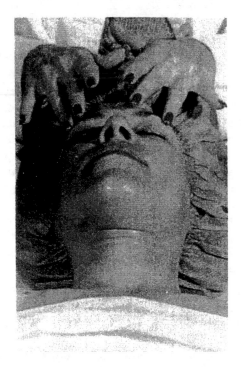 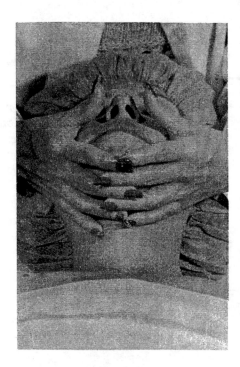

9.13—Massage step 11   **9.14**—Massage step 12

13. Using the index and middle finger of each hand, alternately scissor off the nose wings from the base of the nose to the bridge of the nose. Repeat twelve times using moderate pressure (Fig. 9.15).
14. Using the middle fingers, circle up the sides of the nose, slide up to the forehead and down to the temples. Maintain pressure at the temples for five seconds. Repeat four times (Fig. 9.16).

Ears.

15. Using the thumbs and forefingers, lightly massage the ear lobes and move up the fleshy part of the ear. Repeat four times (Fig. 9.17).

Mouth.

16. Using the index and middle fingers of each hand, alternately scissor horizontally across the mouth and chin. Use moderate pressure and repeat six times with each hand (Fig. 9.18).
17. Using the middle and ring fingers of each hand, apply moderate pressure to the chin using circular motions. Move up the jaw line

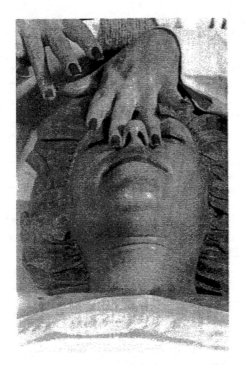

9.15—Massage step 13

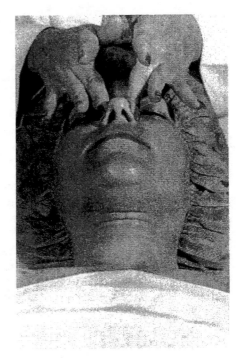

9.16—Massage step 14

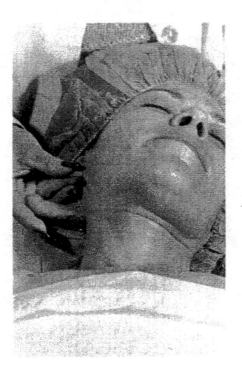

9.17—Massage step 15

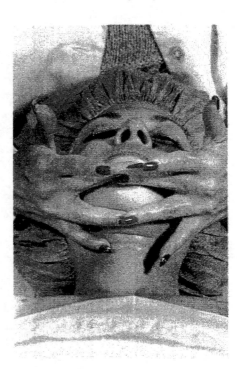

9.18—Massage step 16

to the base of the ear, continuing in small circles. Repeat four times (Fig. 9.19).

18. Make small circles upward from the chin to the sides of the mouth. Use moderate pressure and repeat four times (Fig. 9.20).

19. Using the middle fingers, slide across the top of the mouth and up from the chin to the corners of the mouth. Use moderate pressure. Do only once (Fig. 9.21).

20. Repeat steps 17, 18, and 19 three more times.

Neck, Chest, Upper Arms and Shoulders.

21. Using the hands in a swimming motion, with light pressure, move down the neck from the jaw to the clavicle four times on each side. On reaching the clavicle, slide the hands up to the top of the neck and apply moderate pressure at the point behind the ears (Point GB-11). Maintain pressure for five seconds (Fig. 9.22).

22. Using the hands, move across the upper chest from the sternum to the shoulders in a swimming motion. Use moderate pressure and repeat four times (Fig. 9.23).

23. Using the knuckles, move across the upper chest from the sternum to the clavicles in a swimming motion. Use light pressure to avoid hurting the client, but not so light the client is tickled. Repeat four times (Fig. 9.24).

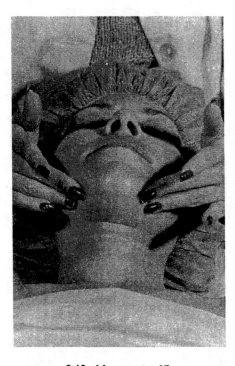 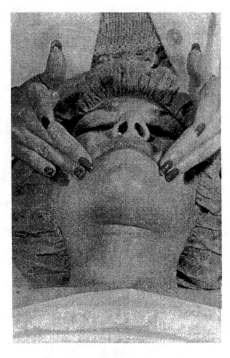

9.19—Massage step 17   9.20—Massage step 18

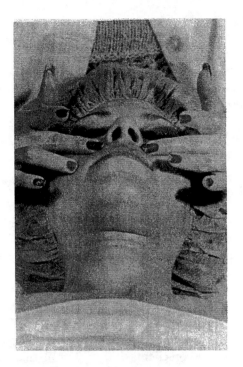

9.21—Massage step 19

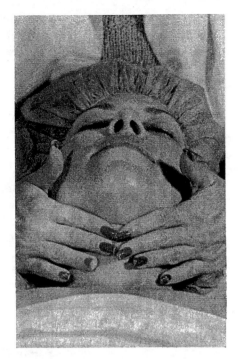

9.22—Massage step 21

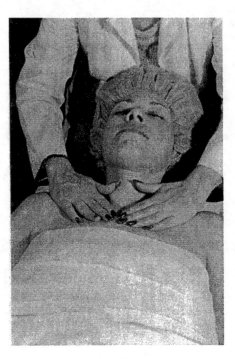

9.23—Massage step 22

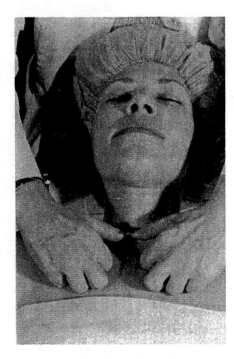

9.24—Massage step 23

24. Moving from the center of the cleavage to the clavicles, swim up and across the chest with the hands. Stop at the clavicles and apply moderate pressure to the point at the hollow of the clavicles (Point LU-2). Repeat four times (Fig. 9.25).
25. Without breaking contact, move the hands from the clavicles to the shoulders. With moderate pressure, massage the shoulders and upper arms with broad circular strokes. Repeat four times (Fig. 9.26).

Back.

26. Stand up for better leverage. Swim in and out from the shoulders to the center of the back in broad circular motions, using moderate pressure. Repeat four times (Fig. 9.27).
27. Using the fingers, make circles up the back of the neck with moderate pressure. Join the middle fingers and pull the back of the neck up with moderate stretching. Slide the hands up to the occipital area and apply moderate pressure to the point at the occipital nerve. Repeat four times (Fig. 9.28).

Phase 2—Stimulation   This phase utilizes slapping movements. This phase may be modified or eliminated on clients with oily or blemished skin.

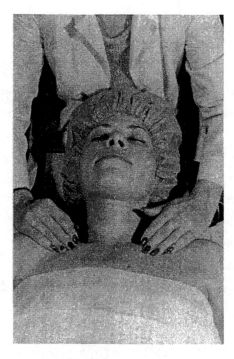

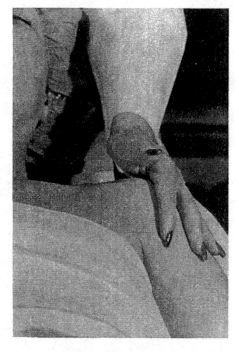

9.25—Massage step 24   **9.26**—Massage step 25

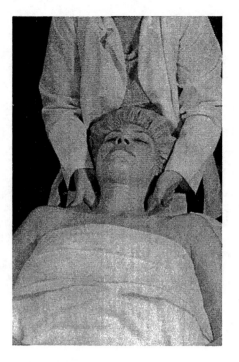 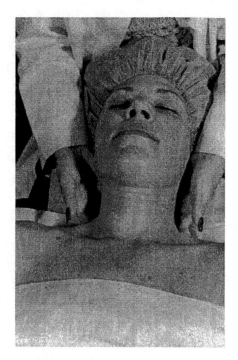

9.27—Massage step 26   **9.28**—Massage step 27

28. Using the hands alternately, slap the chin with moderate force. Repeat twelve times with each hand (Fig. 9.29).
29. Using the same hand motions and pressure, slap upward from the chin to the ear under the jawbone. Repeat twelve times with each hand (Fig. 9.30).
30. Turn the client's head to the right. Using the middle and ring fingers of each hand, slap upward in a rolling, lifting motion with firm force on the cheek near the left ear. Repeat twelve times (Fig. 9.31).
31. Using the same motion and force, slap the cheek. Use three fingers for this step. Repeat twenty-four times.
32. Using the same motion, but with slightly less force, slap the corner of the mouth. Use only the middle finger. Repeat twelve times.
33. Reverse the procedure of steps 30, 31, and 32, working from the corner of the mouth to the corner of the ear.
34. Turn the client's head to the left. Repeat steps 30 through 33 on the right side of the face.
35. Turn the client's head back to center. Using the middle and ring fingers of each hand, alternately slide the fingers from the center of the forehead to the temples. Repeat four times, decreasing the pressure each time until the last is only a feathering touch (Fig. 9.32 and Fig. 9.33).

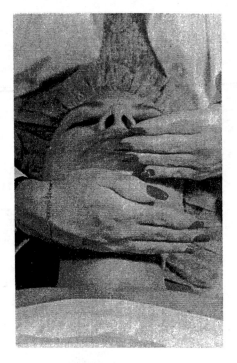

9.29—Massage step 28

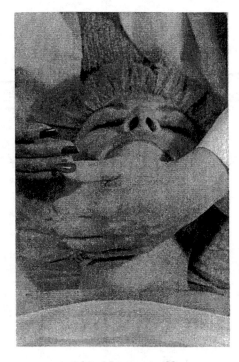

9.30—Massage step 29

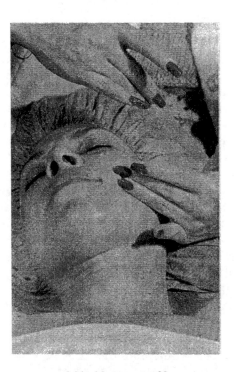

9.31—Massage step 30

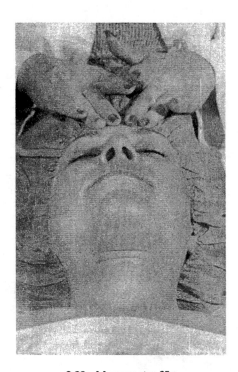

9.32—Massage step 35a

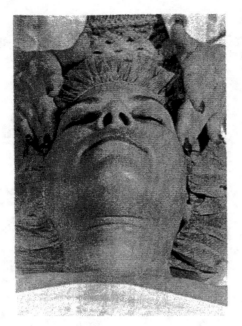 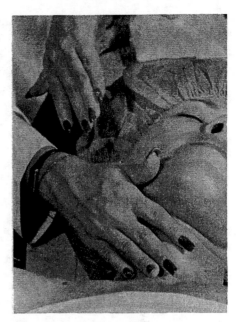

9.33—Massage step 35b   **9.34**—Massage step 36

Phase 3—Molding   This phase utilizes deep friction, pinching, vibration and stroking.

36. Turn the client's head to the right. Using both hands, slowly make long strokes with moderate pressure from the base of the neck all the way up to the cheek. Repeat four times (Fig. 9.34).

37. Turn the client's head to the left and repeat step 36 on the right side of the face.

38. With moderate pressure, slowly slide the hands from the chin to the temples. Pause at the temples for five seconds. Repeat four times (Fig. 9.35).

39. Using two fingers with moderate pressure, slowly slide the hands from the chin, around the corners of the mouth, up to the sides of the nose and across the cheekbones to the temples. Press at the temples for five seconds. Repeat four times.

40. Using the thumbs and middle fingers, using a rapid pinching motion, follow the same path used in step 39. Repeat four times (Fig. 9.36).

41. Using the fingertips, rapidly vibrate up the same path as used in step 39. Repeat four times.

42. Rotate the knuckles of both hands in an inward circular motion over the cheeks. Lift and press under the cheekbones for five seconds. Use moderate pressure and repeat four times (Fig. 9.37).

43. Using the thumbs and middle fingers, make big pinching motions at the jawbone and the sides of the neck. Use moderate pressure and repeat four times (Fig. 9.38).

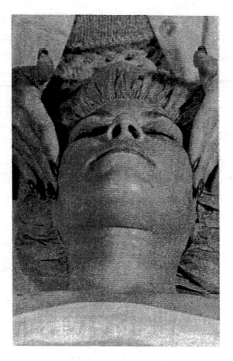

9.35—Massage step 38

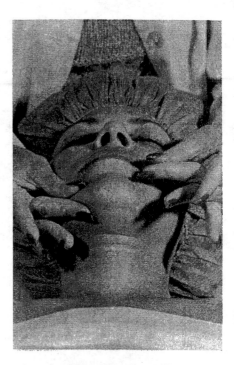

9.36—Massage step 40

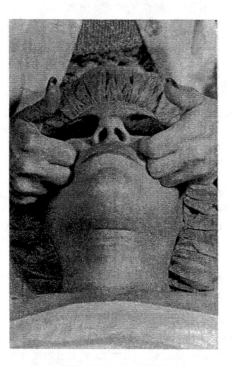

9.37—Massage step 42

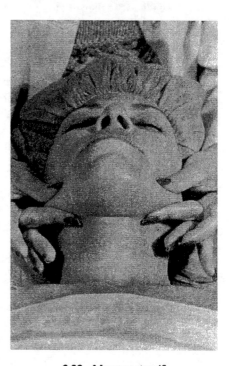

9.38—Massage step 43

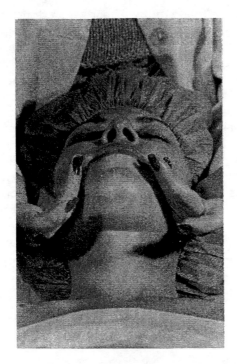

9.39—Massage step 44

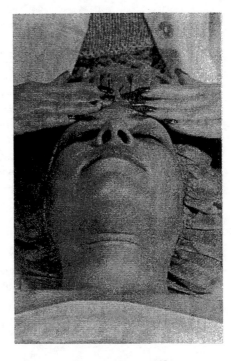

9.40—Massage step 45a

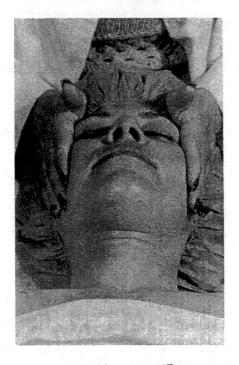

9.41—Massage step 45b

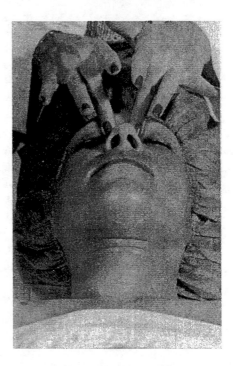

9.42—Massage step 46

44. With the fingers fully extended, start at the index fingers and fan-roll across the cheeks to the little fingers. This is a rapid rotary motion in which each finger touches the cheek in turn. Use light force. Repeat twelve times (Fig. 9.39).

45. Place the palms on the forehead. Lightly caress the forehead and slide down to the temples. Apply moderate pressure to the temples. Repeat four times, decreasing the pressure each time. The last time should have feather-light pressure (Fig. 9.40 and Fig. 9.41).

46. Using the index fingers, press the point at the inner corners of the eyes (Point B-1). Hold for five seconds. Switch to apply pressure at the temples with the middle fingers. Hold for five seconds. Repeat eight times, decreasing pressure each time (Fig. 9.42).

REVIEW QUESTIONS

1. What does massage do?
2. Why is massage important to the facial?
3. What are the two bases for massage?
4. Why is Swedish massage used?
5. What is shiatsu?
6. What is "ki"?
7. What type of massage does the esthetician use?
8. How does massage affect the client psychologically?
9. How does massage help feed the body?
10. How does massage help cleanse the body?
11. What are endorphins?
12. How does massage revitalize the body?
13. What is the difference between yin and yang?
14. What is the energy flow pattern of the meridians?
15. Why is the yin/yang concept important in massage therapy?
16. What are the three planes of the aura?
17. What is effleurage?
18. Why is feathering used?
19. What effect do friction movements have?
20. Why are petrissage movements good for oil-dry skin?
21. What do stretching maneuvers accomplish?
22. What are tsubos?
23. What does pressure on pressure points accomplish?
24. How does massage rely on science and art?
25. What is the right way to give a facial massage?
26. How should contact with the skin be broken?
27. When should massage not be given?
28. What should the esthetician do if the client has had cosmetic surgery within a year?

10 Hair Structure and Removal Methods

OBJECTIVES *After completing this chapter, you should be able to:*

❶ Describe hair structure and function.
❷ Discuss methods of removing unwanted hair through shaving, chemical depilatories, waxing, and electrolysis.

INTRODUCTION

Hair—some call it our "crowning glory"—is a filamentous keratin thread that covers virtually the entire body, although it is most apparent on the top of the head and in the axillary and pubic areas. Men and women spend countless hours and billions of dollars each year on caring for their hair—shampooing, cutting, styling and coloring it. And we undergo considerable anguish when we start losing it. Hair is an important appendage of the skin. At least when it's on the head.

Body hair, however, is another matter. Men's fashions, with respect to body hair, change. Beards and moustaches come and go. The hairy chest, correctly or incorrectly, has long been considered a sign of virility.

On the other hand, body hair on women has never been considered fashionable. Although some cultures tolerate body hair more than others, women spend almost as much time, effort, and money removing unwanted body hair as they do on preserving the hair on their head.

Women want to rid themselves of that unsightly hair and the esthetician can help them do it. Hair removal, whether permanent or temporary, is a valid aspect of skin care and can easily be accomplished in the well-equipped salon.

HAIR STRUCTURE

The hair and the follicles comprise the **pilary system**. Hair is a thread of highly keratinized, closely packed cells. It grows from a **follicle** (FOL-i-kel), a tubular structure of epidermis that extends from deep in the dermis to the surface of the skin. The base of the follicle is bulbous and contains the **dermal papilla**, which is wrapped by a well-developed capillary network that supplies nourishment to the follicle and the papilla. As the cells of the follicle move upward, they become differentiated, enlarge and change shape, paving the way for the growth of the hair (Fig. 10.1 and Fig. 10.2).

Hair follicles undergo three separate, alternating phases of existence. In the **anagen** phase, they are actively growing. As growth slows, the follicle begins to atrophy. The hair separates from the papilla and falls out. This is called the **catagen** phase. In the **telogen** phase, the follicle is inactive and has shrunk to about half its original size. In this resting phase, the follicle has lost its bulb. After a relatively short rest period, it will gradually regenerate itself and hair once again begins growing.

There are two parts to hair—the shaft and the root. The hair shaft extends above the surface of the skin; the root is below the surface. The hair bulb sits at the lower end of the root and covers the papilla, which nourishes the bulb.

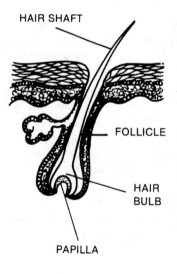

10.1—Hair structure

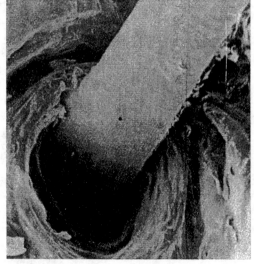

10.2—Electron microphotograph of hair follicle (*Reprinted with permission from* Les Nouvelles Esthetiques—*American Edition*)

The hair shaft consists of three layers of horny cells. The outer layer, the **cuticle** (KYOO-ti-kel), is transparent. The center layer, the **cortex** (KOR-teks), contains the pigment that gives the hair its color. The inner layer is the **medulla** (mi-DUL-ah). Hair grows over the entire body, except for the palms of the hands and soles of the feet. The average life span for healthy hair is four to seven years. Since there are no nerve endings in the hair, it has no sensation, hence, there is no pain when it is cut.

Human hair can be characterized as either terminal or vellus. **Terminal hairs** are the long, coarse, pigmented hairs most prevalent on the scalp and other parts of the body. **Vellus hairs** are very short, soft and unpigmented. These hairs are distributed over most of the body except where there are large concentrations of terminal hairs.

HAIR REMOVAL METHODS

There are four major methods for removing unwanted body hair—shaving, chemical depilatories, waxing, and electrolysis. Only two, waxing and electrolysis, are generally offered as a salon service. Of the four methods, only electrolysis offers permanent hair removal. All other methods are temporary.

Shaving

Shaving cuts hair off at or slightly below the skin line. Within a day or two, normal hair growth lets the cut hair shaft reappear above the skin surface. The short, blunt-ended hairs create a rough stubble that must be removed again by shaving. In addition, the scraping action of the razor can irritate the skin. It is also very easy to cut and nick the skin.

Chemical Depilatories

Chemical depilatories work by caustic action on the hair shaft. They are available as creams, lotions, and powder. A thin layer of the chemical is applied to the skin and allowed to remain on the skin for a short period of time. Then it is wiped off, taking the hair with it. These materials chemically "burn" off the hair. Like shaving, these products remove hair only to the skin line, allowing quick regrowth. The caustic action may also irritate the skin.

Waxing

Waxing is a clean, efficient method of removing unwanted body hair. The procedure is safe, relatively easy, and gives results that last a long time. It is an ideal adjunct to the esthetician's services and doesn't require a separate license, as electrolysis does. Although easy to do, waxing does require practice to build proficiency.

Unlike shaving, waxing pulls the hair out by its roots, without damaging the papilla. Since the papilla is undamaged, hair can continue to grow. Because the waxing process has removed the hair from the root, however, it takes longer to regrow—up to four to six weeks in some cases. And it leaves the skin smooth.

Although not a permanent method of hair removal, with repeated waxing, the follicles tend to weaken and hair growth becomes more sparse.

The procedure for waxing is relatively simple. The skin is cleaned of oil and moisture. A thin layer of warm wax is applied. A cloth strip is rubbed onto the wax, then pulled off. The wax and the hair adhere to the cloth strip and are removed from the skin. It is a relatively painless procedure, although the client will feel a slight stinging sensation.

Any area of the body except for the eyelids may be waxed. The most commonly requested salon waxing services are for the eyebrows, upper lip, chin, bikini line, and legs.

Before starting, make sure the wax is at the proper temperature and a sufficient supply of cloth strips are available. Have all other materials at hand. There are a number of depilatory wax heating machines available. These hold either a jar of wax or special roller applicators at the proper temperature. Generally, these machines are thermostatically controlled and may be left on throughout the entire salon workday.

Line the chair with paper of the type doctors use on examining tables. The paper is available in rolls from medical supply houses. The paper will protect the chair from any wax that is spilled. Have the client change into a smock and drape her with towels to prevent spilling wax on her.

Check the client's skin. Do not wax over pustules, pimples, lesions, or moles. As with any salon service, keep accurate records of the waxing services performed.

Make sure the client is comfortable. Keep the temperature of the room cool enough so the client does not perspire. Perspiration may interfere with the adhesion of the wax. Cleanse the area of the skin to be waxed thoroughly to remove oils, makeup, dirt, and moisture. Wipe the area with an astringent or with witch hazel, dry the skin, and then apply a light dusting of unscented talcum powder. If the hair is long, trim to about ¼ inch before waxing.

Work on small areas of the skin. Using a clean wooden spatula or special roller applicator, apply the warm wax in a thin coat in the direction of hair growth. Don't cover an area larger than the cloth strip. Apply the wax in one smooth motion. Do not go back and forth. As soon as the wax has been applied, place the cloth strip on the wax and rub it firmly in the direction of hair growth to make sure it adheres to the wax. Hold the skin taut and pull the cloth strip off in the direction opposite to hair growth. Keep the strip parallel to the skin. If the strip is removed at too high an angle, the hair may break

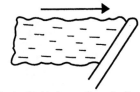

A. Apply thin layer of wax in direction
of hair growth

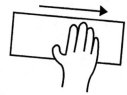

B. Smooth down cloth strip in direction
of hair growth

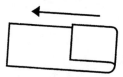

10.3—Waxing procedure

C. Pull off strip at low angle in direction
opposite of hair growth

instead of being pulled out (Fig. 10.3). Dispose of the used cloth strip
in a covered trash receptacle.

Immediately apply firm hand pressure over the area just waxed to
minimize smarting. Remove excess wax with another cloth strip.
Continue the process until the entire area has been waxed. Once
waxing is completed, apply a lotion to the skin to soothe and minimize irritation. In some cases, the client may be able to reduce the
redness and irritation by taking an antacid tablet before waxing.

The procedure is the same no matter what area is being waxed.
However, special care should be taken when waxing eyebrows and
bikini lines. In these two cases, the object is not to remove all hair, but
to shape and form a line. It is possible to remove too much hair.

Waxing is an ideal way to shape and space eyebrows so they act
as a beautiful frame for the eyes. The eyebrow should begin at the
inside corner of the eye and end at the outer corner. The arch should
be at its highest above the outer edge of the iris. The brow should not
have any excess hair outside its lines.

Brush the eyebrows first. Then carefully apply a thin coat of warm
wax at the edge of the desired line, in the direction of hair growth.
Rub on a small cloth strip, also in the direction of hair growth. Hold
the skin around the brow taut with finger pressure and pull off the

strip in the direction opposite to hair growth. Wax the top of the brow first, then the bottom. Finish by waxing the area above the bridge of the nose, if necessary. Make sure no wax is placed on areas where hair should not be removed. Remember, if the eyebrow is removed accidently, it can't be put back. Do not wax the eyelid area. Any superfluous hair in this area should be tweezed.

For best results when waxing the bikini line, have the client wear the bathing suit she'll be using. Line the edge of the suit with paper towels to prevent soiling the suit with wax. If necessary, trim the hair before starting. Establish the desired line, then wax along that line.

Electrolysis

Electrolysis is the only method for permanent hair removal. In this method, radio frequency (RF) current is used to destroy the papilla, cutting off nourishment to the hair bulb. This causes the hair to come out. Since the papilla has been destroyed, no new hair will grow from that follicle.

It is a safe, relatively painless, and effective procedure, but takes a considerable amount of time since hairs are removed one by one. Though simple in concept, electrolysis requires considerable training and practice and, in most states, requires a separate license.

There are two types of electrolysis machinery—the conventional needle type and the newer tweezer type. Both operate on the same general principle, supplying current to the papilla, and use the same radio frequency current of thirteen to twenty-seven megahertz (million cycles per second). There is some doubt, however, about the ability of the tweezer type to provide truly permanent hair removal.

In the more common method of electrolysis, the esthetician inserts a needle into the hair follicle, following the direction of the hair shaft, until the end of the needle touches the hair bulb. A short burst of diathermy (RF) current is applied by stepping on a foot pedal. The high heat produced coagulates the hair germ cells and kills the papilla. The needles vary from .003 inch to .007 inch in diameter and from one quarter to one half inch long.

The tweezer method operates under similar principles, except that instead of applying current through a needle, a specially shielded electric tweezer is used. The esthetician grasps the hair with the tweezer, taking care not to touch the skin with the end of the tweezer. As with the needle machine, current is applied by stepping on a foot pedal. The current is applied for up to twenty seconds. In this case, the high heat generated by the current is transmitted to the hair bulb through the hair shaft.

The tweezer method is more gentle than the needle method, but it takes longer and may not be quite as permanent.

In either case, the general procedures are similar. Sanitation is of paramount importance. All implements should be sterile, especially the needles. Make sure the client is comfortable and at ease. The client should be draped and be comfortably situated in the facial chair. Her eyes should be covered with moist cotton pads to protect them from the light of the magnifying lamp.

Cleanse the client's skin in the area to be treated to remove make-up, oil, or moisture and pat dry. Trim the hair, if necessary.

Using the magnifying lamp, begin the hair removal process. Work on small areas and keep sessions relatively short to prevent over-irritating the client's skin. Be alert to any client discomfort. After the treatment session, apply a soothing lotion to the skin. Sterilize the needles or tweezer and store in a sterile container.

Never give an electrolysis treatment on irritated skin or over pustules or open lesions. If the client is pregnant or has a heart pacemaker, get written permission from her physician before starting treatments. Never remove hair from inside the nose, inside the ears, or the eyelids. Never remove hair from a mole. As with any salon service, keep complete records of the treatments given.

REVIEW QUESTIONS

1. What is hair?
2. What makes up the pilary system?
3. What is a follicle?
4. What are the three phases of hair growth?
5. What are the three layers of the hair shaft?
6. What are vellus hairs?
7. What are the four methods of removing unwanted hair?
8. Which methods of hair removal are valid skin-care salon services?
9. Which method offers permanent hair removal?
10. How do chemical depilatories work?
11. Why is waxing an efficient way to remove hair?
12. What precautions should be taken when waxing?
13. What are the two types of electrolysis machines?
14. How is the tweezer type different?
15. From where should hair never be removed during electrolysis?

11 Chemistry for the Esthetician

OBJECTIVES *After completing this chapter, you should be able to:*

❶ Discuss chemistry for the esthetician from a historical perspective.
❷ Understand how chemical reactions impact skin-care products.
❸ Discuss various branches of chemistry—including organic and biochemistry—and relate them to skin care.

INTRODUCTION Chemistry is the branch of science concerned with matter—the fundamental materials of the world we live in. It is the study of changes in matter, and of the interaction and reactions of different materials. As such, chemistry is central to our daily existence. Modern life depends on this queen of sciences.

Everything we see, touch, smell or feel is a product of chemistry—either natural, as in the air we breathe or the food we eat, or manufactured, as in the plastics and synthetic fabrics we use to make many of our artifacts (Fig. 11.1 and 11.2). Our bodies, in fact, are chemical factories, engaged in countless chemical reactions, including the conversion of food into new tissue and energy.

A basic knowledge of chemistry is important to the esthetician for two reasons. First, the products used in the practice of skin care are chemicals, and it is advisable to understand the nature of the components, how they may interact, and why they have the effects they do.

Second, it is necessary to understand the nature of the biochemical reactions within our bodies and, in particular, their effects on the skin. The biochemical products occurring during the processes involved in nutrition are a good example.

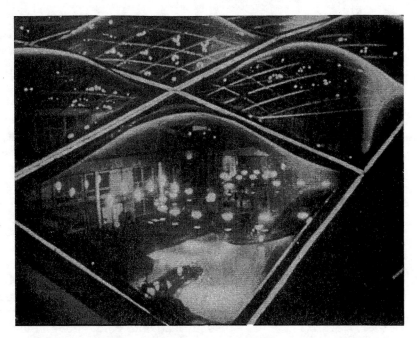

11.1—Plexiglas® acrylic plastic enclosure *(Courtesy of Rohm and Haas Company)*

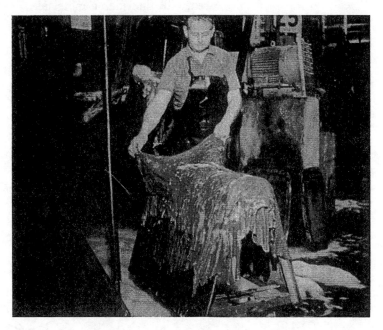

11.2—Leather tanning and finishing operation *(Courtesy of Rohm and Haas Company)*

HISTORICAL PERSPECTIVE

Chemistry, as a craft and as a philosophy, has its roots in antiquity. Undoubtedly, it began in prehistory when early humans discovered fire and the chemical change in meat when it was roasted. Later, as the iron age began, iron-working techniques were developed and used to make more efficient tools. These early discoveries were born of expediency, and were more of a craft than a science.

It was the ancient Greek philosophers who began to develop laws for this craft, thus attempting, through logic, to understand the nature of the changes they observed. They postulated the idea that all nature was composed of four elements: fire, earth, air, and water. These elements had the properties of coldness, hotness, dryness, or wetness. Each element, they believed, shared two of these properties. Fire, therefore, was hot and dry; earth was cold and dry; air was hot and wet; and water was cold and wet. One element could be changed into another element by altering its properties (Fig. 11.3). This theory of matter persisted through the Middle Ages, as the alchemists preoccupied themselves trying to transmute base matter, usually lead, into gold. Though they were never successful in doing this, they did expand the list of materials and properties while discovering new chemical processes.

Out of these ideas grew the idea of a combustible property associated with flammable materials. This property was called "phlogiston," and was necessary to support combustion. According to the phlogiston theory, an object would burn only so long as it contained phlogiston. Once the phlogiston was gone, the object would no longer burn.

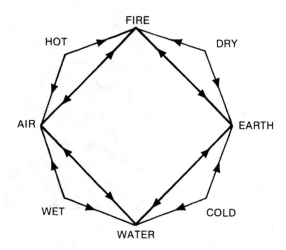

11.3—Four classical elements and their properties

Joseph Priestly (1733–1804), an English clergyman, discovered a gas, which he called "dephlogisticated air," that supported combustion more vigorously than ordinary air.

In 1772, **Antoine Lavoisier** (1743–1794), considered the father of modern chemistry, conducted a series of experiments on combustion using quantitative measurements. His findings could not be explained by the phlogiston theory. He thereby rejected the theory. Instead, he gave Priestly's "dephlogisticated air" a new name, "oxygen," and postulated that oxygen is removed from the air and is incorporated into the object as it burns. Lavoisier relied on quantitative measurements made during carefully controlled experiments as opposed to qualitative observation. This is the basis of the scientific method by which modern science is conducted.

The Scientific Method   In the scientific method, careful observations, and measured results of experiments are used to develop generalized statements that describe and summarize the observed phenomena. These descriptions are called **laws**. The scientist then develops **hypotheses** (hey-PATH-e-seez) to tentatively explain the laws. A hypothesis must be tested by further experimentation so it can be verified. If experimentation shows the hypothesis to be valid, it becomes a **theory** (THE-or-ee), a generalized explanation of a scientific law.

Science progresses as scientists continually test hypotheses and theories through experimentation and observation to verify or refute their validity. A key to this work is careful measurement using standards that allow replication of results. The system of measurement used in scientific study is the metric system. Emphasis is placed on SI units, basic metric units known as **International System Units,** chosen for their precision and reproducibility (Table 11.1).

MATTER

The universe consists of **matter** (MA-ter), any substance that has mass and occupies space. Matter exists in one of three states—gas, liquid, or solid (Fig. 11.4). Gases are readily expandable and compressible. They have neither form nor volume, but expand to fill their containers. On application of pressure, they contract readily. Gases flow readily and diffuse rapidly. Different gases form homogenous mixtures in all proportions. The individual molecules of a gas are far apart and are in great disorder. They have no great attractive force and move about freely.

Liquids are neither expandable nor compressible. They have no form, but have a specific volume, so they take the shape of their containers, but do not expand to fill them. Liquids do not compress

TABLE 11.1—SI Units

MEASURE	SI UNIT
Length	Meter (m)
Mass	Kilogram (Kg)
Time	Second (s)
Temperature	Kelvin (K)
Volume	Cubic Meter (m^3)
Force	Newton (N)
Pressure	Pascal (Pa)
Energy	Joule (J)
Light Intensity	Candela (C)
METRIC/ENGLISH SYSTEM EQUIVALENTS	
1 meter = 1.094 yds.	
2.54 cm = 1 inch	
1 Kg = 2.2 lbs.	
453.6 gm = 1 lb.	
1 liter = 1.06 qts.	
100°C. = 212°F.	
0°C. = 32°F.	

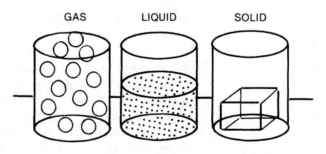

GAS   LIQUID   SOLID

11.4—Properties of gases, liquids, and solids

on application of pressure. They flow freely, but do not diffuse quickly. Different liquids do not necessarily form homogenous mixtures. The individual molecules of a liquid are also disordered and free to move about, but they are much closer together and can exert attractive force on each other.

Solids, like liquids, are neither expandable nor compressible. Unlike liquids, solids have both form and volume and do not take the shape of their containers. They hold their shape under the application of pressure. They do not flow. The individual molecules in a solid are highly ordered and have no free movement, although they can vibrate. The particles are close together and exert considerable attractive force.

Under proper conditions, many substances can change from one state to another. For example, water, a liquid at room temperature, when heated to its boiling point becomes steam, a gas. When frozen, it becomes ice, a solid. Carbon dioxide, a gas, becomes dry ice when frozen. When warmed, dry ice reverts to a gas without going through a liquid phase.

Matter is classified into elements, mixtures, or compounds. **Elements** (EL-e-ments) are the simplest forms of matter. At present, there are 105 known elements, which can be sub-classified into metals or nonmetals (Table 11.2). Of the known elements, relatively few are found in great abundance. The human body, for example, consists mostly of just three elements: carbon, oxygen, and hydrogen. The remaining elements in the body occur in very small amounts.

Mixtures are composed of two or more elements intermingled physically but not chemically. No element in a mixture loses its identity or physical characteristics. Mixtures are capable of being separated into their individual elements by physical means. **Homogenous** (HO-mow-jee-nee-us) mixtures, that is, mixtures that are uniform throughout, are known as **solutions**. Nonuniform mixtures are called **heterogeneous**.

Compounds consist of two or more elements joined together chemically to create a new substance with properties different from those of its components. Each element in a compound loses its identity. The elements cannot be separated by physical means, although they may be separated chemically. In a compound, the atoms of the elements combine in a definite molecular arrangement.

Atomic Theory

Elements differ from one another in their atomic structure. That is, each element is made up of tiny particles called **atoms** (AT-omz), the smallest unit of the element that can combine with other elements. All of the atoms in an element are identical (Fig. 11.5).

Atoms can be subdivided into three subatomic particles: **protons** (PRO-tonz), **neutrons** (NOO-tronz), and **electrons** (ah-LEK-tronz). Protons have a positive charge; neutrons have no charge; electrons

TABLE 11.2—Elements

NAME	SYMBOL	ATOMIC NUMBER	ATOMIC WEIGHT	NAME	SYMBOL	ATOMIC NUMBER	ATOMIC WEIG
Actinium*	Ac	89	227	Mercury	Hg	80	200.6
Aluminum	Al	13	27	Molybdenum**	Mo	42	95.9
Americum*	Am	95	243	Neodymium	Nd	60	144.2
Antimony	Sb	51	121.8	Neon	Ne	10	20.2
Argon	Ar	18	39.9	Neptunium*	Np	93	237
Arsenic	As	33	74.9	Nickel	Ni	28	58.7
Astatine*	At	85	210	Niobium	Nb	41	92.9
Barium	Ba	56	137.3	Nitrogen	N	7	14
Berkelium*	Bk	97	247	Nobelium*	No	102	253
Beryllium	Be	4	9	Osmium	Os	76	190.2
Bismuth	Bi	83	209	Oxygen	O	8	16
Boron	B	5	10.8	Palladium	Pd	46	106.4
Bromine	Br	35	79.9	Phosphorus**	P	15	31
Cadmium	Cd	48	112.4	Platinum	Pt	78	195.1
Calcium**	Ca	20	40.1	Plutonium*	Pu	94	242
Californium*	Cf	98	249	Polonium*	Po	84	210
Carbon	C	6	12	Potassium**	K	19	39.1
Cerium	Ce	58	140.1	Praseodymium	Pr	59	140.9
Cesium	Cs	55	132.9	Promethium*	Pm	61	147
Chlorine**	Cl	17	35.5	Protactinium*	Pa	91	231
Chromium**	Cr	24	52	Radium*	Ra	88	226
Cobalt**	Co	27	58.9	Radon*	Rn	86	222
Copper**	Cu	29	63.5	Rhenium	Re	75	186.2
Curium*	Cm	96	247	Rhodium	Rh	45	102.9
Dysprosium	Dy	66	162.5	Rubidium	Rb	37	85.5
Einsteinium*	Es	99	254	Ruthenium	Ru	44	101.1
Erbium	Er	68	167.3	Rutherfordium*	Rf	104	257
Europium	Eu	63	152	Samarium	Sm	62	150.4
Fermium*	Fm	100	253	Scandium	Sc	21	45
Fluorine**	F	9	19	Selenium**	Se	34	79
Francium*	Fr	87	223	Silicon	Si	14	28.1
Gadolinium	Gd	64	157.3	Silver	Ag	47	107.9
Gallium	Ga	31	69.7	Sodium**	Na	11	23
Germanium	Ge	32	72.6	Strontium*	Sr	38	87.6
Gold	Au	79	197	Sulfur**	S	16	32

(contin

TABLE 11.2—(continued)

NAME	SYMBOL	ATOMIC NUMBER	ATOMIC WEIGHT	NAME	SYMBOL	ATOMIC NUMBER	ATOMIC WEIGHT
Hafnium	Hf	72	178.5	Tantalum	Ta	73	180.9
Hahnium*	Ha	105	260	Technetium*	Tc	43	99
Helium	He	2	4	Tellurium	Te	52	127.6
Holmium	Ho	67	165	Terbium	Tb	65	158.9
Hydrogen	H	1	1	Thallium	Tl	81	204.4
Indium	In	49	114.8	Thorium	Th	90	232
Iodine**	I	53	126.9	Thulium	Tm	69	168.9
Iridium	Ir	77	192.2	Tin	Sn	50	118.7
Iron**	Fe	26	55.9	Titanium	Ti	22	47.9
Krypton	Kr	36	83.8	Tungsten	W	74	183.9
Lanthanum	La	57	138.9	Uranium*	U	92	238
Lawrencium*	Lw	103	257	Vanadium**	V	23	50.9
Lead	Pb	82	207.2	Xenon	Xe	54	131.3
Lithium	Li	3	7	Ytterbium	Yb	70	173
Lutetium	Lu	71	175	Yttrium	Y	39	89
Magnesium**	Mg	12	24.3	Zinc**	Zn	30	65.4
Manganese**	Mn	25	54.9	Zirconium	Zr	40	91.2
Mendelevium*	Md	101	256				

*Radioactive elements.
**Elements important to nutrition.

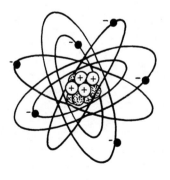

⊕ PROTON   ⊗ NEUTRON

● ELECTRON

11.5—Atomic structure of the carbon atom

have a negative charge. The positive and negative charges are equal, so there is no charge on the atom as a whole. That is, an atom must have the same number of electrons as it has protons. Protons and neutrons are found in the **nucleus** of the atom, a small volume at the center of the atom, while the electrons revolve about the nucleus. Most of the atom consists of empty space. The electrons remain in orbit around the nucleus because of the attraction caused by the opposite charges of the electrons and protons. Because of their location, electrons are most important to chemical reactions.

An element is identified by the number of protons in the nucleus of its atoms, which, as stated earlier, must equal the number of electrons. The number of protons the atom contains is its **atomic (ah-TOM-ik) number**, which is the same for all atoms of the element.

The number of neutrons in an atom of an element may vary. When this occurs, the atom is said to be an **isotope** (EYE-sow-towp) of the element, and will have a different atomic weight, even though the atomic number stays the same. The atomic weight of an atom is the sum of the protons and neutrons in its nucleus.

The **Periodic Table** was developed as an aid to classifying elements by their atomic numbers and by their familial characteristics. The elements are listed in rows by ascending atomic number and in columns by families or groups that have similar properties (Table 11.3).

The members of group 1A, for example, are known as the **alkali (AL-ka-ly) metals**; group 2A are the **alkaline (AL-kah-lyn) earth metals**. These are both considered as **active metals**. The groups in the center of the table are the **transition (trans-IH-shun) metals**, while the **nonmetals** are in the columns to the right and are separated from the metals by a heavy stepped line. The members of group 8A are known as the **inert** or **rare** gases.

Molecules (MAWL-ik-kules) are combinations of atoms bound tightly together. Molecules can consist of a group of like atoms, as in some elements. A molecule of oxygen, for example, consists of two oxygen atoms bound together. Its chemical formula is O_2. Ozone consists of three atoms of oxygen bound together as O_3. Even though they are chemically different, they are still elements.

Compounds (KOM-pownds) consist of molecules formed by binding atoms of two or more elements together. Thus, a molecule of water, H_2O, consists of two atoms of hydrogen and one atom of oxygen.

During chemical reactions, atoms can gain or lose electrons and, thereby, pick up an electrical charge. This creates a charged particle, called an **ion** (EYE-on). The nucleus of the atom remains unchanged during this process, however. Metal atoms generally lose electrons

TABLE 11.3—Periodic Table of the Elements

NONMETALS

TRANSITION METALS

1A	2A		3B	4B	5B	6B	7B		8B		1B	2B	3A	4A	5A	6A	7A	8A
																	1 H	2 He
3 Li	4 Be												5 B	6 C	7 N	8 O	9 F	10 Ne
11 Na	12 Mg												13 Al	14 Si	15 P	16 S	17 Cl	18 Ar
19 K	20 Ca		21 Sc	22 Ti	23 V	24 Cr	25 Mn	26 Fe	27 Co	28 Ni	29 Cu	30 Zn	31 Ga	32 Ge	33 As	34 Se	35 Br	36 Kr
37 Rb	38 Sr		39 Y	40 Zr	41 Nb	42 Mo	43 Tc	44 Ru	45 Rh	46 Pd	47 Ag	48 Cd	49 In	50 Sn	51 Sb	52 Te	53 I	54 Xe
55 Cs	56 Ba		57 La	72 Hf	73 Ta	74 W	75 Re	76 Os	77 Ir	78 Pt	79 Au	80 Hg	81 Tl	82 Pb	83 Bi	84 Po	85 At	86 Rn
87 Fr	88 Ra		89 Ac	104 Rf	105 Ha													

LANTHANIDE SERIES

58 Ce	59 Pr	60 Nd	61 Pm	62 Sm	63 Eu	64 Gd	65 Tb	66 Dy	67 Ho	68 Er	69 Tm	70 Yb	71 Lu

ACTINIDE SERIES

90 Th	91 Pa	92 U	93 Np	94 Pu	95 Am	96 Cm	97 Bk	98 Cf	99 Es	100 Fm	101 Md	102 No	103 Lw

ACTIVE METALS

and become positively charged. These ions are called **cations** (KAT-eye-onz). Nonmetal atoms, on the other hand, generally gain electrons and become negatively charged. These ions are called **anions** (AN-eye onz). The ions have chemical properties that differ greatly from the neutrally charged atoms they came from.

CHEMICAL REACTIONS

When two or more substances are mixed, they react chemically to form one or more completely different substances. The **chemical reaction** is represented graphically by a **chemical equation** in which the **reactants** (re-AK-tant), the original substances, are shown on the left of the equation and the **products** (PROD-ukts), the substances formed as a result of the reaction, are shown on the right. A plus sign means **reacts with** and an arrow represents **produces**.

So, for example, the chemical reaction obtained by adding hydrochloric acid (HCl) to sodium hydroxide (NaOH) to produce salt (NaCl) and water (H_2O) would be shown as follows:

$$HCl + NaOH \rightarrow H_2O + NaCl$$

Chemical equations must be balanced; that is, there must be an equal number of atoms of each reactant and each product. In the above example, there are two atoms of hydrogen (H), and one each of sodium (Na), chlorine (Cl), and oxygen (O) on each side of the equation, so the equation is balanced.

It is important to note that atoms are neither created nor destroyed during a chemical reaction. They only gain or lose electrons. The total mass of the substances involved stays the same before and after the reaction. This is called the **Law of Conservation of Mass**.

The chemical reaction defines the relationship between the electron configurations of the substances as they undergo change. The atoms of each product of reaction bond together. The term, **valence** (VAL-lenz), is used to define the capacity of the atom to combine chemically with other atoms and may be thought of as the charge of a single ion. The sodium ion, for example, Na^+, has a valence of one. The oxygen ion, O^{2-}, has a valence of two.

Atoms can bond ionically, that is, by electrostatic forces, as in salt, Na^+ and Cl^-. Most metals (i.e., elements on the left side of the periodic table) undergo ionic bonding. Ionic substances generally are brittle, crystalline solids with high melting points.

Atoms can also bond covalently, that is, by sharing electrons. Two atoms of hydrogen, for example, H + H, share electron pairs to form the hydrogen molecule, H_2. Most nonmetals, (i.e., elements on the right side of the periodic table) undergo covalent bonding. Gases, liquids, and amorphous solids tend to be formed with covalent bonds. Amorphous solids are more elastic than more rigid crystalline solids and have lower melting points.

All chemical reactions do not necessarily proceed to completion; that is, until all of the reactants are used up. Depending on the conditions under which the reaction occurs, a reaction may stop before that point. When this happens, the reaction has reached **equilibrium** (ee-kwa-LIB-re-um). In many commercial processes, it is desirable to change the equilibrium point to increase the yield of the end product. The equilibrium point can be changed by changing conditions, such as increasing or decreasing temperature or pressure. Often, however, the equilibrium point can be changed by the addition of a **catalyst** (KAT-a-list).

A catalyst is a substance that increases the output of a chemical reaction without undergoing a change in its structure or becoming part of the products of the reaction. Enzymes, for example, are catalysts that allow many of the complicated biochemical reactions in the human body to take place.

Energy is also a product of chemical reactions. Combustion reactions, for example, produce heat. Some produce both heat and light. Burning a magnesium ribbon produces magnesium oxide and heat and light. This describes the chemical reaction in a photographic flash bulb. When a reaction gives off heat, it is said to be **exothermic** (ex-oh-THER-mik). If it absorbs heat, it is **endothermic** (en-doh-THER-mik). Chemical ice packs used in first aid work because the chemical reaction is endothermic.

Combustion reactions are commonly used to produce heat energy. Digestion is a combustion reaction, as the food consumed is ultimately converted to heat energy to power the engine of life.

Chemical reactions can also produce electrical energy, as in the case of battery power. In an automotive battery, the anode is made of lead; the cathode of lead dioxide. Both electrodes sit in sulfuric acid. The chemical reaction uses up the sulfuric acid and produces water while, at the same time, it produces electrical power. In a lead-acid battery, the reaction is reversible. This allows the battery to be recharged.

From the point of view of the esthetician, there are two important types of chemical reaction: oxidation-reduction reactions and neutralization reactions. In the process of **oxidation,** a metal loses electrons; in the process of **reduction,** a nonmetal gains electrons. The flashbulb and lead-acid battery are examples of oxidation-reduction reactions, as are most biological processes. An oxidizing agent takes electrons away from another molecule; a reducing agent gives electrons to another molecule.

Neutralization reactions involve the chemical reaction of an acid and a base during which the properties of both are neutralized. The example given earlier of hydrochloric acid and sodium hydroxide combining to yield salt and water is a typical reaction of this kind. A base takes protons away from another molecule; an acid gives protons to another molecule.

ACIDS AND BASES

The chemical compounds known as **acids** (ASS-eds) and **bases** (BAY-ses) are among the most important to the esthetician. Many of the products used in skin care possess either acidic or basic properties and, in many cases, are used either to enhance or to neutralize the acidity or alkalinity of the skin. **Alkali** (AL-kah-ly) is another word for base.

Acids have a sour taste and react with metals to produce hydrogen. In solution with water, they give up, or **dissociate**, hydrogen. The degree to which they give up their hydrogen ions determines whether they are **strong acids** or **weak acids**. Strong acids become completely dissociated in water. Typical strong acids are hydrochloric acid (HCl) and sulfuric acid (H_2SO_4). Strong acids are good **electrolytes**, that is, conductors of electricity. Weak acids, which do not dissociate completely in water, conversely, are poor electrolytes and don't conduct electricity well. Phenol, a commonly used disinfectant and the product most often used for chemical peels, is an example of a weak acid. The chemical formula for phenol is HOC_6H_5.

It is important to note, however, that the terms "strong" and "weak" refer to the ability of the acid solution to conduct electricity and not to its ability to react chemically with other substances. Hydrofluoric acid (HF), for example, although classed as a weak acid, is highly corrosive and will even dissolve glass.

Acids may be further classified as inorganic acids or organic acids. Organic acids contain carbon. Phenol is an organic acid, as is acetic acid ($HC_2H_3O_2$). Vinegar is acetic acid. The amino acids, the building blocks of protein, are organic acids as are the fatty acids and some vitamins, such as vitamin C, or ascorbic acid ($HC_6H_7O_6$).

Note that all acids, whether strong or weak, organic or inorganic, begin their chemical formulas with hydrogen.

Bases, or alkalies, have a bitter taste and a slippery feel. In solution with water, they give up hydroxide (OH) ions. As with acids, the degree to which bases dissociate determines whether they are considered strong or weak bases. The most soluble bases are strong. Caustic soda, or sodium hydroxide (NaOH), is a typical strong base. Ammonia (NH_3) is considered a weak base because it dissociates in water to yield the hydroxyl radical OH and the ammonium ion NH_4.

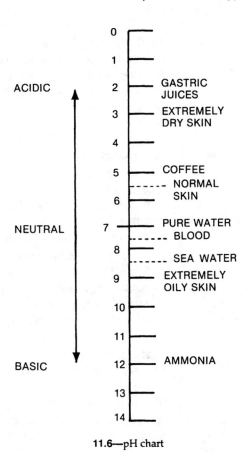

11.6—pH chart

As with acids, the terms weak base and strong base refer to the ability of the hydroxide ions to dissociate and does not refer to the degree of alkalinity of a solution.

Bases may also be classified as organic or inorganic, depending on whether or not they contain carbon. Caustic soda, for example, is an inorganic base. Nicotine ($C_{10}H_{14}N_2$) is an organic base.

The acidity or alkalinity of a solution may be determined by the use of **indicators** (in-de-KAYT-ors), substances that change color when exposed to the solution. The most common indicator is **litmus** (LIT-mis), an organic material derived from lichens. Litmus paper turns red in acid solutions and blue in basic solutions. Most indicators, however, give qualitative indications rather than quantitative indications. That is, they tell whether a solution is acidic or basic, but not the degree to which it is acidic or basic.

The degree of acidity or alkalinity is measured by the pH of the solution. The pH, or hydrogen potential, is defined as the negative log of the hydrogen-ion concentration, using base 10, and measured on a scale of 0 to 14. Thus, a solution with a pH value of 7 is neutral. If its pH is lower than 7, it is acidic; if its pH is higher than 7, it is alkaline. The pH scale is logarithmic rather than linear. That is, the degree of acidity or alkalinity doubles with each rise or lowering of number. So, for example, a solution with a pH of 5 is twice as acidic as a solution with a pH of 6 (Fig. 11.6).

Pure water has a pH of 7, and is neutral. Sea water, because of the dissolved minerals, has a pH of about 8.4 and is basic. Blood, with a pH of 7.4, is slightly basic. Household ammonia, with a pH of almost 12, is strongly basic. Coffee has a pH of 5, and is mildly acidic. Gastric juices, with a pH of 2, are strongly acid. The pH of human skin varies between 3 and 9, depending on the skin type. Extremely oily skin has the highest pH value, that is, is most alkaline; extremely dry skin has the lowest pH value, that is, is the most acidic. Normal skin is slightly acidic, with pH values between 5 and 6. In general, pH is a good measure of skin type. Unfortunately, however, pH is difficult to measure without technically sophisticated and highly expensive equipment.

The pH of a solution can be changed by adding an acid or base. In many substances, however, it is important to maintain a specific pH value. Blood, for example, must maintain a pH of 7.4. Any significant change in this value could cause death. For this reason, blood is buffered, that is, it contains substances that resist changes in pH when acids or bases are added. A **buffer** (BUF-er), then, is a solution that reacts with either acids or bases to limit pH changes in substances to which it is added. Buffers are used whenever it is important to maintain a given pH level in a product.

SOLUTIONS

Few of the substances encountered are pure. Most are either compounds or mixtures, as discussed earlier. When the mixture is homogeneous, that is, the molecules of the components are uniformly intermingled, the mixture is called a **solution** (SA-loo-shun). A solution can be a gas. Air is a solution of gaseous substances. It can be a solid, as in an alloy of different metals. Or it can be a liquid. The esthetician will be most concerned with liquid solutions, since most skin-care products take this form.

Solutions consist of the **solute**, the substance being dissolved, and the **solvent**, the substance that dissolves the solute. Water is the most common solvent, especially in skin-care products. Other commonly used solvents are alcohols, acids, and oils. The concentration of the solution is a measure of the relative amount of solute it contains. A **dilute solution** contains a relatively small amount of solute. A **concentrated solution** contains a relatively large amount.

The solubility of a solution is a measure of the ability of the solute to be dissolved in the solvent under a certain set of conditions. Some substances have relatively low solubility; others have high solubility. Ethyl alcohol, for example, has almost unlimited solubility in water. Whether the drinks are strong or weak, the whiskey mixes completely with the water. Vitamins B and C are soluble in water. Vitamins A, D, E, and K are not soluble in water, but are soluble in the fatty oils of the body. Oils are not generally soluble in water, meaning that oil and water do not mix.

When two liquids mix readily, they are said to be **miscible** (MIS-e-bel). Liquids that do not mix readily are said to be **immiscible** (IM-MIS-e-bel). Oil and water, then, are immiscible; whiskey and water are miscible.

When the solution has reached **equilibrium**, that is, when it contains all the dissolved solute it can hold, the solution is said to be **saturated**. The solubility of a solute can be increased by increasing the temperature or the pressure. When this happens, the solution is **supersaturated**. If the temperature or pressure is then decreased, the excess solute will come out of solution.

In **heterogeneous** (het-er-oh-GEE-nee-us) mixtures, which are not solutions because the molecules of the various components do not intermingle but stay separate, the particles stay suspended in the liquid phase. If the particles are relatively large, the mixture is called a **suspension** (sus-PEN-shun). If they are relatively small, the mixture is a **colloid** (KO-loyd). In colloidal mixtures, the particles may be too small to be seen, but the mixture looks cloudy.

The undissolved particles gradually settle to the bottom of the container. When this happens in a skin-care product, it makes the product unusable, or in the case of a retail product, makes it unsalable. To prevent this, manufacturers add chemical agents to the products that will hold the undissolved particles in suspension and will disperse them evenly throughout the product.

Products that contain oil and water phases require the addition of agents called **emulsifiers** (ee-MUL-si-feyers). These agents keep the phases from separating. When the mixture contains oil particles suspended in water, it is called an **oil in water** mixture (O/W). When it contains water particles suspended in oil, it is called a **water in oil** mixture (W/O). Many skin-care products are either O/W or W/O mixtures.

Because of its usefulness as a solvent, and since it is the major component of many skin-care products, water deserves separate mention. Water has been called the universal solvent. Pure water, H_2O, is a neutral substance with a pH of 7. Most natural water, however, contains dissolved minerals. The specific mineral content of the water depends on the place from which it comes. When the water contains a high percentage of dissolved minerals, it is referred to as **hard water**. Hard water does not allow the formation of suds in detergents and soaps and is responsible for the ring left around bathtubs after a bath.

Before water can be used to make skin-care products, it must be softened, that is, the minerals must be removed to make the water pure. This is accomplished by **distillation** (dis-te-LAY-shun), in which the water is boiled and the steam is collected on plates and cooled back to the water phase. The condensed water is purified. Water is also purified by **deionization** (dee-eye-en-eye-ZAY-shun), in which the water is passed through beds of ion exchange beads. The ion exchange beads do just what their name implies. They exchange the metallic mineral ions from the water for harmless hydrogen or hydroxide ions.

BRANCHES OF CHEMISTRY

Organic Chemistry

Chemistry may be rather loosely divided into inorganic and organic disciplines. Organic chemistry is concerned with substances that contain the element carbon, which is found in all life forms. Only carbon, of all the known elements, is able to form single, double, or triple bonds to produce long chains of atoms.

Among the important organic compounds are the **hydrocarbons** (hy-dro-KAR-bonz), which contain hydrogen and carbon. Even though the hydrocarbons contain only these two elements, they may be arranged in almost infinite numbers to form a great variety of different materials because of the unique bonding ability of carbon. There are four groups of hydrocarbons: **alkanes**, **alkenes**, **alkynes**, and **aromatics**. The first three groups are called, collectively, the **aliphatics** (al-i-FAT-iks) (Table 11.4).

A carbon atom of an alkane is connected to hydrogen or other carbon atoms by four single bonds. Methane, (CH_4), the principal component of natural gas, is the simplest alkane. Structurally, the carbon atom is in the center; the four hydrogen atoms in the four corners of an imaginary rectangle.

An alkene has at least one carbon atom double bonded to another carbon atom. Because of the double bond, an alkene has two fewer hydrogen atoms than an alkane, and is more chemically reactive. The simplest, and probably the most familiar, alkene is ethylene, (C_2H_4), which is the material used to make the widely used plastic, polyethylene. Polyethylene is a major packaging material. Alkenes are also called **olefins** (OH-le-fins).

An alkyne has at least one triple carbon to carbon bond and is highly chemically reactive. These compounds are not found as readily in nature as the other aliphatic compounds. The simplest alkyne is acetylene, (C_2H_2), a flammable gas used for welding.

TABLE 11.4—Hydrocarbon Structures

GROUP	HYDROCARBON	FORMULA	STRUCTURE
ALKANE	METHANE	CH_4	H H C H H
ALKENE	ETHYLENE	C_2H_4	H H $C{=}C$ H H
ALKYNE	ACETYLENE	C_2H_2	$H{-}C{\equiv}C{-}H$
AROMATIC	BENZENE	C_6H_6	

In the aromatic hydrocarbons, the carbon atoms are bonded together in a ring structure. Because of this, the aromatics are highly stable compounds. The simplest aromatic is benzene, (C_6H_6), used as a solvent in varnishes and lacquers.

Crude oil, or petroleum, contains a mixture of alkanes, alkenes, and aromatics, along with other organic compounds. The proportion varies depending on the source of the oil. The crude oil must be refined; that is, separated according to boiling point, to produce commercially useful products, including gasoline, fuel oil, lubricating oil, paraffin wax, and asphalt.

The hydrocarbons react readily with many other substances, either through oxidation, addition or substitution reactions. **Oxidation reactions** release large amounts of energy in the form of heat. This makes refined hydrocarbons, such as gasoline and heating oil, ideal fuels. Modern civilization, in fact, depends to a great extent on the availability of petroleum and petroleum products.

In **addition reactions**, the double or triple bonds of alkenes, alkynes and aromatics are broken so other elements can be added to produce different compounds. **Polymerization** (po-LIM-er-eye-zay-shun) is an important addition reaction. In the polymerization process, individual alkene molecules (**monomers**) bond together into long chains (**polymers**). This is the way almost all plastics are made.

In **substitution reactions**, one or more hydrogen atoms are replaced by atoms of other elements. This type of reaction is most effective with alkanes or aromatic hydrocarbons, which are less reactive than alkenes and alkynes. When benzene, for example, is reacted with nitric acid (HNO_3), with sulfuric acid as a catalyst, a hydrogen atom is replaced with a nitro group (NO) to yield nitrobenzene, a chemical used to give a pleasant odor to cheap soaps.

Through such chemical reactions, many hydrocarbon derivatives are manufactured. **Hydrocarbon derivatives** are substances that are basically hydrocarbons, but contain one or more functional groups of other elements. The nitro group (NO) was discussed earlier. Other important functional groups are the chloro (Cl) and hydroxo (OH). The functional group attached to the hydrocarbon often determines its chemical characteristics.

Alcohols (AL-ke-holz) are hydrocarbon derivatives. They are formed by replacing one or more hydrogens with a hydroxo group. Alcohols formed from aliphatic hydrocarbons are classified according to how many other carbon atoms are bonded to the carbon atom containing the hydroxo group. In a **primary alcohol**, there is only one other carbon atom. A **secondary alcohol** has two; a **tertiary alcohol** has three. Alcohols are important compounds for the esthetician.

Ethanol, a derivative of the alkane, ethane (C_2H_6), is produced naturally by the fermentation of sugar or starch through the action of yeast. Isopropyl alcohol, rubbing alcohol, is produced by hydrating propylene, an alkene, with sulfuric acid as a catalyst. Phenol is produced by substituting one hydrogen in the benzene ring with a hydroxo group, and is an example of an aromatic alcohol.

Aldehydes (AL-da-hyds), a class of chemical compounds with wide use in the manufacture of cosmetics, are made from the oxidation of primary alcohols. The most familiar of the aldehydes is formaldehyde, formed by the oxidation of methyl alcohol. Formaldehyde is used extensively as a preservative and bacteriocide and as the principal ingredient of embalming fluid.

Ketones (KEE-tonz) are made from the oxidation of secondary alcohols and are similar to aldehydes but are less reactive. Acetone, the most widely used of this class of hydrocarbon derivatives, is formed by the oxidation of isopropyl alcohol. Acetone is used as a solvent in nail polishes and polish removers.

If a primary alcohol is oxidized with an excess of oxygen, the result is a **carboxylic acid** instead of an aldehyde. Acetic acid, present in vinegar, is one such organic acid. When a carboxylic acid is reacted with an alcohol, the result is an **ester** (ES-ter). Ethyl acetate, a common solvent in nail polish removers, is produced by the reaction of acetic acid and ethanol.

Biochemistry Many organic compounds are produced commercially and used extensively in skin-care and cosmetic products because of the characteristics they impart to the product. Many others are found in nature, produced by both plants and animals. The human body is, in fact, a complex chemical factory, utilizing plant and animal materials to produce energy and chemical products for the life processes.

The elements of primary importance to human life are carbon, hydrogen, oxygen, nitrogen, phosphorus, and sulfur. Other elements are also important, but are required in far smaller quantities. These elements are combined in a variety of ways to form the materials needed to sustain life and support growth of the system. The materials can be classified as proteins, carbohydrates, fats and oils, and nucleic acids. In this chapter, these materials will be discussed as chemicals. Their role as nutrients was discussed more thoroughly in Chapter 8.

Proteins (PRO-teenz) are the major component of animal tissue, including skin, nails, muscles and bones. Some, the **simple proteins**, are made up entirely of **amino acids** (ah-MEE-no ASS-ids), the building blocks of the body. Others, the **conjugated proteins**, are bonded to other biochemicals. Half or more of each protein consists of carbon. The other components, in descending order, are oxygen, nitrogen, hydrogen, and sulfur. Phosphorus is not usually present.

Structurally, proteins exist in long chains of amino acids in various combinations. The number of possible arrangements is almost infinite. The sequence of amino acids in the chain gives the protein its characteristics.

There are twenty-two known amino acids. Fourteen of these can be synthesized in the body. The other eight, the essential amino acids, must be supplied through food. The amino acids have the general formula

$$\underset{\underset{NH_2}{|}}{R-\overset{\overset{H}{|}}{C}}-\overset{\overset{O}{|}}{C}=OH$$

They differ in the R group.

Enzymes are another type of protein that act as catalysts in the biochemical reactions of the body. The more than 1,000 known enzymes in the body are highly efficient in controlling many thousands of biochemical reactions. Without enzymes to speed up the reactions, many of the processes would proceed at such slow rates that life would be impossible to sustain. They are also very selective. Many enzymes control the biochemical reaction of only one type of molecule. Enzymes are closely related to **vitamins**, which are also catalysts and help form the enzymes. Few of the twenty known vitamins are synthesized in the body, so they must be supplied in the diet.

Carbohydrates (kahr-bow-HY-drates), occurring as sugars, starches and cellulose, are important as fuel for the body processes. Chemically, the carbohydrates are polyhydroxy aldehydes and ketones. Glucose is an aldehyde; fructose is a ketone. Both are simple sugars or **monosaccharides**. When two monosaccharides are joined together, the result is a **disaccharide**. The most common of these is sucrose, ordinary table sugar.

Starches (STAR-chez) are polysaccharides found in plants. The plant starches are converted to glucose in the body through the action of enzymes. **Cellulose** (SEL-yoo-loos) is the major structural component of plants. The molecular structure of cellulose is similar to that of starch. Enzymes, however, cannot convert cellulose to glucose. Therefore, while starches are important foods, cellulose is useless as a food source in humans. Some animals, such as cattle, can digest cellulose.

Fats and **oils** are esters of long chain carboxylic acids and are used to store energy. They are called **triglycerides** (treye-GLI-sir-ides) because they contain three groups of hydrocarbon chains. If the compound is liquid at room temperature, it is an oil; if it is solid, it is a fat. These compounds are found in both plants and animals. The carboxylic acids formed from the hydrolysis of a triglyceride are known as **fatty acids** (ASS-ids). In the body, the triglycerides are hydrolyzed by the enzyme **lipase** to form glycerol, which is converted to energy, and the fatty acids. Fatty acids are produced commercially as ingredients in soaps and detergents.

The **nucleic acids** are **nucleotide** polymers. A nucleotide consists of a phosphoric acid, a ring-form sugar, and a ring-form organic base containing nitrogen. These compounds fall into two groups: **deoxyribonucleic** (dee-ox-i-RY-bow-noo-KLAY-ik) **acids (DNA)** and **ribonucleic** (RY-bow-noo-KLAY-ik) **acids (RNA)**.

DNA contains deoxyribose as the sugar. RNA contains ribose. DNA is found in the cell nucleus, while RNA is found in the cell cytoplasm. Structurally, DNA takes the form of a double-stranded helix. Both of the nucleic acids carry the genetic information that determines how the body will grow.

REVIEW QUESTIONS

1. With what is chemistry concerned?
2. What is chemistry?
3. Why is a knowledge of chemistry important to the esthetician?
4. What was the ancient Greek idea of nature?
5. What is the scientific method?
6. What is a theory?
7. What is matter?
8. What are the three states of matter?
9. What are elements?
10. What are the three most common elements in the body?
11. What is a mixture?
12. What is a compound?
13. What is an atom?
14. What are the parts of an atom?
15. What is the Periodic Table?
16. What are molecules?
17. How are chemical equations balanced?
18. What is a catalyst?
19. What two types of chemical reactions are most important to the esthetician?
20. Why are acids and bases important to the esthetician?
21. What are indicators?
22. What is pH?
23. What is the pH of skin?
24. What is a solution?
25. What are the parts of a solution?
26. What is the most common solvent?
27. What are immiscible liquids?
28. What is an emulsifier?
29. What is organic chemistry?
30. What are the four groups of hydrocarbons?
31. How is the body a type of chemical factory?
32. What are amino acids?
33. What are enzymes?
34. Why are RNA and DNA important?

CHAPTER
12 Skin-Care Products

OBJECTIVES   *After completing this chapter, you should be able to:*

❶ Put to practical use the information presented about chemistry in Chapter 11 and understand product forms.
❷ Describe the kinds of ingredients used in different skin products, gaining an understanding of how the ingredients work to make the products effective.
❸ Read and understand product labels.
❹ Summarize product categories.

INTRODUCTION   The correct choice of products is the key to the successful practice of skin care. Skin-care treatments may be given without the aid of machinery, but they cannot be given without the use of some type of chemical product. To a large extent, the esthetician's ability to pick the right product for the right application will determine the success or failure of the treatment.

There are many excellent products on the market, as well as many that are not so good. Making the right choice from among the seemingly bewildering numbers and types of products currently on the market can be difficult. The esthetician should try a variety of brands, then choose those that seem to work best. As with equipment, it pays to use the best products available. Even after choosing, the esthetician must continually test new products as they come on the market.

Skin-care products can be grouped by type. The categories are cleansers, toners, moisturizers, masks, and treatment products. Within each category, the products must be further differentiated by the type of skin for which they are formulated. Thus, there are cleansers, toners, etc. developed for dry skin, others for oily skin, others for normal skin, and so on.

It is important to use the correct formulation for the skin type. Using the wrong formulation is ineffective at best and, under some conditions, may worsen the problem the esthetician is trying to correct. For example, a moisturizer for dry skin may contain certain emollients and other ingredients that will add oil to the skin to alleviate dryness. Using this same moisturizer on oily skin may make the skin even oilier. Astringents, which are used on oily skin, generally contain alcohol to help dry up excess oil. If used on dry skin, however, an astringent will dry the skin even more.

Before using any product, read the manufacturer's literature. Know what the product is supposed to do, how it is supposed to work, and how it is meant to be used. Know what ingredients are in the product and be familiar with what each ingredient does. And be aware of potential side effects of particular ingredients. For example, some products contain algae. This may cause an allergic reaction in clients who are allergic to shellfish.

During the consultation, the esthetician should ask about the client's food or drug allergies and keep these in mind when determining which products to use. If in doubt about a possible allergic reaction, conduct a patch test first. If an allergic reaction occurs while using a product, discontinue use of that product immediately.

If the client has an allergic reaction, the culprit will most likely be the fragrance contained in the product. FDA studies indicate that fragrance and fragrance ingredients are the most common causes of cosmetic allergies. Other potential allergy-causing ingredients include preservatives, lanolin, and propylene glycol. If the client shows an adverse reaction to a product, it may be necessary to use products listed as hypoallergenic. This generally means the product does not contain a fragrance. Bear in mind, however, that hypoallergenic does not guarantee there will be no allergic reaction. It only means that such a reaction is less likely.

PRODUCT FORMS

Skin-care products come in different forms. They may be packaged as aerosols, liquids, creams, gels, or solids.

Aerosols allow the product to be applied as a fine spray mist or as a foam. With mists, the product is broken into tiny droplets and dispersed by a propellant, either a chemical under pressure or air pumped manually or mechanically. With foams, the product mixes with the propellant to form a fluffy, light, aerated mass.

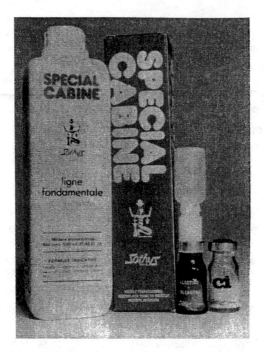

12.1—Typical product packaging *(Courtesy of Sothys, USA, Inc.)*

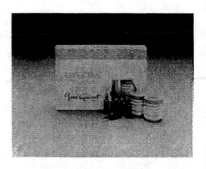

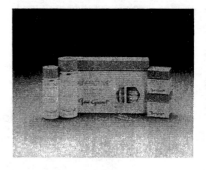

12.2—Typical product packaging *(Courtesy of Lachman Imports, Inc.)*

Liquids flow freely and are pourable, with a watery consistency. They tend to be clear or transparent. **Creams** tend to be thicker in viscosity than liquids and are usually emulsified. They vary from pourable to spreadable and are generally opaque.

Gels are thick and sticky, and have a jellylike consistency. They are not emulsified and vary from clear to translucent.

Solids can be loose and free-flowing, like powders, or bound particles, like sticks. They vary in consistency and texture. Some solid skin-care products are used in their solid state; others are meant to be mixed with water or other products for use.

Packaging is an important part of the product. The package, whether it be a bottle, jar, or can, must keep the product clean, let the product be readily identified, yet allow easy access to the product. And the package should be attractive, especially for products intended for retail sale (Fig. 12.1 and Fig. 12.2).

To keep the product clean, the package should be relatively impermeable to outside elements. It should not let air, moisture, or other contaminants in, and should not let the product leak out. If the product is sensitive to light, the package should be opaque or trans-

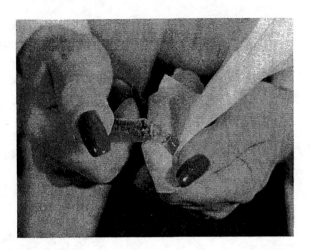

12.3—Ampoule in use

parent dark brown or green. The package should be reclosable and should be kept covered whenever the product is not being used.

The label on the container should be legible and understandable so that the product can be readily identified. All necessary information for the safe use of the product should be contained on the label. An empty container should never be refilled with a different product.

The container should allow ready access to the product. That is, it should be easy to get the product out of the container when it is needed and in the proper amount needed.

The package must also project a professional image. The container and its label should be attractively designed. An attractive package helps instill confidence in the professionalism of the esthetician and also helps impel the client into making a purchasing decision on the products he or she will take home.

Most skin-care products are packaged in glass or plastic bottles or jars. Bottles are used for pourable liquids and creams; jars for spreadable creams and solids. One of the more recent developments in packaging is the use of ampoules. **Ampoules** are small hermetically sealed glass tubes that contain a concentrated active ingredient. Since the sealed ampoule is sterile, there is usually little or no preservative added to the product. However, once the ampoule is broken, the entire contents must be used at once (Fig. 12.3).

INGREDIENTS

Skin-care products consist of one or more ingredients. Each ingredient in a product plays an important role in the product's effectiveness, either directly or indirectly. Thus, an ingredient may be active, that is, work directly on the skin, as with a moisturizer or cleansing agent, or it may work indirectly, giving the product stability, color, or texture, as, for example, a preservative.

The ingredients used in skin-care products are derived from a number of sources. They may derive from plant materials, animal products, vitamins, or minerals. In addition, they may be synthesized from chemicals or from any of the previously named sources.

Plant materials can include herbs, such as aloe, chamomile, balm mint, or yarrow, to name only a few. They can include algae or plants from the sea, as kelp or seaweed. Fruits, in the form of juices or pulps, are often used. Oranges, avocados, and strawberries are among those that form essential ingredients. Exudates from trees, such as gum arabic, are also important, as are many vegetable oils, such as peanut oil, safflower oil, olive oil, and others.

Animal products also play an important role in the formulation of skin-care products. Lanolin, from sheep wool, is widely used, as is albumin, from egg whites. Collagen, derived from the connective tissue of cows, is an important active ingredient of many products.

Vitamins are used extensively for a number of different purposes. Biotin, vitamin H, is used as a texturizer. Inositol, a vitamin B complex, and retinol, vitamin A, help treat acne. These are just a few examples.

Minerals, such as kaolin, silica, and zinc, along with many others, serve many varied purposes in skin-care products.

Then there are the chemical products. These are derived from many of the natural materials, such as the fatty acids and alcohols. Or they may be the oxides of minerals, such as zinc oxide, or aluminum oxide. Or they may be hydrocarbons, petroleum derivatives, such as mineral oil or kerosene. Some are synthesized from coal, such as benzene; or coal tar, such as the aniline dyes used widely as colorants.

The number of substances that can serve as ingredients in skin-care products is virtually endless. Almost any plant material, most minerals, and many animal products and synthetic materials can play a part in the formulation of a product. To list all of the products that could be used is beyond the scope of this chapter. For more complete information on this topic, the esthetician should consult one of the many excellent reference works on cosmetic ingredients available.

While it is important for the esthetician to be familiar with the names and derivations of at least the most common ingredients, it is more important to be aware of what those ingredients do, and to be able to discuss these functions with the client.

Each ingredient in a skin-care product has a specific function. Many substances serve more than one function. For example, tetrasodium pyrophosphate (TSPP) is used as a sequestering agent, a clarifying agent, and a buffer. The more important functions of ingredients include:

- **Antioxidants** prevent spoilage caused by exposure to oxygen. Commonly used antioxidants include tocopherol (vitamin E) and benzoic acid.
- **Binders** hold the ingredients in the product together and increase the consistency of the formulation. Commonly used binders include sorbitol and glycerin.
- **Buffers** control the level of acidity or alkalinity in the product by preventing wide swings in the pH of the product when acids or bases are added during formulation. Commonly used buffers include citric acid and calcium carbonate.
- **Clarifiers** remove unwanted materials from liquid products to make them clear. Citric acid and tannin are often used for this purpose.
- **Cleansing agents** do the actual work of cleaning the skin. They may consist of either soaps or detergents. Sodium laureth sulfate is a commonly used detergent.
- **Colorants** give the product its characteristic color. Vegetable, mineral, or animal dyes or pigments may be used without specific government approval. Coal tar derivative dyes, however, must undergo a long and expensive certification process before they can go into skin-care products. Certified colorants are listed as FD&C (Food, Drug and Cosmetic) colors, D&C colors or ext. D&C colors. FD&C colors can be used in food, drugs and cosmetics. D&C colors are only for use in drugs and cosmetics. Ext. D&C colors are for external use only in drugs and cosmetics.
- **Defoaming agents** keep the ingredients in the product from foaming during formulation. Simethicone is one of the chemicals used for this purpose.
- **Deodorizers** eliminate unpleasant or unwanted smells from the product. Chlorophyll and urea are used as deodorizers.
- **Emollients** soften and soothe the skin. There are many different emollients used in skin-care products. They may be greasy or nongreasy, depending on whether the melting point is low or high. And they may be natural, for example, aloe vera, coconut oil, or lanolin, or they may be synthetic, for example, acetylated lanolin alcohol, cetyl acetate, or myristal myristate.
- **Emulsifiers** let oil and water be mixed together in a product without separating on standing. The oil/water mixture is called an emulsion. If a smaller amount of oil is mixed with a larger amount of water, the emulsion is called an oil-in-water, or O/W emulsion; conversely, if a smaller amount of water is mixed with a larger amount of oil, the emulsion is called a water-in-oil, or W/O emulsion. Commonly used emulsifiers include glyceryl stearate, polysorbate 80, and triethanolamine (TEA).

- **Extenders** are added to the product to increase its volume. They may also serve to dilute the product. Water and petrolatum are two examples.
- **Fixatives** retard the vaporization of the components of fragrances, so that the desired odors last longer. Musk and civet are commonly used as fixatives.
- **Foaming agents** are added to products, usually cleansers and shampoos, to make them foam during use. Dodecylbenzene sulfonic acid is one example.
- **Fragrances** give the product its characteristic odor. Many different substances, both natural and synthetic, are used for their ability to provide a pleasant aroma in skin-care products. Most fragrances added to products are complex blends of ingredients, whose compositions are kept secret by the manufacturers. Because of their proprietary nature, the FDA does not require that the ingredients in fragrances be listed on the label. Only the word, "fragrance," is necessary.

  A good quality fragrance operates on three levels, or **notes**. The **top-note,** or first impression, is the most volatile portion and vaporizes first. This leaves the **body-note,** or the major characteristic of the fragrance, which vaporizes more slowly. Finally, after all the volatile components have vaporized, the fragrance is left with the **bottom-note.**
- **Healing agents** promote healing or soothing of the skin, provide antiseptic properties and reduce or help prevent inflammation. Many herbs, such as aloe, yarrow, and chamomile, are used because of their healing powers, as are some vitamins, such as biotin and retinol. Minerals, such as zinc oxide, and chemicals, such as urea, are also used for their healing and soothing properties.
- **Humectants** retard moisture loss in the product, especially if the container is left open. When the product is put on the skin, the humectants in the product help trap moisture and hold it in the skin. Commonly used humectants include glycerin, sorbitol, and propylene glycol.
- **Lubricants** provide a coating on the skin to reduce friction and wear. Mineral oil, cocoa butter, and isopropyl myristate are among the substances used for lubrication.
- **Moisturizing agents** help the skin absorb and retain moisture. Aloe is a widely used moisturizing agent, as is safflower oil.
- **Opacifiers** (oh-PASS-i-feyers) make the product milky, so that light is not transmitted through it. Cetyl alcohol and stearyl alcohol are often used for this purpose.
- **Preservatives** are chemical or natural agents that kill harmful bacteria, fungi, and yeasts, to prevent discoloration, putrefaction,

or property changes in the product. They also help prevent infection. They help insure the long-term stability of the products and keep them safe to use. The parabens are the most commonly used preservatives in skin-care products. Methyl paraben is used for the water phase elements; propyl paraben is used for the oil phase elements. Imidazolindyl urea is also used widely as a preservative. Most skin-care products contain a number of different preservatives, since no single preservative protects against all types of microorganisms. Isothiazolone, however, a relatively new microbicide, is gaining wide application in skin-care and cosmetic products because it controls a greater variety of bacteria, fungi, and yeasts than other microbicides.

- **Sequestering agents** retard changes in the appearance of the product, especially its color or texture. In this respect, sequestering agents are a type of preservative. However, they work by chemical reaction rather than by attacking microorganisms. Tetrasodium pyrophosphate (TSPP) and ethylenediamine tetraacetic acid (EDTA) are common sequestering agents.

- **Solvents** are used to dissolve or disperse the other ingredients in a product. Water is the most common solvent. Other solvents include alcohol, acetone, and methyl ethyl ketone.

- **Stabilizers** maintain the equilibrium of the product, keeping it in balance and preventing its characteristics from changing. Among the many stabilizers used in skin-care products are borax, polysorbate 80 and cetyl alcohol.

- **Surfactants** (sur-FACK-tunts) reduce the surface tension of the product, allowing it to spread and penetrate more easily. Surfactants are also known as wetting agents. Sodium laureth sulfate and dioctyl succinate are two surfactants used in skin-care products.

- **Texturizers** are added to products to enhance their texture, that is, to make them smoother. Calcium chloride and biotin (vitamin H) are texturizers.

- **Thickeners** give body to the product. Among the commonly used thickeners are bentonite, carbomer 934, stearic acid, and cellulose gum.

- **Vehicles** are the carriers for the other ingredients and, in most cases, account for the largest portion of the product. Water is the most commonly used vehicle, although alcohol or other solvents may also be used.

LABELING

By law, under the jurisdiction of the Food and Drug Administration, all cosmetic products must list all ingredients on the label. The ingredients are listed in descending order according to the amount of the ingredient contained in the product. It is not necessary, however, to list the actual amount of each substance.

A typical cleanser, for example, lists the following ingredients: deionized water, sodium laureth sulfate, aloe extract, lauramide DEA, polysorbate 80, cetyl acetate, acetylated lanolin alcohol, hydrolyzed animal protein, allantoin, chickweed extract, chapparal extract, methylparaben, imidazolidinyl urea, propylparaben, FD&C yellow no. 5, fragrance.

Deionized water, the ingredient present in the greatest quantity, is the vehicle. The water carries the rest of the ingredients, dispersing them evenly throughout the product. Deionization removes minerals from the water and makes it softer. All water used in cosmetic products is sterile.

Sodium laureth sulfate is the major cleansing agent in this product. It is also a surfactant. This substance is the salt of lauryl alcohol, which is synthesized from cocoanut oil.

Aloe extract is an emollient and healing agent to soothe and soften the skin. This is the juice from the aloe vera plant, a member of the lily family from South Africa.

Lauramide DEA is a foaming agent and a softener. This chemical comes from lauric acid, a fatty acid of cocoanut oil.

Polysorbate 80 is an emulsifier and stabilizer and comes from the reaction of sorbitol and oleic acid.

Cetyl acetate is also an emulsifier and stabilizer. This compound is the salt of cetyl alcohol, a waxy solid.

Acetylated lanolin alcohol is an emollient and emulsifier, and is derived from lanolin, a product of sheep wool. Acetylated means that the lanolin has been treated with acetic anhydride to remove all of its water, making it repel water and stay on the skin.

Hydrolyzed animal protein is used to smooth and protect the skin. Hydrolysis partly turns the protein to water, allowing it to penetrate the skin more readily.

Allantoin is a healing and soothing agent taken from the herb comfrey. Chickweed is an anti-inflammatory agent and antiseptic. Chaparral is also an antiseptic and a cleansing agent.

Methylparaben is a preservative used as a bactericide for the water phase of an emulsion. It is an ester of hydroxybenzoic acid.

Imidazolidinyl urea is also a preservative, effective against a wide variety of bacteria and useful over a broad pH range. This substance is derived from urea.

Propylparaben is another preservative used as a fungicide and as a bactericide for the oil phase of an emulsion. It is also an ester of hydroxybenzoic acid. The two parabens are the most often used preservatives in skin-care products.

FD&C yellow no. 5 is a colorant. As a coal tar derivative, it must be certified by the FDA as acceptable for use on a batch to batch basis.

Fragrance gives the product a pleasant aroma. As mentioned earlier, because of their complexity and their proprietary nature, the components of fragrances do not have to be listed.

PRODUCT CATEGORIES

The products with which the esthetician works are cleansers, toners, moisturizers, night creams, masks, and treatment products. Each of these categories plays an important role in skin care. And each is available in numerous formulations from a number of manufacturers.

Cleansers are used to rid the skin of dirt and other impurities, such as dead cells, makeup and excess sebum. An effective cleanser cleans both the surface of the skin and the pores. Soaps, which are highly alkaline, dry the skin and strip it of its acid mantle. Cleansers, however, are not so alkaline. They cleanse the skin thoroughly, removing dirt and impurities without drying the skin or stripping it of its protective oils. Unlike soaps, which can leave a dulling film on the surface of the skin, properly formulated cleansers rinse off the skin easily (Fig. 12.4).

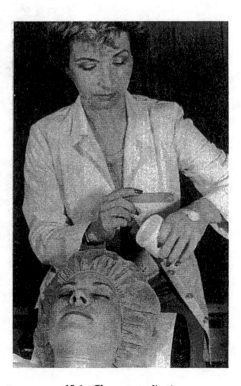

12.4—Cleanser application

Toners are used to complete the cleansing process. They remove all traces of the cleanser and help restore the acid mantle. And they refresh the skin. There are three types of toner. **Astringents** (a-STRINJ-ents) are designed for oily skins and generally contain alcohol to dissolve excess oil. **Toners** are used on dry skin and do not contain alcohol or other drying ingredients. **Fresheners** are for normal skin (Fig. 12.5).

Moisturizers help prevent the loss of moisture from the skin and help protect the skin from the environment. They also soften the skin, and by keeping it moist, slow the effects of aging. To be effective, a moisturizer must contain oils and emollients as well as water.

Developed primarily for daytime use, moisturizers deposit a thin film on the surface of the skin. This film, consisting of the oily component of the product, stays on the surface and has no ability to penetrate to the deeper layers. The barrier formed by the film holds the moisture in the skin. But oil has no ability to soften skin, so the emollients and water phases of the product actually do the softening.

Night creams are similar to moisturizers in that they also help retard moisture loss. Unlike moisturizers, however, which are designed to protect the skin, night creams are designed to help repair

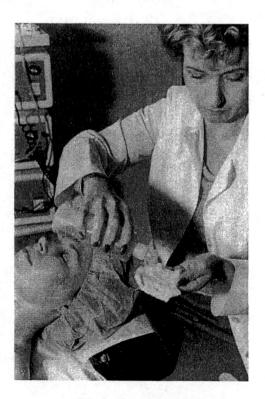

12.5—Application of toner

skin damage. Night creams contain relatively high levels of healing agents and are formulated to penetrate into the skin. The ingredients in these products soothe, help restore cellular function, and nourish the skin.

In contrast to day moisturizers, which are used while the client is active and can be worn under makeup, the more powerful night creams are meant to be used while the client is at rest and should not be covered with other cosmetics.

Masks are among the most important tools the esthetician has at his or her disposal. There are many different types of facial masks available, each with a specific purpose. There are tightening masks, which help tighten and tone sagging skin; drawing masks, which absorb excess oils; and moisturizing masks, which add moisture to the skin. Depending on the formulation, a mask can soothe the skin, oxygenate, improve the circulation, nourish, help clear blemishes, or reduce fine lines and wrinkles for a short time. Masks can be hard or soft. Masks are covered thoroughly in the next chapter.

Treatment products actually cover a wide variety of products having many different purposes. What they all have in common, however, is their use to treat specific skin conditions. They are the special purpose tools in the esthetician's repertoire (Fig. 12.6).

The **exfoliation products,** the **scrubs** and **peels,** may be considered as "super cleansers." These products remove impurities from the pores and slough off dead surface cells, while stimulating and improving the circulation of the skin. The scrubs contain small granules that are mild abrasives. The abrasive action, when the granules are rubbed off, removes the dirt and dead cells, leaving the skin

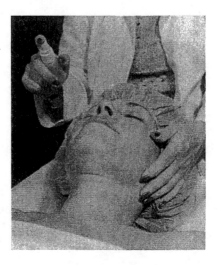

12.6—Application of treatment product

clean and glowing. The peels, on the other hand, contain enzymes that "digest" the dead skin cells. They have little or no abrasive action. Unlike chemical peels that may be used only by dermatologists or plastic surgeons and remove layers of living skin, these peels work only on the surface of the skin and are safe.

Eye and throat creams provide nutrients and lubrication to these areas, which have little natural oil of their own. These products are useful on clients with dry or aging skin.

Oil absorbers are formulated to absorb excess oil and are useful on clients with oily or blemished skin. They may be used in place of moisturizers on these types of skin.

There are many other treatment products, as well. Some are "super moisturizers." Others provide nutrients, increase oxygenation, help rejuvenate skin, or help in the formation of new cells. They may contain a variety of ingredients, including collagen, elastin, vitamins, herbs, essential oils, or proteins. They contain high levels of the active ingredients for maximum potency and are available as creams and lotions or, in some cases, in ampoule form where they are highly concentrated.

REVIEW QUESTIONS

1. Why must the esthetician know about skin-care products?
2. Why is it important to use the correct formulation for the client's skin type?
3. Why should the esthetician ask the client about food or drug allergies?
4. When the esthetician is not sure about using a product on a client, what should he or she do first?
5. What ingredient is the most likely cause of allergic reactions in skin-care products?
6. What is the difference between a cream and a liquid?
7. What functions does the package perform?
8. What are ampoules?
9. What is an active ingredient?
10. From where do ingredients in skin-care products derive?
11. What is an antioxidant?
12. What is a FD&C colorant?
13. What is an emollient?
14. What are the three levels on which a fragrance operates?
15. What is a humectant?
16. What is a sequestering agent?
17. What is the vehicle?
18. What is the FDA labeling law?
19. What kinds of products does the esthetician work with?
20. What is the function of a moisturizer?

13 Facial Masks

OBJECTIVES   *After completing this chapter, you should be able to:*

❶ Discuss functions and types of facial masks.
❷ Describe the ingredients utilized and how masks are used in the salon.
❸ Provide information on facial masks for home use.

INTRODUCTION   T he facial mask can be considered a transition step between the cleansing aspect of the facial and the normalization aspect. Masks, depending on the type, perform both functions. Masks are used to remove impurities from the skin, to absorb oils, to tighten, to nourish, to soothe or to stimulate the skin.

Facial masks are one of the world's oldest beauty aids, having been used since antiquity. Women have long used clays, muds, and creams on their faces to cleanse and tone their skin. In *The Arts and Secrets of Beauty,* Madame Lola Montez, the noted nineteenth-century courtesan, spoke of her contempories who "used to bind their faces, every night on going to bed, with thin slices of raw beef, which is said to keep the skin from wrinkles, while it gives a youthful freshness and brilliancy to the complexion."

In these modern times, the esthetician still relies on many of the substances used in facial masks since antiquity—muds and clays, herbs, essential oils, milk, etc. Now, however, up-to-date production techniques and the scientific application of chemical principles have added many refinements to the old materials and have introduced many new materials to the esthetician's tool kit. Today, the esthetician has an almost staggering number of commercially available products to use as facial masks, making it a relatively simple matter to choose a mask best suited to the client's needs.

Even though there are a large number of commercially available masks, many are similar in formulation and function. The esthetician cannot use them all. He or she should read the manufacturer's literature to determine which masks may be most suitable for use, then test as many of them as possible. Finally, the esthetician should settle on those few that match specific requirements and methods of working.

Although it is possible for the esthetician to make facial masks from a number of natural products, it is almost always better to use commercially available masks. There are a number of sound reasons for this:

1. It draws on the vast research and knowledge of the manufacturers and their formulation expertise.
2. Batch-to-batch variations in the product are eliminated.
3. It reduces the likelihood of contamination due to spoilage of the raw materials.
4. It lessens the risk of infections or adverse reactions.
5. It, therefore, lowers the risk of liability suits against the esthetician.
6. It places the burden of product liability on the manufacturer.
7. It shows the client a more professional approach to skin care.

FUNCTIONS OF FACIAL MASKS

Depending on type, facial masks perform a variety of functions. Masks can be loosely classified as either tightening or conditioning. Most, but not all, tightening masks are hard; that is, they are applied as a paste, which dries and hardens. The primary action occurs during the drying phase. Most, but not all, conditioning masks are soft. That is, they are applied as a soft, moist paste and do not dry. The primary action occurs because of the active ingredients in the mask. Masks that harden are usually more difficult to remove than soft masks.

Hardening masks are generally used for cleansing and for toning up skin. They are most often used with normal to extremely oily skin types. Soft masks are generally used to nourish and normalize skin and are most often used with normal to extremely dry and mature skin types. It is important to remember, however, that any given facial mask may perform both hard and soft mask functions.

Tightening masks improve skin tone and texture and temporarily remove wrinkles and fine lines. They also refresh the skin. As the mask is applied, it has an initial cooling effect because of its moisture content. This cooling effect soothes the skin, which has just undergone a thorough cleansing. As the moisture evaporates, the materials in the mask form a film, which contracts as it dries. This contraction tightens the skin. At the same time, since the mask doesn't let the skin breathe, perspiration and sebum are kept from escaping and stay in the skin. This plumps up the skin. As a consequence, wrinkles and fine lines are removed, although this effect lasts only a relatively short time.

Excess oils, dead surface cells, and dirt, which have been loosened by the previous cleansing procedures, are absorbed by the mask material to provide additional cleansing. In addition, the action of the mask stimulates the circulation of blood in the blood vessels closest to the surface. This increased blood flow brings additional oxygen and nutrients to the skin. The mask treatment is also soothing and relaxing psychologically, since the client lies back and rests during the mask treatment.

As a result of all these effects, when the mask is removed, the skin has a radiant glow, it feels tighter, it looks better, and the client feels better.

Conditioning masks, which include tightening masks with added active ingredients, nourish the skin. They add minerals and vitamins to the skin, in addition to increasing the circulation. Some active ingredients help fight blemishes and soothe irritations and reduce inflammation. Others draw out impurities, while still others add moisture to the skin surface. These masks also have psychological benefits for the same reasons as discussed earlier. They also make the client look and feel better.

FACIAL MASK INGREDIENTS

Commercially available facial masks contain a wide variety of ingredients. The most commonly used ingredients are:

Clays   **Clays** are used as absorbing and tightening agents. They absorb excess oils, dirt, and surface debris and exert a drawing action for impurities. They also help form the film that contracts to tighten the skin. Some clays contain minerals that help remineralize the skin. The most commonly used clays are kaolin, bentonite, diatomaceous earth, and Fuller's earth.

Kaolin (KAY-oh-lin) is a yellowish-white powder composed of hydrated aluminum silicate. **Bentonite** is a white silicaceous clay. **Diatomaceous** (DY-ah-tow-may-shus) **earth**, also known as **kieselguhr** (KY-zel-goo-er), is a porous silica composed of the remains of diatoms, a single-celled form of algae. **Fuller's earth** is a brownish-white powder composed of aluminum magnesium silicate.

Gums
Gums are used as emulsifiers, binders and film formers. These materials form the tightening film as the mask dries on the face. They also hold the other ingredients together. The most commonly used of these agents are gum tragacanth, albumin, polyvinylpyrrolidone, and cellulose gums.

Gum tragacanth is a gel-forming exudate from a plant common to the Middle East. Albumin is a water soluble protein derived from egg whites. Polyvinylpyrrolidone is an albumin-like synthetic plastic resin. Cellulose gums are derived from the cell walls of plants. The forms used in commercial products, however, are produced synthetically.

Herbs
Herbs have many uses in skin care (Chapter 14). They perform the same detoxifying, normalizing, and building functions when used as an active ingredient in facial masks. Although almost any herb can be used, some of the more commonly found herbs and herbal extracts in commercial masks are aloe vera, camphor, chamomile, coltsfoot, comfrey, juniper tar, sage, and witch hazel.

Lubricants
Oils and creams are used in facial masks to lubricate the skin and also to act as emollients, softening dry skin. Commonly used lubricants include lanolin, vegetable oils, cod liver oil, and petrolatum. Lanolin is a water-absorbing wax derived from sheep oil. Vegetable oils include safflower oil, avocado oil, and corn oil. Cod liver oil is derived from fish. Petrolatum (pet-tro-LAT-tum) is derived from petroleum.

Minerals
In addition to clays, minerals used in facial masks include sulfur and zinc oxide. Sulfur is an antiseptic used in masks for blemished skin. Zinc oxide is also an antiseptic and is used in many masks to soothe the skin and tone down redness.

Moisturizers
Among the ingredients used in facial masks to moisturize the skin are glycerine, paraffin, and collagen. Glycerine is a humectant (hyoo-MEC-tant) derived as a by-product of soap manufacture and absorbs moisture from the air and holds it on the skin. Paraffin is a wax by-product of petroleum distillation and traps water and holds it on the skin. Collagen is a super moisturizer and comes from animal tissue.

Nutrients
A number of ingredients used in facial masks nourish the skin. Among these are vitamins, enzymes, wheat germ, and algaes. Vitamins A, B and E are especially good for the skin. Enzymes used

include **papain** (pay-PAHN), derived from papaya. **Wheat germ**
and **algaes** nourish and remineralize the skin.

FACIAL MASK APPLICATION

The facial mask is normally applied as the last step in the cleansing
process after brushing, steaming, massaging, disincrustation, and
manual extraction. At this stage of the facial, the skin is at its most
receptive to the action of the mask. As a transition step, the mask
completes the cleansing process and starts the process of normalization and treatment. The type of mask chosen depends on the needs
and skin type of the client. For combination skins, it may be necessary to use two different types of mask at the same time—one on the
oily areas and the other on the dry areas.

The amount of time the masks are left in place varies with the
type. In general, the hardening masks are left on slightly longer than
soft masks because of the time needed for them to dry. The normal
duration for a mask is seven to ten minutes. Some masks require
much longer time. Except when using the contour mask, the esthetician need not stay with the client while the mask is working. This
offers an opportunity to take a short break or catch up on
paperwork. Or the esthetician may perform an added service, such
as a hand treatment or a reflexology massage.

Commercially available facial masks may be classified in a number of types. Their ingredients may vary, but there is wide overlap in
the functions performed by the different types. By the same token,
the method of application of these different types of masks varies.
Regardless of type, however, the manufacturer's directions for use
should be followed.

Algae Masks   Algae masks nourish and remineralize the skin and are excellent for
use on dry and normal skin. Some variations may be used on oily
skins. Algae masks should not be used on clients who are allergic to
shellfish. These masks are available commercially as a prepared
creamy paste or as a powder, which is mixed with a small amount of
water or vegetable oil to make a paste.

The esthetician's hands should be clean before starting. A small
amount of the paste is removed from the jar or from the mixing bowl
with a spatula and placed on the back of the hand. The materials
should never be taken from the container with the hands. Starting at
the chin, a small quantity of mask material is transferred from the
back of the hand to the face with the fingers and spread evenly over
the face. The mask is applied by spreading upward. The face should
be covered thoroughly, but the mask should not be placed near the
eyes or on the lips. The neck should also be coated with mask

material. The mask should be allowed to dry. Once visibly dry, it may be removed by wiping gently with a warm, damp towel.

Clay and Mud Masks

Clay and mud masks absorb oil, draw impurities and tighten the skin. These masks are good for use on oily skin. With the addition of active ingredients such as sulfur, camphor or other herbs, they are also good for blemished skin. As with algae masks, they are commercially available as creamy pastes or powders and are applied the same way (Fig. 13.1).

Once they have dried, the clay masks are removed by softening them with the application of a hot, damp towel. The softened mask is then removed carefully by wiping the clay off with damp towels. Care must be taken not to stretch the skin while removing the mask. The mask must be removed thoroughly. Masks that harden, such as clay masks, are the most difficult types of mask to remove (Fig. 13.2).

Collagen Masks

A relatively new development in skin-care technology, collagen masks are super-moisturizing facial masks that add moisture to the skin and help smoothe fine lines and wrinkles. They are excellent for use on dry or dehydrated skin and are especially beneficial for mature skin.

The masks are available in the form of dried sheets of collagen.

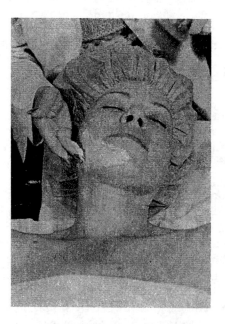

13.1—Application of clay mask

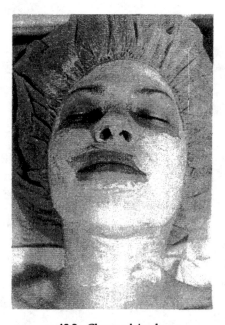

13.2—Clay mask in place

While dry, the collagen sheets have a long shelf life. For use, they are moistened with tepid water or with a treatment product and placed over the face. Once moistened, the sheets soften into a gel-like mass that can be molded to the exact contours of the face. The mask is left in place for twenty to thirty minutes, then peeled off. This type of mask comes off easily and leaves no residue.

The sheets are also available in pre-cut form with holes for eyes, nose and mouth already in place. As with virtually any mask, this material should not be placed directly over the eyes. Liquids other than tepid water can be used to moisten the mask. For example, essential oils, herbal extracts or other active ingredients may be used in conjunction with the collagen for added effect. Strips can be cut from the sheets for local application to selected areas of the face and neck.

The collagen sheets are more expensive than other types of masks and require more time to use. For these reasons, additional charges are warranted for their application.

Contour Masks

Contour masks firm and tighten the skin and remove fine lines and wrinkles on a temporary basis. These masks usually have a gum base for film forming and may contain enzymes and herbal extracts, as well. They are available in powder form and are mixed with water to form a gel. They are suitable for use on most skin types but should not be used on couperose areas or on skins that are sensitive.

The gel is applied to the face and neck with a soft brush, taking care to avoid the eye area. A thin line of skin at the top of the neck should also be left free of the mask material because of the contracting action of the mask. Once the mask is applied, the client should lie still and will be unable to talk while the mask is in place. Any movement of the mouth or excessive head movement will cause the mask to crack and diminish its effectiveness.

As the gel dries, the client will feel a pulsating action as the film tightens and contracts. The mask is left in place until this pulsating action stops. The time varies from client to client and may last from ten to thirty minutes. When the client no longer feels the mask working, the mask material is softened and removed with mild skin cleanser. Contour masks are somewhat difficult to remove.

It is important that the esthetician stay with the client while the mask is drying. As with the collagen masks, the added time and effort required to use this type of mask warrant additional charges for its application.

Cream Masks

There are many different kinds of cream masks, varying in their active ingredients. Most contain emollients, herbal extracts, and minerals for softening, nourishing, and moisturizing the skin. These are generally designed for use on dry, mature, and sensitive skins.

Some cream masks are medicated, containing antiseptics and healing agents. These include camphor, sulfur, juniper tar, or zinc oxide which soothe the skin and fight blemishes. These are generally designed for use on oily, blemished skins.

Cream masks are available as soft creams and remain soft after application. They are applied the same way as clay and algae masks. Since they don't harden, however, they are much easier to remove. They are removed by wiping off with a damp towel.

Paraffin Masks

Paraffin masks are used to tighten the skin and temporarily remove fine lines and wrinkles. They may be used on any type of skin except couperose and sensitive skins, but work best on dry and mature skin types.

About the only piece of equipment that may be required for facial masks is the paraffin bath. Paraffin bath tanks melt and hold paraffin wax at the proper temperature for use in hand and foot treatments or for paraffin facial masks (Fig. 13.3). The larger tanks are designed to let the client dip his or her hands or feet into the molten paraffin, letting it coat the extremity and trapping heat and moisture inside the wax glove thus formed. These tanks hold the paraffin at a temperature of about 134°F.

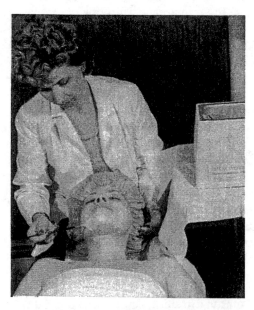

13.3—Application of paraffin mask

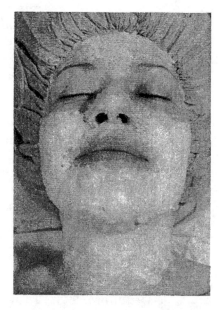

13.4—Paraffin mask in place

The smaller tank, used for paraffin facial masks, is designed to hold the molten wax in a semi-liquid state so it can be transferred to the client's face by brush. Because some heat is lost during the transfer, this tank operates at a slightly higher temperature, about 136°F.

At this temperature, the wax flows easily but is not too hot for the skin. The wax is applied by brushing it onto the face and neck, adding coat after coat until it is about ¼ inch thick. Wax should not be placed over the eyes or lips. The wax remains on the face until it cools. The time may be extended by shining a low intensity infrared lamp on the mask (Fig. 13.4).

The wax keeps the skin from breathing and prevents moisture loss from the skin to the atmosphere. At the same time, the heat causes perspiration. Since the moisture can't escape, it is reabsorbed into the skin, plumping the skin and filling in fine lines and wrinkles. The heat also causes the blood vessels near the surface of the skin to dilate, bringing increased blood flow and a greater supply of oxygen and nutrients to the skin.

Treatment creams may be applied to the skin before coating it with wax. The wax mask will increase the penetration of the creams. The wax may also be applied over a piece of gauze that has been cut in the shape of the face and has holes for the eyes, nose, and mouth. The gauze is dampened and molded to the contour of the face and neck and serves as a base to keep the melted wax from flowing too readily.

Once the paraffin has cooled, it may be removed by carefully stripping the wax from the skin. If gauze has been used as a base, the mask may be removed by simply lifting up the gauze. Wax masks are relatively easy to remove. The added time and effort required to use paraffin masks warrant additional charges for their application (Fig. 13.5).

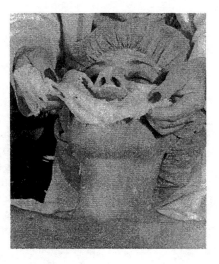

13.5—Paraffin mask removal

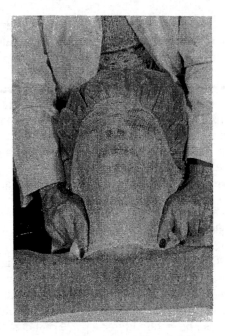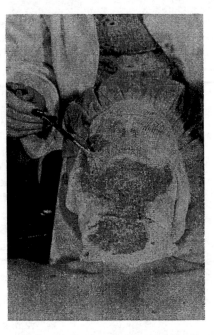

13.6—Use of gauze as mask base　　**13.7**—Application of wheat-germ mask

Wheat-Germ Masks

Consisting of powdered wheat germ and other ingredients, wheat-germ masks are used on all types of skin to nourish and revitalize the skin. They are commercially available in powder form and are mixed with equal parts of tepid water to form a paste that is applied to the skin.

Because of the runny consistency of the wheat-germ mask, it is best applied over gauze that has been cut to the shape of the face, dampened and molded to the facial contours. The gauze holds the wheat-germ paste in place, yet allows it to penetrate the skin (Fig. 13.6).

After the gauze is in place, the wheat-germ paste is spread over the entire face and neck in a thick layer. The paste should be applied with a soft bristle brush. As the wheat germ is mild and nourishing, it is just about the only type of mask that can be used over the eyes and lips. It is an excellent opportunity to revitalize and nourish these areas (Fig. 13.7 and Fig. 13.8).

The mask is left in place for five to ten minutes. The wheat-germ mask may be used in conjunction with gentle heat by steaming or by using an infrared lamp. The mask is removed simply by lifting up the gauze. Any residue may be removed by wiping with a damp towel (Fig. 13.9).

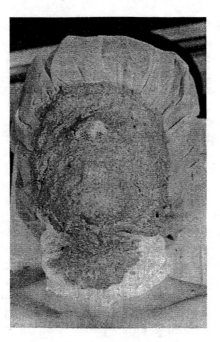

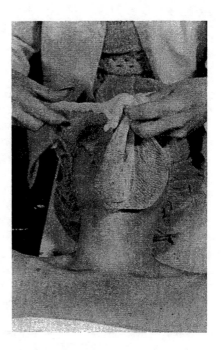

13.8—Wheat-germ mask in place   **13.9**—Wheat-germ mask removal

MASKS FOR HOME USE

Except for contour masks and paraffin masks, which should be applied only by estheticians trained in their application and use, most types of facial masks discussed here are also suitable for home use. The manufacturers of these masks usually package them in smaller sizes for retail sale as well as in the larger professional sizes. For the same reasons commercial masks should be used in the salon, the esthetician should have the client use commercially available masks as part of the home care regimen.

There may be occasions, however, when this cannot be done. For these occasions, the client may use a variety of fruits, vegetables, and herbs as masks for home use. The esthetician should be aware of these in order to advise the client on their proper use if the client insists on them.

Fruits and vegetables should be mashed to a pulp. They may be applied in that form or may be mixed into a paste with a small quantity of light vegetable oil, with wheat germ, brewer's yeast, or oatmeal. Pulps with a runny consistency should be applied over gauze to keep the mess to a minimum. Herbs may be made into a tea and applied to the skin with cloth compresses.

Most fruits and vegetables contain high levels of vitamins and nourish the skin. Acidic fruits such as strawberries, plums, grapefruit, and oranges are astringent and are good for use on oily skins. Lemons are beneficial, but may be too acidic for use at home. Other fruits, such as avocados, apricots, bananas, and peaches, are soothing and moisturizing and are most suitable for use on dry skin. Papaya and pineapple contain enzymes that help dissolve dead surface cells and remove surface impurities. In general, acidic fruits and vegetables are best used on normal to oily skin; nonacidic fruits and vegetables are best used on normal to dry skin.

Vegetables suitable for homemade masks include cucumbers, carrots, potatoes, spinach, and tomatoes. Cucumbers and potatoes are both hydrating and oil-absorbing and are suitable for both oily and dry skin. Carrots are hydrating and soothing and are best used on dry skin. Spinach and tomatoes are astringent and are best used on oily skin. Spinach is good on blemished skin.

Many of the herbs found in the home kitchen may be made into strong teas or poultices for use as home facial masks. These include fennel and celery seeds, which are soothing and cleansing; parsley and sage, which are astringent; rosemary and peppermint, which are stimulating and refreshing; and sesame and thyme, which are soothing and softening. Other herbs of value for home facial masks include aloe vera, comfrey, and chamomile.

Other products found in the kitchen are also beneficial when used on the skin. These include wheat germ, oatmeal, and brewer's yeast, which are nourishing and cleansing and can also be used as a base to carry fruit and vegetable pulps and herb teas. Yogurt and buttermilk are softening and cleansing as well as nourishing. Egg whites are tightening; egg yolks are nourishing and soothing. Honey is a natural moisturizer. Vinegar, especially cider vinegar, helps normalize skin functioning and restores the acid mantle of the skin. It is also astringent, yet can help soften skin.

Although the esthetician can inform the client of the possible benefits of these homemade facial masks, they cannot be guaranteed to be effective or even safe because their purity and use by the client are beyond the esthetician's control. The client should be warned to use any of these products carefully and to avoid those that may cause an allergic reaction. If an allergic reaction occurs, the client should discontinue use immediately.

REVIEW QUESTIONS

1. What is the relationship between the facial mask and the rest of the facial?
2. Why are masks used?
3. What are two reasons that estheticians should use commercially available masks in the salon?
4. What are the two classifications of masks?
5. Why are hardening masks used?

6. What do tightening masks do?
7. What do conditioning masks do?
8. What are some commonly used ingredients in masks?
9. How are clays used in masks?
10. What are some of the most commonly used herbs in masks?
11. Why is sulfur used in masks?
12. Why is the mask used after most cleansing operations have been finished?
13. What are the functions of algae masks?
14. What are collagen masks?
15. What are the functions of contour masks?
16. On what kinds of skin are herb-based cream masks generally used?
17. How do paraffin masks remove wrinkles?
18. What kinds of ingredients may be used for masks at home?
19. Why are pineapple and papaya effective ingredients?
20. What warnings should the esthetician give the client regarding the use of homemade masks?

14 Supplemental Techniques

OBJECTIVES *After completing this chapter, you should be able to:*

❶ Understand herbals and aromatherapy as they are used in the field of esthetics.

❷ Provide information about water therapy techniques, such as thalassotherapy and balneotherapy.

❸ Describe the practice of iridology.

INTRODUCTION

Skin care, to be practiced on a truly professional level, is a balance of many disciplines. It is no longer enough for the esthetician to merely know how to give a facial. Today's professional must be conversant with a number of supplemental techniques in order to take full care of the client's needs. The more the well-trained esthetician knows and understands these alternate disciplines, the better able he or she will be to practice and prosper in this exciting profession.

The esthetician may use such supplemental techniques as herbals, aromatherapy, thalassotherapy and balneotherapy, iridology, and advanced massage techniques, including accupressure, lymphatic drainage, and shiatsu. Although each will be discussed separately, it is important to remember that many of these alternate treatments overlap and are used in combination.

This chapter serves as an introduction to all of the disciplines except the massage techniques, which were discussed in Chapter 9. In practice, some of these treatments border on medical applications, and as such, may not be utilized by the esthetician. It is important, however, for the esthetician to have a basic understanding of the principles involved in these treatments, because of their impact on the care of the skin, even though they may not be applied personally. The information presented in this chapter is intended to provide a basis for that understanding.

HERBALS

The use of **herbs** (ERBS), i.e. plant materials, has its roots in antiquity. Every culture, even the most primitive, has a history of herbal medicine. Today, herbs are widely used throughout the world. Whether used as spices, as cosmetics, or as medicine, herbs play an important part in everyday life. Although the medical use of herbs has declined in our modern technological societies in favor of **allopathic** medicine, which relies on synthetic drugs, herbs remain valuable **homeopathic** remedies.

There are hundreds of different herbs used both singly and in combinations. Collectively, these herbs have a variety of properties. They soothe or stimulate, moisten or dry, tighten or ease. They heal, alleviate pain, dispel gas, cleanse, purify the blood. They arouse or diminish sexual desire. They are antiseptic, antibiotic, and disinfectant. They increase perspiration or decrease it. The list could go on and on.

As medicines, herbs **detoxify, normalize,** or **build.** Detoxifying herbs eliminate poisons from the body and help purify it. Normalizing herbs help correct imbalances in bodily functions that result in illness; thus, they let the body heal itself as opposed to synthetic drugs, which alleviate symptoms but may not eliminate the underlying cause of the illness. The building herbs strengthen the various organs of the body to help prevent further illnesses.

As homeopathic remedies, herbs work slowly. Allopathic remedies (i.e. synthetic drugs) work quickly. As an analogy, consider an illness as a mountain. There are two ways to level a mountain. It can be eroded by the action of rain and the elements slowly but gently, with no traces left or it can be blasted apart with dynamite, quickly but roughly, with rubble strewn about. Although they work slowly, herbs are thorough yet gentle and, for the most part, have few undesirable side effects. Synthetic drugs, on the other hand, work rapidly, but are rougher on the body's systems and can have a number of undesirable side effects.

Retinol A, for example, a widely used drug for treating acne, controls blemishes rapidly and effectively but has potentially harmful side effects, such as headache, nausea, and possible destruction of sebaceous glands. By careful use of skin-care products that contain a variety of herbs, the esthetician can control acne effectively, albeit more slowly, without side effects to the client. The drug treats the symptom of acne, the excess sebum. The herbs treat the underlying causes of acne and bring the body functions into balance so the reasons for the excess sebum are eliminated.

Admittedly, this example is overly simplified. It is important to remember that allopathic remedies are valuable and should be used when warranted. The esthetician should never suggest that the client stop taking medication prescribed by a physician and use herbal remedies instead.

Herbs are available from many sources. They may be picked in the wild, but this requires considerable time and expertise. Similarly, they may be grown in home gardens. This also requires time. For the esthetician, the more practical sources are the herb specialty stores and some manufacturers of skin-care products.

Herbs are most effective when they are used fresh. The fresh plant consists of the root, stem, leaf, and in the case of the flowering plants, flower and fruit; in the case of woody plants, bark. For a given herb, one or more parts of the plant may contain the active, or medicinal, ingredient. Fresh herbs must be used soon after they are picked since their effectiveness diminishes rapidly. For this reason, fresh herbs are harder for the esthetician to use.

To maintain long-term stability, herbs are often dried, then ground into powders for use. Although they lose some activity when dried, they remain efficacious for longer periods of time. They should be stored in dark, air-tight containers to prevent moisture absorption that could cause them to spoil.

Herbs may be prepared in a number of ways: as infusions, decoctions, poultices, fomentations, tinctures, or ointments.

- An **infusion** (in-FYOO-shun) is made by steeping the herb in boiling water, just as in making tea. (Herb teas are infusions.) The process of steeping extracts the vitamins and volatile ingredients from the plant. The liquid is then strained and can be taken internally or used externally.

- A **decoction** (de-COK-shun) is similar to an infusion, except the herb is boiled in the water instead of being steeped. This process extracts the mineral salts and bitter principles from the plant. As with infusions, the liquid must be strained before using.

- A **poultice** (POWL-tez) is made by bruising or crushing the herb and mixing the pulpy mass with a hot liquid or gummy substance to make a paste. The paste can be applied directly to the skin or wrapped in a hot, moist towel and wrapped around the body part to be treated.

- A **fomentation** (FO-men-ta-shun) is made by soaking a towel in a hot infusion or decoction and applying it to the body part to be treated. Fomentations are less effective than poultices because the application of the active ingredient is less direct.

- A **tincture** (TINK-chur) is made by soaking the herb in alcohol. The alcohol extracts the active ingredient from the plant. Tinctures keep for long periods of time. Tinctures meant for internal use must be made with grain alcohol. Those meant for external use only may be made with other alcohols.
- An **ointment** (OYNT-ment) is made by mixing the herb with a hot fat or petroleum jelly to make a thick cream or salve. The salve is spread on the area of the body to be treated. Ointments are for external use only.

Although herbs may be used both internally and externally, the esthetician will be concerned only with the external applications. Except for serving various herb teas in the salon, for purposes of refreshment only, the esthetician should never administer any herb preparation internally to a client.

There are literally hundreds of herbs that have application in skin care. It is beyond the scope of this chapter to cover any but the most commonly used plants. Different herbs have different properties and affect the skin in different ways. Some are astringent, some cleansing, some purifying, some healing. Some herbs tighten skin; others ease tightness. Some stimulate; others soothe (Table 14.1).

Many herbs perform more than one function. Also, many herbs work in synergy. Combining herbs produces effects far in excess of the effect of each herb individually. The sum of the herbal effectiveness is greater than the total of the parts. Because of their effectiveness, a number of herbs are used in commercial skin-care preparations. Among the most commonly used herbs are:

- **Acacia** (ah-KAY-she-a), also known as **gum arabic,** is a small tree common to tropical Africa. The useful part of the plant is the gum that exudes from the stem. Acacia soothes and softens skin. As a gum, it often serves as a binder for other ingredients in skin-care preparations.
- **Almond** is a tree grown in many parts of the world. The kernels of the nut are the most useful part of the plant. Almonds are emollients that help smooth rough skin while moisturizing. Ground almond meal makes a good cleansing scrub.
- **Aloe vera** is a spiny, cactus-like plant native to east and south Africa, although it is cultivated in other tropical areas. The gel is extracted from the leaves. Aloe is healing and soothing. It helps reduce inflammation. It moisturizes the skin and helps slow the outward appearance of aging. This herb has become one of the most popular herbs used in skin care.
- **Arnica** is a **perennial** (pe-REN-ee-al) plant found in the northern latitudes. The flowers and roots are the useful parts of the plant. Arnica helps skin function normally by stimulating circulation

TABLE 14.1—Commonly Used Herbs

HERB	PROPERTIES	REMARKS
Acacia	astringent, healing, tightening, stimulating, nourishing	also known as gum arabic
Almond	cleansing, moisturizing	good anti-wrinkle agent, blackhead remover
Aloe	healing, soothing, moisturizing, softening	good for all types of skin especially dry skin
Arnica	astringent, healing	good for circulation
Balm Mint	soothing, stimulating	
Birch	astringent, healing	good on damaged and blemished skin
Chamomile	astringent, soothing, cleansing, anti-inflammatory	good for blackhead removal, good anti-wrinkle agent
Coltsfoot	healing, soothing	good on couperose skin
Comfrey	healing, softening, cell regenerator	good for blackhead removal, good for damaged skin
Cucumber	astringent, drying, tightening	good for oily skin
Echinacea	astringent, healing	
Grape	soothing, healing	good for dry skin
Horsetail	astringent, tightening, drying, stimulating	good for oily skin
Houseleek	healing, nourishing	good for blackhead removal, good on blemished skin
Lady's Mantle	astringent, drying, healing, cleansing, anti-inflammatory	good for oily skin, good anti-wrinkle agent
Lemon	astringent, drying, healing, soothing	good for oily skin, good for blackhead removal
Marigold	healing, moisturizing, softening, soothing	good for circulation, good anti-wrinkle agent, good for couperose skin
Marshmallow	healing, soothing, softening	good on damaged skin
Rosemary	astringent, cleansing, stimulating, antiseptic	good for circulation
Sage	astringent, healing, tightening, soothing	good for oily skin
St. John's Wort	astringent, healing, antiseptic	
Witch Hazel	astringent, drying, antiseptic	
Yarrow	astringent, drying, stimulating	good for oily skin, good for blackhead removal

and helping remove waste materials. It is an astringent and aids in the healing process.

- **Balm,** also known as **balm mint,** is a perennial plant found in the Mediterranean and Near East countries as well as in the United States. The leaves are the most important part, although most of the plant may be utilized as well. A member of the mint family, balm is, at the same time, both soothing and stimulating to the skin.

- **Birch,** also called **white birch,** is a tree common to the northern United States and Canada. The bark is the most important part, although the young leaves may also be useful. The herb is soothing and healing and acts as an astringent. The active ingredient in birch bark is **salicylic acid,** which is the major component of aspirin.

- **Chamomile** (KAM-e-myl) is a perennial plant found throughout Europe. The flowers are the important part of the plant. Chamomile softens and heals the skin and is an astringent. The active ingredient in chamomile is **azulene,** an anti-irritant and anti-inflammatory agent.

- **Coltsfoot** is a perennial plant found in wet areas in the United States and Europe. The leaves and the flowers are the important parts. Coltsfoot soothes and heals the skin. It acts on the capillaries near the surface of the skin, making it good for use on couperose skin.

- **Comfrey** is a perennial plant common to the United States and Europe. The roots are the most important part of the plant. Comfrey softens the skin and helps heal wounds and bruises. It also helps stimulate tissue growth. The active ingredient of comfrey is **allantoin.**

- **Cucumber,** the fruit of the common garden plant, is an important plant for skin care. Cucumber juice is an astringent that softens, moisturizes, and nourishes the skin.

- **Echinacea,** a mid-western perennial plant, has antiseptic properties and is useful as a blood purifier. Like all herbs that purify the blood, echinacea can be effective for use on skin conditions such as eczema and acne. The root is the part of the plant used.

- **Elder,** a shrub native to many parts of the world in a variety of forms, has healing properties. An astringent, it stimulates circulation and tightens skin. Roots, leaves and flowers all contribute to skin care.

- **Horsetail** is an annual plant native to North and South America. The leaves have astringent properties. Horsetail is stimulating and drying and helps tighten the skin. It helps promote elasticity and rejuvenates the skin.

- **Houseleek,** a perennial European plant, is astringent and cooling. Juice from the leaves is healing and soothing for a number of skin conditions.
- **Lady's Mantle,** a perennial plant found in damp areas in North America and Europe, is healing and anti-inflammatory. It is an astringent and natural cleanser. The entire plant can be used.
- **Lemon,** the citrus fruit common to Florida and California, is an effective astringent and cleanser for the skin. It has healing and drying properties and helps hydrate surface cells. Pure lemon juice may be too acidic for direct application to the skin and should be diluted with water.
- **Marigold,** also known as **calendula,** is an annual garden plant. The leaves and flowers have antiseptic and healing properties and help soften skin. Marigold helps detoxify and nourish skin cells.
- **Marshmallow** is a plant found in waste areas in Europe and North America. It is a lubricant and softener for the skin, and has healing and soothing properties. The entire plant can be used.
- **Rosemary,** a cultivated shrub, is an antiseptic and stimulant for the skin. It decongests surface tissue and helps heal the skin.
- **Sage,** a perennial plant found in the Mediterranean area, is an astringent and antiseptic. It is healing and is effective in reducing perspiration. The leaves are the parts of the plant used medicinally. Sage and rosemary are common kitchen spices.
- **St. Johnswort,** a perennial shrub native to the East and West Coasts of the United States, is an astringent and antiseptic with healing properties. It is useful on irritated or injured skin. The entire plant is used.
- **Wild Oregon grape** is an evergreen shrub found in lower mountainous areas of the Pacific Northwest. The roots are effective as a blood purifier and, as such, can be effective with a number of skin conditions, including acne, eczema, and psoriasis.
- **Witch hazel,** a shrub that grows in wooded areas in Canada and the eastern part of the United States, is one of the best known herbs used in skin care. The leaves and bark are astringent and antiseptic and have healing properties.
- **Yarrow,** also known as **milfoil,** is a perennial plant found throughout the world. It is astringent and drying and stimulates the circulation, thus is used to help improve the functioning of the skin tissue.

AROMATHERAPY

Aromatherapy (ah-ROW-ma-ther-ah-pee) is akin to herbal therapy in that it is a branch of plant medicine. Like herbal therapy, aromatherapy is based on the use of plant materials. Rather than using the various parts of the plant, however, aromatherapy utilizes the essential oils derived from those plants. Aromatherapy is easier for the esthetician to utilize in practice than herbal therapy, since the essential oils are concentrated and penetrate the skin. As with herbs, the esthetician should only use essential oils externally.

An **essential oil** is a **phytohormone** (fy-tow-HOR-mone), or plant hormone, and serves the same function in the plant that animal hormones serve in the human body. In the plant, the essential oil functions as a bactericide; it assists in photosynthesis; it repels pests; and it assists in cross-pollenization. The characteristic smell of the plant comes from the essential oils it contains. The purpose of the odor is to attract insects that carry pollen from other plants. Once the plant is pollenated, it stops emitting the scent, since it no longer needs to attract insects. The essential oils are then reabsorbed into the plant to serve other purposes.

Essential oils are soluble in fats or alcohols. They are highly volatile and aromatic. Oils are obtained from the plant in a number of ways. The most common method is **steam distillation**, in which the plant is steamed to separate the oil from the rest of the plant. Oils may also be extracted with solvents or they may be pressed out of the plant by applying pressure. Since essential oils are soluble in fats, two methods of extraction with fat are used. These are **enfleurage**, in which the plant is placed on beds of fat, where the oils are absorbed, and **maceration**, in which the plants are bathed in hot fat.

Essential oils have four basic properties that make them important in skin care. They are germicidal; they stimulate or calm; they penetrate; and they contain phytohormones. Essential oils contain aldehydes, esters, and phenols. They are natural antiseptics, germicides, and fungicides. All essential oils, regardless of their other characteristics, have this ability to kill bacteria and fungi. In many cases, they are more effective than manufactured chemical antiseptics; yet, unlike the chemical substances, are generally harmless to human tissue.

Approximately 20 percent of all essential oils are soothing. These oils act as **vasoconstrictors**, causing the blood vessels to constrict, thus slowing the flow of blood and oxygen. About 80 percent of all essential oils are stimulating. These act as **vasodilators**, causing the blood vessels to expand, thus increasing the flow of blood and oxygen. Because of their effect on the circulatory system, essential oils are helpful in correcting skin problems associated with poor circulation.

Essential oils also have the ability to penetrate the skin and be absorbed throughout the body. Thus, aromatherapy massage affects not only the skin, but also the organs beneath the skin in the areas in which the oils are placed. The essential oils can also act as carriers for other molecules the esthetician may want to penetrate the skin.

TABLE 14.2—Commonly Used Essential Oils

OIL	PROPERTIES	REMARKS
Basil Oil	antiseptic, stimulating, decongesting	
Benzoin	soothing, healing	useful on red, dry, itching skin
Cajuput	antiseptic, soothing, healing	useful for acne and psoriasis
Chamomile	soothing, healing, anti-inflammatory	useful with sensitive skin
Eucalyptus	antiseptic, germicide	
Geranium	soothing, healing, anti-inflammatory, decongestant	useful on sores, burns, and dry eczema
Hyssop	healing	useful with eczema
Juniper	antiseptic, healing, stimulating	useful for acne, weeping eczema, and psoriasis
Lavender	soothing, healing, anti-inflammatory	useful for acne, eczema, and psoriasis
Neroli	soothing, healing	
Rosemary	healing, germicide	useful for sores and burns
Sandalwood	soothing, healing, anti-inflammatory	
Ylang-Ylang	soothing, antiseptic	

The phytohormones contained in the essential oils supplement the natural hormones in the body, helping them work more effectively (Table 14.2).

Just as there are many herbs of use to the esthetician, so are there many essential oils of value in skin care. And, like herbs, many essential oils work best in combination, so that synergy comes into play. Essential oils may be purchased individually or in pre-mixed combinations designed for use on various types of skin. Among the essential oils of value to the esthetician are:

- **Basil** oil is greenish-yellow in color and contains the active ingredient, **linalol.** It is a general antiseptic and, like all essential oils, has disinfectant properties. It stimulates the skin and helps decongest pores.
- **Benzoin,** from the gum of an east Indian tree, is reddish-brown in color and contains **benzoic acid** as its active ingredient. Benzoin soothes the skin and helps promote healing for red, dry or itching skin.

- **Cajuput** oil, from a tree common to the Philippines and Malaysia, contains **cineol** and **terpineol.** It is a general antiseptic and healing agent and helps calm the skin. It is useful against acne and psoriasis.
- **Chamomile** oil, blue to greenish-blue in color, contains **azulene** as its principal active ingredient. Chamomile oil soothes the skin and helps promote healing. It is an excellent anti-inflammatory agent and is useful on sensitive skin.
- **Eucalyptus** (yoo-ka-LIP-tus) oil, a clear liquid, contains **eucalyptol** and **tannin** as its principal active ingredients. It is an effective bactericide and parasiticide and helps disinfect sores and wounds.
- **Geranium** oil, a clear to light green essence, contains terpenes and linalol as its active ingredients. It is an anti-inflammatory agent and soothes and helps heal the skin. It is useful against sores and burns and is effective against dry eczema. Geranium oil can be used with any type of skin but is especially good on congested, oily skin.
- **Hyssop** (HIS-ep) oil, a light yellow essence, contains borneol and cetone. It is a healing agent and is useful for various skin disorders, including eczema.
- **Juniper** oil, light greenish-yellow in color, contains borneol and terpineol. It is an effective antiseptic and healing agent, and stimulates the circulation. Juniper oil is useful against acne, weeping eczema, and psoriasis. It is also good for cleansing and toning oily skin.
- **Lavender** oil, a clear liquid containing linalol and geraniol among its principal active ingredients, is one of the most useful essences. Lavender oil is a soothing and healing agent and has anti-inflammatory properties. It is useful for many skin disorders, including acne, eczema and psoriasis. This essence is also effective in promoting cell regeneration and is often used in skin-rejuvenating agents. It may be used effectively on all skin types.
- **Neroli** oil, also known as orange blossom oil, is a pale yellow liquid extracted from seville orange flowers. Its principal active ingredients are linalol and geraniol. It has soothing and healing properties and is useful on all types of skin. Like lavender oil, neroli helps cell regeneration.
- **Rosemary** oil, a clear liquid, contains pinene and cineol among its ingredients. It is a healing agent and parasiticide. It is useful as an astringent and toner for the skin, and is effective against burns and sores.
- **Sandalwood** oil, a thick greenish-yellow liquid, contains terpenes. This oil is one of the most useful essences for skin care and may be used on all skin types. It is an antiseptic and healing agent and is effective in relieving itching and inflammation. It also acts as an astringent.

- **Ylang-ylang** (ee-lanj-EE-lanj) oil, a light yellow liquid, contains geraniol, linalol and salicylic acid. It is antiseptic and soothing to the skin. Although it can be used with any skin type, it is especially effective on oily skin.

THALASSOTHERAPY

Thalassotherapy (tha-lass-o-THER-uh-pee) is the technique of using sea water and sea products for the care of the skin. In its most broad form, thalassotherapy is concerned with whole body care and, by its extensive practice in health spas around the world, is primarily a medical specialty. Thus, spa treatments include Scotch hose treatments, tub treatments, reeducation pool treatments, and algae packs (Fig. 14.1). **Balneotherapy** (bal-nee-o-THER-uh-pee) is similar to thalassotherapy, except it utilizes fresh water instead of sea water.

Scotch hose treatments involve the use of high pressure hoses, from which jets of hot (i.e., body temperature) sea water are played along the main lymphatic channels. The hot water dilates the blood vessels while the pressure massages the deep muscle tissue and promotes lymphatic drainage.

The **thalassotherapy tub** is filled with hot sea water. While the client relaxes in the tub, air bubbles gently massage the lymphatic system and water jets massage the deeper tissues. The **reeducation pool** is used for physical therapy in which the client performs various exercises in the pool of hot sea water. The water displaces body

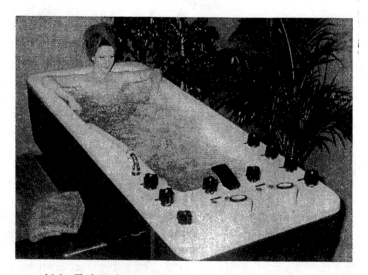

14.1—Thalassotherapy tub *(Courtesy of Etablissements Doyer)*

TABLE 14.3—Composition of
sea water

ELEMENT	AMOUNT (g/l)
Chlorine	19.00
Sodium	10.50
Magnesium	1.35
Sulfur	0.89
Calcium	0.40
Potassium	0.38
Bromine	0.07
Carbon	0.03
Strontium	0.008
Boron	0.005
Silicon	0.003
Fluorine	0.001

weight. The hydrostatic pressure of the water allows penetration of the marine ions from the sea water.

In the **algae pack treatment,** algae is mixed with sea water to make a thick paste. The paste is spread along the client's spine and covered with paraffin. The client then lies under heat lamps for 30 to 45 minutes. The spinal column is chosen as the site of the treatment because the spine contains the bones closest to the surface of the body and major arteries and veins pass along the column. The marine ions diffuse quickly and penetrate more rapidly into the body from this area.

All of these treatments promote detoxification of the tissues and remineralize the body. In the spas, these treatments are conducted by highly trained and skilled technicians.

While thalassotherapy at the spa level is beyond the scope of most estheticians, the use of sea water and sea products still has a valuable place in skin care. Marine clays, algaes, and sea plants can be used effectively to cleanse and revitalize skin tissue (Table 14.3).

All life came from the sea. The composition of sea water is identical to the composition of the natural fluids of the body. Sea water contains, in the same proportions, all of the trace elements, vitamins, amino acids, and minerals that are necessary to sustain life. Dr. Rene Quinton, a French physician, proved this in 1904 by bleeding a German shepherd to near death, then replacing the blood plasma with sea water. The dog survived with no apparent ill effects. Today, paramedics transfuse saline solution into accident victims during transport to hospitals.

The human body contains sixty to eighty-five percent water, depending on age. Children's bodies contain up to eighty-five percent water; older peoples' bodies, down to 60 percent, as aging is partly a process of drying out. The body fluids consist of **blood** (about five percent); **lymph** (about fifteen percent); **intercellular fluid** (about twenty-five percent); and **interstitial fluid** (about twenty-five percent). All cells continually bathe in water. And this water closely resembles sea water.

The products of the sea—seaweed, algae and sediments—also have beneficial properties, and are generally more readily available to the esthetician than sea water. Seaweed and algae accumulate and concentrate all of the materials contained in the ocean. One kilogram of seaweed (2.2 pounds) contains the same mineral wealth as 10,000 liters (2,500 gallons) of sea water. Sediments, such as clays and **peloids,** a blend of mud and oyster secretions, also contain many trace elements and minerals.

The marine plants, as used in skin care, perform a number of vital functions. They remineralize and rehydrate the skin, helping to retain moisture. They contain phytohormones, which are compatible with human hormones, and, thus, work in the same manner as essential oils and herbs. They are rich sources of **iodine**, which acts on the thyroid gland, helping it secrete more **thyroxin,** important to the body's immune system. Seaweed is very helpful in treating acne. Because of its iodine content, however, seaweed should not be used with clients who are allergic to shellfish.

Seaweed and algae stimulate circulation, thus aiding nutrition and detoxification of the cells. Clays and peloids, on the other hand, have a soothing and calming effect and help decongest pores. Sea products work especially well when used in conjunction with essential oils. Seaweeds and algae are also excellent dietary supplements.

IRIDOLOGY

Iridology (eye-ri-DOL-o-jee), unlike the other subjects covered in this chapter, is not a method of treatment, but a diagnostic tool. Iridology is the analysis of the iris of the eye to determine the state of health of the individual. This practice was initiated in the early nineteenth century by Ignatz von Peczely, a Hungarian physician, who observed that changes in the eyes of his patients mirrored changes in the tissues of the organs of their bodies. In the United States, its best known practitioner is Dr. Bernard Jensen, whose comprehensive iris charts are reproduced here. Iridology is a highly controversial discipline, which has not been accepted by the medical community. Its practitioners, however, can point to many successful uses of the techniques. The esthetician should form his or her own judgments as to the value of iridology.

According to the theory of iridology, the iris contains thousands of nerve endings, blood vessels, and other tissues and is connected to the organs and tissues of the body. Through the various nerve reflexes, the state of every part of the body is reflected in the iris. Thus, a change in an organ manifests itself with a corresponding change in a part of the iris (Fig. 14.2).

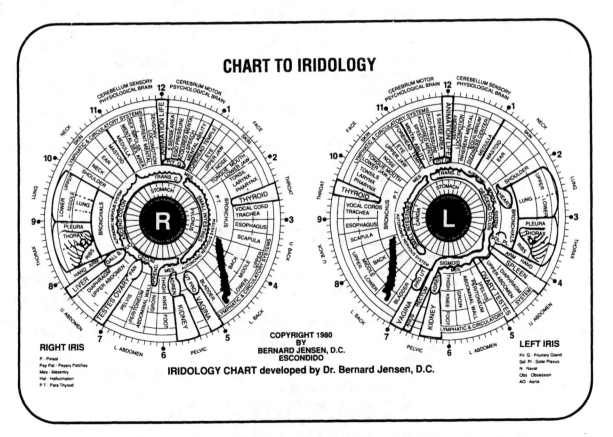

14.2—Iridology chart (*Chart reproduced courtesy of Dr. Bernard Jensen, D.C., Iridologists International*)

The chart is a map that shows the correspondence of nerve endings in the iris to specific organs and systems. The iris is divided into seven zones, rings around the pupil that correspond to various systems. The organs are mapped on radials, or spokes, from the center of the eye and are located by reference to the clock. So, for example, the skin and sensory nerves are located in the seventh, or outermost ring; the stomach, in the first, or innermost ring. The temple and forehead nerves are located at the eleven o'clock position of the left iris and the one o'clock position of the right iris.

The most important sign, as far as the practice of skin care is concerned, occurs in the seventh zone, the outer ring of the iris, which covers the integumentary system. Darkness in part or all of this area may indicate the accumulation of waste materials due to an underactive skin. The dark area, called a **scurf ring,** shows that the skin is not eliminating wastes properly.

White, yellow, or brown spots occurring in the sixth zone, the second ring from the outside, which covers the lymphatic system, may indicate toxic accumulation of waste materials in the lymphatic glands. These spots are known as the **lymphatic rosary.**

For the esthetician, a general knowledge of iridology may be useful in confirming other observations on the state of the client's skin. Such confirmation, however, should not be shared with the client. Although it is not expected that the esthetician have complete mastery of this complex and controversial discipline, an understanding of those areas concerned with skin health may be helpful.

REVIEW QUESTIONS

1. Why must the esthetician be aware of many advanced techniques in skin care?
2. What medical uses do herbs have?
3. How do normalizing herbs work?
4. How are herbs prepared for use?
5. How is an infusion made?
6. How is a tincture made?
7. What restriction must the esthetician follow when using herbs?
8. What are some uses of aloe vera?
9. What is the active ingredient in birch bark?
10. What functions does chamomile have in skin care?
11. What is aromatherapy?
12. What is a phytohormone?
13. What are the four basic properties that make essential oils important in skin care?
14. What do all essential oils have in common?
15. What does benzoin do?
16. On what kind of skin is geranium oil especially good?
17. What is thalassotherapy?

18. What is a thalassotherapy tub?
19. What do all spa treatments accomplish?
20. Why is sea water useful?
21. What are peloids?
22. What do seaweed and algaes do in skin care?
23. What do peloids do in skin care?
24. What is iridology?

15 Physics for the Esthetician

OBJECTIVES   *After completing this chapter, you should be able to:*

❶ Provide a background on physics and esthetics.
❷ Discuss the various forms of energy, including mechanical, heat, light, sound, and electrical.
❸ Discuss color theory.
❹ Understand the physical principles that regulate the operation of the various machines used in the practice of skin care.

INTRODUCTION

Physics (FIZ-iks), like chemistry, is one of the natural sciences. Unlike chemistry, which focuses on chemical changes in matter, physics focuses on the physical changes in matter. The physicist seeks to explore the laws that define and measure material phenomena. Among these material phenomena are force, energy, and motion. Like the chemist, the physicist relies on careful observations, experimentation and precise measurement.

An understanding of the basic laws of physics is important to the esthetician because these laws are behind the operating principles of much of the equipment used in the practice of skin care. This includes electrical apparatus, such as motors and galvanic current machines, mechanical equipment, such as facial chairs, and optical apparatus, such as magnifying lamps and Wood's lamps. Every piece of equipment the esthetician uses relies on one or more principles of physics. Generally, these principles of physics include some form of energy, whether mechanical, heat, light, or electrical.

HISTORICAL PERSPECTIVE

Human beings have studied their world and its phenomena since the beginning of time, looking for the whys and hows to explain their observations. As with all the natural sciences, modern physics has its roots in antiquity. Prehistoric man developed fire, one of the first useful tools in the march toward civilization. Later, still in prehistory, the search for tools to make life easier led to the development of the wheel.

As civilizations developed, new explanations for various phenomena were discovered. Some physical laws were found in the search for easier methods of building monuments, as the Egyptian discovery of the inclined plane, used in the construction of the pyramids. Others were discovered as the result of observation and speculation, as the discovery by **Archimedes** (287–212 B.C.) of the laws of buoyancy and flotation.

Each age, from prehistory to the present, contributed to the increase of knowledge about the physical universe. **Galileo** (1564–1642) discovered the laws of accelerated motion through his observations of falling objects. He also developed the telescope. **Christian Huygens** (1629–1695) developed the wave theory of light. In that same era, **Isaac Newton** (1642–1727) postulated the three laws of motion and the law of gravity. **Benjamin Franklin** (1706–1790) produced many practical inventions, from bifocals to the Franklin stove. He also experimented extensively with the nature of electricity. The list of discoveries could go on and on.

ENERGY

Energy (EN-ur-gee) is the capacity of an object, regardless of its size, to do work. This capacity for work may be classified either as **potential** energy, that is, stored by virtue of the position or state of stress of the object, or **kinetic,** or released energy because of motion in the object. Energy can be stored or released from objects as small as atoms and molecules to objects almost infinitely large (Fig. 15.1).

There are a number of different forms of energy. **Mechanical energy** develops from the movement of relatively large masses of matter, for example, simple machines such as pulleys and levers.

Heat and **light** energy develop from the rapid movement of molecules within the object. The friction caused by the molecules rubbing together manifests itself as both heat and light. **Sound** energy develops from the vibration of molecules formed into longitudinal waves. **Electrical** and **electromagnetic** energy develop from the movement of electrons in the atom. **Chemical** energy, discussed in Chapter 11, is released by chemical changes.

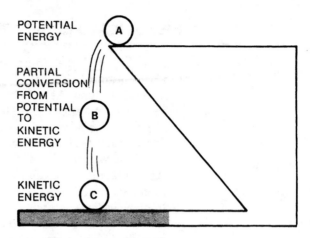

15.1—Potential and kinetic energy

According to the **Law of Conservation of Energy**, energy can neither be created nor destroyed. It can, however, be changed from one form to another. Potential energy is converted to kinetic energy, for example, when a ball is dropped from a window. Mechanical energy is changed to electrical energy in generators or to heat energy in air conditioners. Electrical energy is changed to heat and light energy, as in incandescent light bulbs, or to mechanical energy, as in motors.

If energy is defined as the ability to perform work, **work** can be defined as the product of the force applied to the object times the degree of movement, or displacement, of the object. Thus, the work done on a ten pound object lifted up five feet is:

$$10 \text{ lbs (force)} \times 5 \text{ ft (displacement)} = 50 \text{ ft-lbs (work)}$$

Once the object is at rest at the five-foot height, it has a potential energy of fifty foot-pounds. If the object is dropped, the potential energy is converted to kinetic energy. At the instant the object hits the ground, the kinetic energy is fifty foot-pounds.

Power (POW-er) is defined as work divided by the time it takes to do the work. If it took five seconds to raise the object five feet, the power is:

$$50 \text{ ft-lbs (work)} / 5 \text{ sec. (time)} = 10 \text{ ft-lbs (power)}$$

Mechanical Energy

Mechanical energy develops from the movement of relatively large masses of matter, so work, power and potential and kinetic energy are important concepts in the discussion of this form of energy. For moving small objects, as in the examples above, the amount of work involved is relatively small and not particularly hard to accomplish. For moving larger objects, however, or for moving objects for great distances, the work increases. Machines assist by making it easier or faster to do the work by transferring the force from one point to another.

A machine can multiply either the force or the distance without multiplying the work. According to the **Law of Machines**, the output of work must equal the input of work, if friction is ignored. By this equation, if there were no friction, a machine would be 100 percent efficient.

Friction, a force that opposes free motion of objects sliding or rolling over other objects, however, does exist and must be considered. The amount of friction is determined by a number of factors such as the type of materials used, the roughness or smoothness of the materials, the load the materials must carry, and the type of motion involved. In many machines, friction is reduced and the efficiency of the machine increased by polishing the sliding surfaces, by lubrication, or by the use of ball bearings.

The better quality rotating brush machines, for example, utilize ball bearings to reduce friction. This allows more efficient use of the energy provided. By the same token, the esthetician uses the cleanser as a lubricant on the brush. Using a dry brush on the client's skin would create too much friction and burn the client.

There are a number of different machines. The simple machines include the inclined plane, the pulley, and the lever. The screw and the wedge are types of inclined planes. The complex machines found in industry today do nothing more than utilize the physical principles behind one or more of these simple machines.

Inclined Planes. The **inclined plane**, or ramp, is one of the oldest machines utilized by man. It is nothing more than a flat surface raised to the height required. The length of the surface determines the angle, which determines the force required to raise an object to the required height. The longer the surface, the less the angle and the easier it is to raise the object (Fig. 15.2).

Suppose, for example, the salon has a two-foot high set of steps. For a 200-pound handicapped client to gain entry, it would be necessary to lift her up two feet. The work required would be:

$$200 \text{ lbs} \times 2 \text{ ft} = 400 \text{ ft-lbs}$$

The effort would require a lifting force of 200 pounds. If a six-foot ramp was installed, the work would still be 400 foot-pounds. The effort required now, however, would be:

$$200 \text{ lbs (force)} / 3 \text{ (length/height)} = 66.7 \text{ lbs}$$

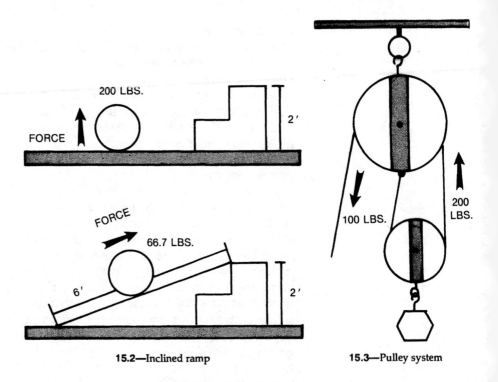

15.2—Inclined ramp   **15.3—Pulley system**

A **screw** is nothing more than an inclined plane wrapped around a cylinder. The load is moved as the cylinder is rotated. The height adjustment control on many estheticians' stools is an example of the uses of the screw.

A **wedge** is actually two inclined planes placed back to back. In the case of a wedge, the load is stationary and the inclined planes are moved. A knife blade is an example of a wedge.

Pulleys. A **pulley** is a grooved wheel rotating in a frame. The frame is called a **block**; the grooved wheel, a **sheave**. This simple machine is used for lifting heavy weights for long distances. Pulleys are often used in multiples to reduce the effort needed for lifting. The mechanical advantage, that is, the amount of reduction in effort, can be determined simply by counting the number of rope segments around the pulleys (Fig. 15.3).

If, for example, a pulley system with one fixed and one moveable pulley was installed over the facial chair to hoist the 200-pound handicapped client, the effort required to lift her would be 100 pounds (200 lbs / 2 rope segments = 100 lbs). If the pulley system had two fixed and one moveable pulley, the effort would drop to 66.7 lbs (200 lbs / 3 rope segments = 66.7 lbs).

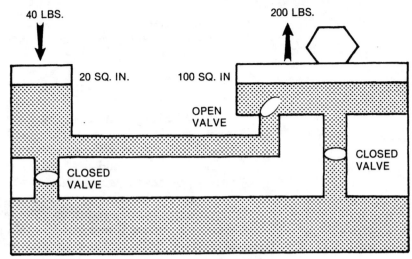

40 LBS.

200 LBS.

20 SQ. IN.

100 SQ. IN

OPEN
VALVE

CLOSED
VALVE

CLOSED
VALVE

OIL RESERVOIR

15.4—Hydraulic chair principle

Levers. A **lever** consists of a bar rotating around a fixed point. The fixed point is called the **fulcrum**. Adjusting the distance from one end of the bar to the fulcrum changes the effort required to lift a load at the other end of the bar. A bottle opener is an example of a simple lever. Tweezers are a form of lever in which both ends of the bar are folded back around the fulcrum.

The simple machines discussed thus far are examples of the mechanical principles of solids. Liquids and gases follow mechanical principles as well. These principles are also utilized in machinery used by estheticians.

In Chapter 11, it was shown that liquids take the shape of their containers and are not compressible. Liquids exert pressure in their containers. The pressure exerted by the liquid depends on its density and its depth, but does not depend on the shape of the container. Pressure increases with density and with depth and is the same in all directions. According to **Pascal's Law**, pressure in an enclosed liquid is transmitted undiminished throughout the entire liquid. It is this principle that allows the operation of hydraulic presses.

The hydraulic salon chair is an example of Pascal's Law in action. The small cylinder is operated by light foot pressure. The pressure is transmitted to the large lifting cylinder and is multiplied according to the difference in area between the two cylinders (Fig. 15.4).

For example, if the piston on the foot pedal has an area of twenty square-inches and is pressed with a foot pressure of forty pounds, the pressure produced will be two pounds/square-inch.

40 lb / 20 sq-in = 2 lb/sq-in

If the large piston has an area of 100 square-inches, the two pounds/square-inch pressure transmitted to it produces a lifting force of 200 pounds.

$$100 \text{ sq-in} \times 2 \text{ lb/sq-in} = 200 \text{ lbs}$$

Thus, the 200-pound client can be lifted by the application of only forty pounds of pressure. The small piston must travel a much greater distance than the large piston, however.

Gases, unlike liquids, can be compressed. According to **Boyle's Law**, as long as the temperature remains constant, the volume of the gas will vary inversely with the pressure. That is, as the pressure rises, the volume decreases and vice versa. This explains the operation of the suction pump on certain skin-care equipment. As a piston is raised, it draws air from an attached chamber past a valve. This causes a decrease in pressure, causing the valve to close. As the piston lowers, it compresses the air in the piston chamber, causing a second valve to open to the outside air (Fig. 15.5).

With the operation of the pump, the vacuum attachment on the chamber side of the pump creates the suction used to remove impurities from the skin. The compressed air released on the compression side of the pump operates the spray bottles. The combination of

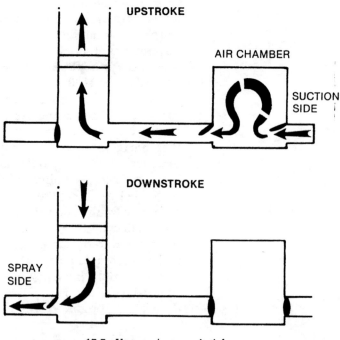

15.5—Vacuum/spray principles

suction pressure and compression pressure lets both instruments be operated by one device.

The mechanics of solids, liquids, and gases involve both force and motion, which are governed by a number of physical laws. **Force** has both quantity and direction and is, therefore, a **vector** (VEK-tor) quantity. This means a force can be represented graphically by a line, or vector. The length of the vector indicates its size; the way it points, its direction. A force will either promote or retard motion, i.e., it will make an object move or prevent it from moving. Except when the force is either straight up or straight down, there will be more than one component of the force. One component will be useful; it will promote the desired effect. One will be useless; it will hinder the desired effect. The actual force applied will be the **resultant** force and will be determined by the angle formed by the two component force vectors.

Suppose, for example, it is necessary to drag the facial chair across the floor. The esthetician ties a five-foot-long rope to the bottom of the chair and pulls with a force of fifty pounds. The top of the rope is held three feet above the ground. Gravity exerts a downward force. This is the vertical component of the force. The horizontal component of the force is parallel to the floor. The resultant force is formed by the angle of the rope. Drawing a vector graph shows that the horizontal component is forty pounds and the vertical component is thirty pounds. The horizontal component is the useful component; the vertical component is the useless component (Fig. 15.6).

All objects on earth are subject to the **Law of Universal Gravitation,** as formulated by Sir Isaac Newton. The Law states, "Every object in the universe attracts every other object with a force directly proportional to the product of their masses and inversely proportional to the square of the distance between them." An object's **weight** is a result of the earth's gravitational pull and varies slightly from one part of the earth to another. Its **mass** is the amount of

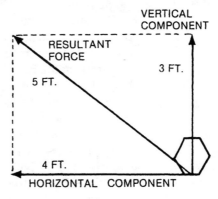

15.6—Vector diagrams

matter it contains and never varies. As Galileo showed, in a vacuum, all objects, regardless of mass, fall at the same rate, thirty-two feet/second/second.

Newton also formulated his three laws of motion to explain some of the relationships between force and motion. Newton's **First Law of Motion** states that an object at rest tends to stay at rest; an object in motion tends to stay in motion. This means that any object will remain at rest or in motion until some external force changes its state. This is known as **inertia** (in-ER-she-ah). In rotating objects, inertia causes parts to fly off in a tangent. That is why an overly wet rotating brush splashes the client and the esthetician.

Newton's **Second Law of Motion** states that a change in an object's velocity is directly proportional to the force applied to it and inversely proportional to the mass of the object. This law explains **momentum** (mow-MEN-tum), which is the product of the mass times the velocity of the object. The larger the object, the more force is required to change its state of motion.

Newton's **Third Law of Motion** states that there is an equal and opposite reaction for every action. So, a facial chair that weighs fifty pounds pushes down (gravity) on the floor with a force of fifty pounds. The floor pushes up with a force of fifty pounds as well. A bullet fired from a gun causes the gun to recoil.

Heat Energy

The application of heat is an important tool in the esthetician's tool kit. The heat can be either wet, as in the steamer, or dry, as with heat lamps. Regardless of the type of heat, however, the energy generated is governed by physical principles.

Unlike mechanical energy, which involves the movement of large masses of matter, heat energy derives from the rapid movement of tiny masses of matter—molecules—within the object generating the heat. The hotter the object, the faster the molecules within it are moving.

The **intensity** (in-TEN-si-tee) of the heat of an object is measured by its temperature. The two temperature scales in common use today are the Fahrenheit scale and the Celcius scale. The device used to measure temperature is the thermometer. Thermometers are calibrated using the freezing point of water, 0°C. or 32°F. at one end, and the boiling point of water, 100°C. or 212°F. at the other end.

The amount of heat in an object is measured by the number of **calories** or the number of **British Thermal Units (BTU's)** it contains.

Precise control of temperature is an important consideration with many products the esthetician uses. Paraffin used in wax masks, for example, should be heated to approximately 136°F. Hotter temperatures would burn the client's face. Cooler temperatures would prevent proper flow of the paraffin. A number of commercially available devices are designed to heat the wax to its most efficient temperature and maintain that temperature.

The sun is our most pervasive source of heat. Radiant heat energy from the sun warms the surface of the earth and allows the existence of life. Fossil fuels, which provide heat through chemical energy, are indirect products of the sun. Coal and oil are the fossilized remains of plants and animal life of millions of years ago, which, like all other life on this planet, owed their existence to the sun.

Chemical energy produces heat through burning of fuels. The chemical reaction from the oxidation of the fuels releases heat energy. Electrical energy is also converted to heat energy as demonstrated by the vaporizer. Electrical current is applied to a metallic heating element such as nichrome wire. The heating element becomes red hot and transfers heat to distilled water, boiling it and converting it to steam.

Mechanical energy can be converted to heat energy through friction caused by rubbing two objects together. Heat is generated during a massage, for example, because of the friction of the hand being rubbed over the face.

Materials expand when heated and contract when cooled. Gases expand and contract more than liquids, which in turn, expand and contract more than solids. Different materials expand and contract at different rates. The thermostat used to control temperature in the paraffin bath tank, for example, operates because of differential expansion. The thermostat consists of a bar made of two different metals. When the bar is heated, one metal expands more than the other, causing the bar to bend. The bar is calibrated to activate a switch or relay when it reaches a preselected point.

Heat is transferred from warmer objects to cooler objects by **convection, conduction,** or **radiation.** In convection heat transfer, a heat source causes movement in liquid or gas molecules. A pan of water on the stove boils because the gas flame heats the layer of water at the bottom of the pan. The hot water rises to the surface, causing the cooler water to sink to the bottom and become heated in turn. This convection current continues until all the water in the pan reaches the same temperature. A radiator heats the room by convection by heating the air closest to it. The warmer air rises and displaces cooler air at the ceiling, moving it near the radiator, where it becomes warmed. The constant movement of air maintains the heat in the room.

Heat in solid objects is transferred through conduction. As one part of the conductor, for example, a frying pan, is heated, the molecular motion travels from the point of heating throughout the pan, until the entire pan is heated. Metals are good conductors of heat. Wood and most plastics are poor conductors. This is why frying pans often have plastic or wood handles.

Heat is also transferred by radiation. The sun heats the surface of the earth by radiation. Radiated heat, unlike convection or conduction, relies on the wave motion from electromagnetic vibration rather than on molecular vibration. The radiant heat waves are absorbed by an object, which is heated. The heat may then be transmitted to another object. The solar collector works on this principle. Radiant heat from the sun heats water held in a shallow network of tubes. The hot water is pumped through pipes in a house to provide heat. The most common source of radiant heat encountered by the esthetician is the infrared heat lamp used in some facial treatments.

Dark objects absorb radiant heat better than light objects, which tend to reflect the radiant energy.

Light Energy

Light, like heat and sound, is a form of energy. And, like other forms of energy, many aspects of the physical principles of light are important to the esthetician. The magnifying lamp, used in the analysis of skin and during manual extraction, illustrates the use of visible light and the lens. The Wood's lamp utilizes the fluorescence of the ultraviolet spectra for analysis. The heat lamp utilizes the radiant energy of the infrared portion of the spectrum. A knowledge of the physics of color is invaluable to the esthetician, as is an understanding of the psychology of color.

James Maxwell (1831–1879) proposed the **electromagnetic theory** of light, which holds that particles of energy vibrate in an undulating, or wave, motion. The speed with which the waves form, that is, their frequency, determines the form of energy in the electromagnetic spectrum. Visible light is only a small portion of that spectrum. However, the wave theory does not fully explain the action of light. In 1900, **Max Planck** (1858–1947) developed the **quantum theory** of light. According to the quantum theory, energy is transmitted in small packets, or **quanta**. The amount of energy contained in any of these packets is proportional to its frequency. Planck's quantum theory is the basis of modern physics.

Light travels at an amazingly high speed, 186,000 miles per second in a vacuum. It is slightly slower in air and slower still in water. Thus, it takes the light from the sun, which is 93 million miles away from earth, approximately eight minutes to reach this planet. The distance to other stars is measured in light years, that is, the time it takes their light to reach us. The star we see tonight is not that star's present, but its past. A star that is five light years away, for example, is seen tonight as it was five years ago.

Light lets us see. We see an object because light coming from that object reaches our eyes. When an object reflects light from another source, it is **illuminated**. The client's face is illuminated by the magnifying lamp. When the object passes most of the light through it, it is **transparent**, as in the magnifying lens. When only part of the light passes, the object is **translucent**, as in the diffuser over the ceiling light. If the object emits its own light, it is **luminous**. The bulb in the magnifying lamp is luminous.

The intensity of a light source is measured in **candlepower**. The intensity with which an object is illuminated is a function of both the candlepower of the light source and the distance of the light source from the object, and is measured in **foot-candles**. According to the **Law of Intensity of Illumination**, intensity varies directly with the candlepower of the source and inversely with the square of the distance from the source. Thus, doubling the candlepower of the source will double the intensity of illumination of the object. But doubling the distance of the object from the light source will reduce the intensity of illumination four times.

Light travels in a straight line in a given medium, that is, vacuum, air, liquid or transparent solid. Because of this, shadows are formed when opaque objects interrupt light rays. However, when a ray of light reaches a transparent medium of different density, it bends. This phenomenon is known as **refraction** (re-FRAK-shun). The degree to which the ray bends depends on the density of the substance and the angle with which the ray strikes the surface of the substance. The ratio is called the **index of refraction** of the substance.

Refraction is the physical principle that governs the functioning of lenses. Light rays pass through the lens, which is shaped to bend the rays in a precise manner so that the image will be enlarged or reduced, depending on the shape of the lens.

Lenses are generally either converging (convex) or diverging (concave). Convex lenses, in which the middle is thicker than the edges, bring rays of light together. Magnifying lenses are of this type, as are camera lenses and lenses used to correct farsightedness. Concave lenses, in which the edges are thicker than the middle, move rays of light farther apart. Lenses used to correct nearsightedness are of this type (Fig. 15.7).

Not all light passes through the medium its rays strike. Even in transparent objects, some light rays are reflected. In opaque objects, some light rays are reflected; others are absorbed. Light colored objects reflect more light; darker colored objects reflect less. Mirrors operate on the principles of reflection.

Flat mirrors typically show an object and its reflected image as the same size, although the image appears to be as far behind the mirror as the object is in front of it. The image, however, is reversed left to right. Like lenses, mirrors can be either concave or convex. Light reflecting from such mirrors converges or diverges in the same manner as light transmitted through lenses. The magnifying makeup mirror is concave. The rearview mirror on an automobile is convex.

As mentioned previously, visible light is part of the electromagnetic spectrum. Specifically, it covers the range of wavelengths from about 380 to 760 nanometers. The visible spectrum is divided into

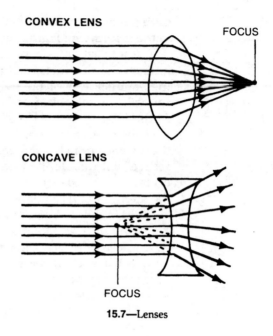

15.7—Lenses

seven distinct colors. From the longest wavelength to the shortest, these are: red, orange, yellow, green, blue, indigo, and violet. (A simple **mnemonic device** to remember the name is ROY G. BIV). All of the colors mixed together produce white light (Fig. 15.8).

The wavelengths to the left of red, that is, longer than 380 nanometers, are in the infrared range. Wavelengths to the right of violet, that is, shorter than 760 nanometers, are in the ultraviolet range. The infrared spectrum provides heat energy, as demonstrated by heat lamps used in the salon. The red glow from these lamps is from light within the visible spectrum. The ultraviolet spectrum is divided into the long wave ultraviolet, which is relatively harmless, and short wave ultraviolet, which can be harmful. The Wood's lamp utilizes long wave UV light to make blemishes fluoresce. (Note: even though long wave UV light is relatively harmless, the client should not look directly into the Wood's lamp.) Short wave UV light is used in germicidal lamps to kill bacteria.

Color Theory. Different light sources have different color casts, depending on the color temperature of the source. Incandescent lamps, for example, tend towards the red end of the spectrum; fluorescent lights tend toward the blue end. Even daylight changes color.

An object's color depends on the wavelength of the light reflected from it or transmitted through it. A red dress, for example, appears

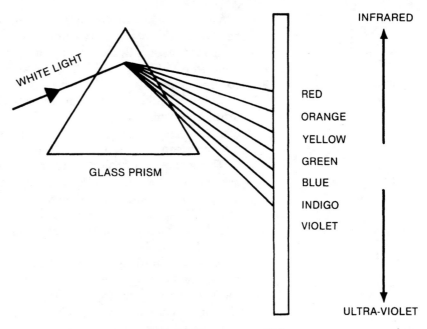

15.8—Visible spectrum of light

red because it absorbs all **wavelengths** of visible light except for red, which it reflects back to the eye. A piece of yellow stained glass transmits only the yellow wavelengths and absorbs the rest. If the object absorbs all of the visible light, it will be black. If it reflects all of the visible light, it will be white.

White light is produced by mixing all seven colors of the visible spectrum. However, white light can also be produced by mixing only the three **primary** colors of light—red, green, and blue-violet. Mixing two primary colors of light produces a **complementary** color. Therefore, mixing a complementary color with a primary color produces white light. This discussion applies only to mixing colors of light. The process is somewhat different when mixing pigments together.

Unlike the colors of light, the primary colors in pigments are red, yellow and blue. Complementary colors are made by mixing two primary colors in equal quantities to produce green (yellow + blue), orange (yellow + red), and violet (red + blue). **Tertiary** (TER-she-air-ee), or intermediate, colors can be created by mixing an equal amount of a primary color and a complementary color. An almost unlimited number of colors can be produced by mixing primary, complementary and tertiary colors in various ratios.

Colors are discussed in terms of their hue, value, and intensity. **Hue** (HYOO) refers to the color itself, e.g., green, yellow. **Value**

(VAL-yoo) refers to lightness or darkness, e.g., light green, dark yellow. Darker values are sometimes called shades; lighter values are sometimes called tints. Intensity refers to a color's brightness or dullness. Shiny colors appear more intense than matte finish colors.

Colors also have temperature, that is, they can be thought of in terms of warm, neutral or cool. Colors containing a predominance of red or yellow tend to be warm; those containing a predominance of blue or green tend to be cool. White, gray and black are neutral.

These aspects of color—hue, value, intensity, and temperature—are important to the esthetician when advising the client on cosmetic colors and fashion colors that will enhance his or her skin and hair tones. While colors can be combined in almost limitless numbers, not all combinations are pleasing. Some combinations are harmonious; others clash.

A color wheel, available from art supply stores, can help the esthetician choose appropriate color schemes, whether they are monochromatic, complementary, analogous, or triadic. A **monochromatic** color scheme consists of one color with varying values. A complementary color scheme consists of two hues directly opposite each other on the color wheel. An **analogous** color scheme consists of three colors next to each other on a color wheel. Each of these colors will contain some of the primary color. A **triadic** color scheme consists of three equidistant hues on the color wheel.

There is also a definite psychology of color, both in how colors are perceived and in the moods they evoke. Color is as much a factor of human perception as it is a physical concept. People see colors differently. A shade of red, for example, will look different to a person with blue eyes than it does to a person with brown eyes. In addition, a given color is seen differently depending on the context in which it is viewed. Thus, a bright red dot on a lighter red field would appear more intense than it actually is. The same bright red dot on a darker red field would appear less intense than it actually is.

Light or bright colors appear to come forward, or advance. Dark or dull colors appear to move backward, or recede. This perception of color is sometimes used to create the illusion of more or less space. Likewise, some colors reflect their hue into adjacent areas, giving those areas overtones of that hue.

The psychological effect of color has long been known. Different colors are associated with different states of emotion. We are "blue" when we feel sad; we are "green" with envy; we refer to a coward as "yellow"; or we "see red" with anger. The color used in the immediate environment can have subtle effects on mood and behavior. Green, for example, is soothing and tranquil and is appropriate for use in treatment rooms and reception areas. Blue promotes a feeling of spaciousness and can be used in smaller, more confined areas such as rest rooms. Yellow is cheerful and stimulating and can be used in consultation rooms and retail areas.

Sound Energy

Sound is also a form of energy and is the effect of the vibration of molecules in some form of matter and transmitted by some form of matter, which carries the sound waves. Sound is most often transmitted through air, a gas, but can also be transmitted through liquids and solids. Sound is not transmitted in a vacuum, however.

Like light, sound is both a physical and a perceptual concept. It is a physical concept in that sound waves are produced whenever matter is made to vibrate. And it is perceptual in that sound is heard when the waves strike the ear and stimulate the auditory nerves. Sound energy is not as directly useful to the esthetician as the other forms of energy discussed in this chapter. Although some forms of sound energy, for example, ultrasonics, or ultra-high frequency sound, are gaining in utility in the medical profession, there is, at present, no use for sound waves in the profession of esthetics.

The major value the esthetician derives from understanding the nature of sound is in the ability to distinguish the difference between music, that is, pleasing sounds, and noise, or unpleasant sounds. Noise control is an important aspect of the salon environment.

When molecules start to vibrate, they set up a wave motion by which the sound energy is transmitted. The wave can be classed as **pulsed** or **periodic**. A pulse is a single vibration that travels through the transmitting medium away from the source of the vibration. Periodic vibrations are recurring back and forth vibrations. Thus, one hand clap would constitute a pulse; applause constitutes a periodic vibration. Sound waves are **longitudinal**, that is, the molecules vibrate back and forth in the same direction as the energy travels. They also consist of a series of alternating peaks or **condensations**, areas where the molecules are packed together, and valleys or **rarifications**, areas where the molecules are spaced farther apart (Fig. 15.9).

A sound wave is characterized by its wavelength, amplitude, and frequency. The **wavelength** is the distance between two corresponding points along the wave or one vibration consisting of one complete peak and one complete valley. The time it takes for one complete vibration to occur is known as the **period**. The **amplitude** of a wave is the height reached by a peak above the average or equilibrium point of the wave. The depth of the valley will be equal to the height of the peak. The **frequency** (FREE-kwen-see) of the wave is the number of complete vibrations that occur in a given unit of time, usually one second. The common unit of frequency is the **hertz** (HERTS) (Hz). One hertz equals one cycle per second.

The speed of sound depends on both the medium through which it is transmitted and the temperature. Sound travels through room

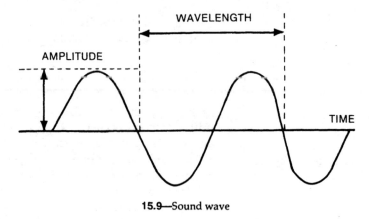

15.9—Sound wave

temperature air at about 760 miles per hour. It is slower in cooler air; faster in warmer air. A supersonic aircraft traveling faster than the speed of sound produces a shock wave of compressed air in front of it, causing the familiar "sonic boom." Thunder is nothing more than the sonic boom caused by a flash of lightning. Air is much cooler at high altitudes than at ground level. Since the speed of sound is less in cool air, high flying aircraft break the sound barrier at lower speeds than lower flying aircraft. Because of this variability, supersonic speeds are given in Mach numbers, named after the Austrian physicist, **Ernst Mach**. The Mach number is the ratio of the speed of the object to the speed of sound in the given medium. The speed of sound is Mach 1. An object traveling at twice that speed would be at Mach 2.

Because of the stronger intermolecular forces in liquids and solids, sound travels faster in these media than in gases, such as air. Sound travels through water at 3200 miles per hour and through steel at more than 11,000 miles per hour.

A sound, as heard, can be either musical or noisy. If the vibrations are regular, the sound will be musical; if they are irregular, the sound will be noise. Noise is irritating. But, as William Congreve said, "Music has charms to soothe a savage breast." Noise must be minimized during a facial treatment to avoid discomfort and promote relaxation. The judicious use of relaxing music also helps promote relaxation.

Music is characterized by pitch, loudness, and quality. Pitch is determined by the frequency. Low frequency sounds are low pitched; high frequency sounds are high pitched. A bassoon, for example, produces low pitch notes while a piccolo produces high pitch notes. The human ear can detect sounds from about 16 hertz to 20,000 hertz. Some animals can detect even higher frequencies. Bats, for example, rely on their ability to generate and detect very high frequency sound, their own built-in sonar, to navigate in the dark.

Loudness is dependent on the amplitude of the vibration. The greater the amplitude, or the greater the amount of energy imparted to cause the vibration, the louder the sound. The loudness of the sound, as perceived by the ear, also depends on its distance from the ear. Sound intensity varies inversely with the square of the distance. Quality depends on the harmonics that are part of the fundamental note, and is the characteristic that differentiates the identical note played on two different instruments.

Sound waves, like light rays, reflect from smooth surfaces. The reverberations thus produced are called **echoes** (eh-KOZ). These echoes can interfere with the direct sounds and cause unpleasant noises. To avoid this phenomenon, sound absorbing materials, such as acoustic ceiling tile, can be placed in the treatment room.

Electrical Energy

Electrical energy is virtually indispensable to the esthetician. Almost all other forms of energy utilized in the skin-care salon are derived from electrical energy. Electricity is converted to heat energy in the vaporizer to produce steam. It is converted to light energy in the magnifying lamp and to mechanical energy in the rotating brushes. It is even turned to sound energy in the audio tape system or radio used in the treatment room.

Static electricity, produced by friction, has been known since the time of the ancient Greeks. Experiments have shown that a glass rod, rubbed with silk, acquires a positive charge, while a rubber rod, rubbed with wool, acquires a negative charge. The glass rod gains electrons; the rubber rod loses electrons. The positively charged rod will attract the negatively charged rod but will repel another positively charged rod, showing that like charges repel and unlike charges attract.

Lightning is the most spectacular manifestation of static electricity, with electrical discharges of up to 10 million volts. A more familiar manifestation of static electricity occurs when someone walks across a wool rug on a dry day and touches a doorknob, setting off an electrical discharge.

Electrons flow from a negatively charged pole to a positively charged pole, establishing a current. The intensity of the current depends on the number of electrons that move past a point in a conductor in a given period of time and is measured in **amperes** (AM-peers). The device used to measure current flow is the **ammeter**. For electrons to flow, there must be a difference in the charges between the two poles. The greater the difference in charge, the greater the electromotive force, or **voltage** (VOLT-ej). This is measured with a **voltmeter**.

Current flows only through **conductors** (KON-duc-tors), substances that allow free movement of electrons. Metals are good conductors

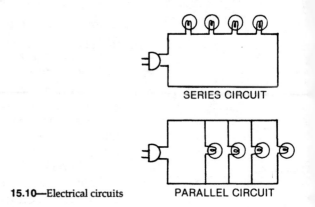

SERIES CIRCUIT

15.10—Electrical circuits

PARALLEL CIRCUIT

of electricity. Current does not flow through **insulators** (IN-sol-ay-tors), substances that restrict the free movement of electrons. Air is an insulator, as is rubber. Some metals are better conductors of electricity than others. The ability of the metal to conduct electricity is a function of its **resistance** (re-ZISS-tans). By **Ohm's law**, intensity varies directly with voltage and inversely with resistance or:

$$I \text{ (amperes)} = E \text{ (voltage)} / R \text{ (resistance)}$$

Electrical power, the rate at which electrical energy is utilized, is measured in **watts**, determined by multiplying volts by amperes:

$$P \text{ (watts)} = E \text{ (voltage)} \times I \text{ (amperes)}$$

To form an electric circuit, there must be a source of voltage and a path for the current to flow through. The current flows through conductors, some of which have a designed resistance. These are called **resistors**. The circuit may also have a switch to open or close the pathway. The voltage source may be a battery or generator.

In a **series circuit** the resistors are connected in a chain and there is only one path for electron flow. These circuits maintain the same current flow throughout the entire circuit, but fail completely if there is an interruption at any point in the circuit. Inexpensive strings of Christmas lights are an example. If one bulb burns out, all of the lights go out (Fig. 15.10).

In a **parallel circuit** each resistor is connected across the terminals of the voltage source, providing multiple paths for the current. These circuits maintain the same voltage across all the resistances. The failure of one resistor does not cause the entire circuit to fail. House current is typically a parallel circuit.

REVIEW QUESTIONS

1. Why is the study of physics important to the esthetician?
2. How does physics differ from chemistry?
3. Match the person to the discovery.

1. Archimedes	a. quantum theory
2. Galileo	b. bifocal lenses
3. Huygens	c. electromagnetic theory
4. Newton	d. buoyancy
5. Franklin	e. accelerated motion
6. Maxwell	f. gravity
7. Planck	g. wave theory of light

4. What is energy?
5. What is the Law of Conservation of Energy?
6. What is friction?
7. What is a screw?
8. What is Pascal's Law?
9. Why is Pascal's Law important?
10. What is Boyle's Law?
11. Why is Boyle's Law important?
12. What is Newton's Third Law of Motion?
13. What are the two temperature scales in common use?
14. What are three ways heat is transferred?
15. What is the speed of light?
16. How do we see an object?
17. What is candlepower?
18. What are the colors of the visible spectrum?
19. What two spectra are on either side of the visible spectrum?
20. What determines an object's color?
21. What are the primary colors in pigments?
22. What are complementary colors?
23. What three terms are used in discussing color?
24. Why is color important to the esthetician?
25. What is the psychological effect of the color, green?
26. How are soundwaves characterized?
27. What is frequency?
28. How is music characterized?
29. What is the most important form of energy to the esthetician?
30. How is the intensity of an electrical current measured?
31. What is an insulator?
32. What is Ohm's Law?

16 Skin-Care Equipment

OBJECTIVES   *After completing this chapter, you should be able to:*

❶ Describe the various machinery and equipment used in skin care.
❷ Describe both electrical and nonelectrical devices.
❸ Discuss the qualities that make each suitable for use in the salon.

INTRODUCTION

Except for a suitable chair for the client, facials can be given without the use of equipment or machinery. The proper equipment, however, makes the procedure more efficient and more effective. There is a wide array of specialized machinery for the esthetician. Each type serves a particular purpose. The esthetician should be familiar with the equipment used in the profession. He or she should know what equipment to use, when to use it, and how to use it to its maximum effectiveness.

There are a number of different manufacturers of skin-care machinery. As with the chemical products, it pays to use the best equipment available. Before choosing which equipment to get, the esthetician should read the literature available from the various manufacturers. If possible, the equipment should be tested.

It is not necessary to get all of the equipment at one time. If capital is limited, the esthetician can get the most important pieces first, then add other pieces as business warrants or the need arises.

Many manufacturers provide the equipment as a package in self-contained racks. These racks hold the equipment together and allow more efficient access to the various pieces during the facial (Fig. 16.1).

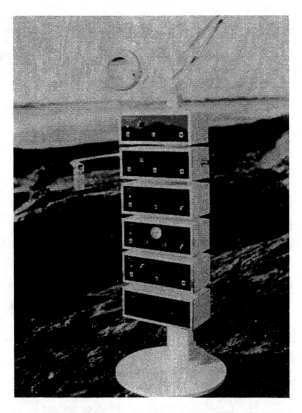

16.1—Typical rack of equipment *(Courtesy of Proteus, Inc.)*

THE FACIAL CHAIR

A suitable treatment chair should be the first piece of equipment acquired. It should be sturdy and well-padded. The padding should be plush, so the chair is comfortable, and it should be made of a material that is easy to clean and sanitize. The chair should be adjustable from fully upright to fully reclined, and the controls should be easy to work. When the chair is in the fully reclined position, the arm rests should be even with the padding. Or they should be removable.

It is important that the chair be as comfortable as possible, since the client will be spending an hour or more in it during the facial. And comfort is the first step toward the relaxed feeling that is necessary to the success of the treatment (Fig. 16.2).

It is also important that the esthetician be comfortable, with a comfortably padded, adjustable stool. The stool should ride on casters so the esthetician has free movement around the facial chair.

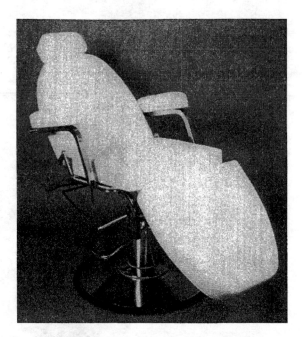

16.2—Facial chair *(Courtesy of Pibbs Industries)*

THE MAGNIFYING LAMP

The magnifying lamp is used during skin analysis and manual extraction. Typically, the lamp consists of a circular fluorescent bulb around a four to five power magnifying lens. The lens and lamp assembly are attached to an articulating arm, so it can be moved to any desired position. Knobs on the arm lock the lamp into position (Fig. 16.3).

The lamps are available with floor mounts on casters for easy mobility or with clamps so they can be mounted on the wall or on equipment trolleys. The choice is a matter of the esthetician's personal preference.

During the facial, the lamp is placed very close to the client's face. If the light bothers the client's eyes, they may be covered with moist cotton pads to shield them from the light.

THE WOOD'S LAMP

The Wood's lamp is a valuable tool for skin analysis. It is a long wave ultraviolet (black light) lamp with a magnifying lens and is usually hand held. The lamp must be used in a totally dark room (Fig. 16.4).

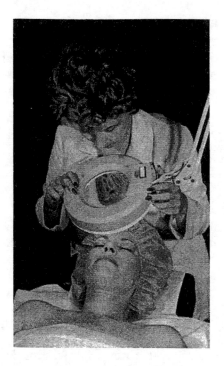

16.3—Magnifying lamp

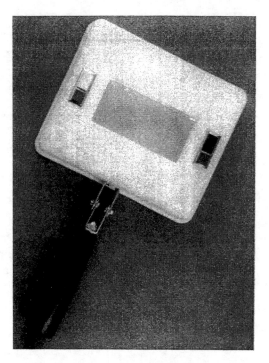

16.4—Wood's lamp *(Courtesy of Pibbs Industries)*

The Wood's lamp works on the principle that different skin conditions fluoresce differently. Under the black light, blemishes and other conditions that are hard to see under normal light show up very easily, giving the esthetician positive visual clues to the client's skin problems. The most common indications on the Wood's lamp are as follows:

Skin Condition	Indication
Normal skin	blue-white
Dry skin	light to deep purple
Oily skin	orange
Dead cells	white
Freckles or other pigmentation	brown
Clogged pores and comedones	orange
Dandruff	white

Neither the esthetician nor the client should look directly into the Wood's lamp during the analysis.

THE VAPORIZER

The vaporizer, or steamer, is one of the most useful machines at the esthetician's disposal. This equipment disperses steam onto the client's face. The steam offers a number of benefits.

1. It expands the blood vessels and increases circulation.
2. It softens the skin and loosens dead surface cells.
3. It softens embedded dirt, oils, and blackheads.
4. It relaxes the pores.
5. It helps moisten and revitalize the skin.
6. It relaxes the client.

Vaporizers are available in a number of forms, ranging from free standing floor models to small, portable units. Regardless of their configuration, however, they all have certain common features. They have a water reservoir, either glass for direct viewing of the water level or metal with a water level gauge. They have a heating element, to boil the water to produce the steam. And they have a nozzle and an adjustable arm to allow the steam to be directed where it is wanted (Fig. 16.5).

Some models also have a timer to measure the treatment time, and some have an automatic low water shut-off to prevent running the unit dry. If there is no automatic shut-off, the water level must be continually monitored to avoid running out of water, as this will damage the unit.

Some manufacturers place a removable felt ring around the nozzle, so that essential oils or other substances can be placed on the felt

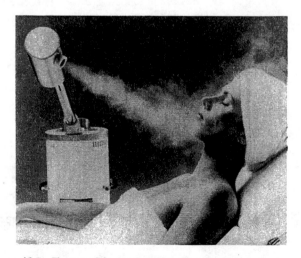

16.5—Floor model vaporizer *(Courtesy of Nemectron, Inc.)*

to mix with the steam and be diffused over the skin.

Ionization units are also added to some models of vaporizers. The ionization unit imparts an electrical charge to the water droplets as they pass the nozzle, forming a finer, more evenly distributed mist. In addition, the ionization unit produces ozone, a form of oxygen, that acts as a disinfectant.

Ozone is poisonous in high concentrations and there is some controversy over its use by estheticians. Some manufacturers, out of concern that the FDA may ban the units, will not sell vaporizers with ionization units to estheticians. Other manufacturers, however, continue to sell the units.

Before starting a facial treatment, the vaporizer should be filled with distilled water. Ordinary tap water contains minerals that will form deposits in the machine and clog the nozzle. It takes at least ten minutes for steam to start coming out of the nozzle once the machine is turned on, so it is necessary to start the machine well before the time it will be needed. While the machine is heating, the nozzle should be kept away from the client's face.

THE ROTARY BRUSH

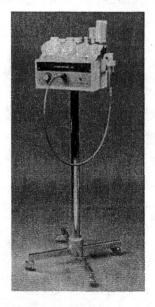

The rotary brush machine is used for deep cleansing, surface peeling and light massage. These machines are available in a number of forms, ranging from hand-held portable units to floor units. The floor units are driven by a flexible shaft arrangement or by direct drive motors. The larger, more sophisticated units have speed controls to vary the brush speed from 0 to 700 or more revolutions per minute. The brushes, which are detachable, come in a variety of sizes for use on different areas of the face or body. They are generally made from natural bristles, such as goat hair, and vary from coarse, for use on oily skin, to soft, for use on dry or mature skin. Other attachments, such as sponges and abrasive stones, are also available (Fig. 16.6).

Brushing also gives a gentle, soothing massage that helps relax the client. For additional massage effect, the brushes can be used dry. With this method, however, avoid extended contact with the skin to avoid irritation.

The rotary brush treatment should take place early in the facial process. Typically, it will be the first step after the analysis of the skin. However, it may be done after the steaming step. After brushing, remove excess product from the client's skin with tepid water, so it will be ready for the next step in the facial.

Clean the brushes and other attachments with soap and hot water, then sanitize them with alcohol. Store in an ultraviolet sterilizer or in a clean, dry, covered container or cabinet.

16.6—Rotary brush machine *(Courtesy of Nemectron, Inc.)*

THE VACUUM/SPRAY MACHINE

Although used for different purposes, the vacuum machine and the spray machine are part of the same piece of apparatus. The vacuum side is used to help remove excess oils and dirt from the skin, while the spray side is used to apply lotions or other skin-care products in a fine, even mist. The machine has an intensity control to regulate the suction or spray volume to suit the client's needs. Some units also have a removable filter to capture debris vacuumed from the skin so it won't clog the machine (Fig. 16.7).

Accessories for the vacuum side include glass ventouses, vessels used for cupping different areas of the skin. The larger ventouses are used on the chin or forehead, while the smaller ventouses are used around the nose area.

For best results, the vacuum treatment should be done after steaming and disincrustation when the pores have been opened and embedded oils have been softened. Except for very slight amounts of disincrustation solution or water, the skin should be free of any cleansers or lotions while it is being vacuumed. Any preparations on the skin will be sucked into the machine and may clog or otherwise damage it.

Clean the ventouses with hot, soapy water and sanitize in alcohol. Store them in a dry sterilizer.

The spray side of the machine is equipped with one or more bottles with fine mist spray nozzles. Although only one bottle can be attached to the machine at one time, there is usually a quick release

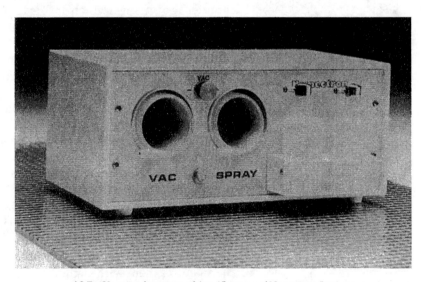

16.7—Vacuum/spray machine (*Courtesy of Nemectron, Inc.*)

mechanism so bottles can be interchanged rapidly. This lets the operator fill bottles with different solutions so the correct product can be used without needing to empty and refill the spray bottle for each client. The product is usually diluted 2 to 1 with distilled water.

The spray can be used at a number of points during the facial. It can be used to rinse traces of cleanser from the face to help restore the acid mantle, after manual extraction to soothe and refresh the skin, or after removing the mask.

THE ELECTRIC PULVERISATOR

The pulverisator, or Dr. Lucas spray, is a hand-held spray machine capable of combining herbs, herb teas, or essential oils with water and applying them in either a warm or cool spray, depending on the distance the unit is held from the face. The unit, which resembles an old time plumber's blowtorch, has an internal water tank and two external containers made of glass. The glass containers are connected to the machine's spray nozzle with flexible tubing (Fig. 16.8).

The tank is filled with distilled water, which then boils. The crushed herbs, herb teas, or other substances to be used for the treatment are placed in the larger glass container. The smaller glass container is used to catch any dripping. The spray starts when the flexible plastic tube is dipped into the large glass container. The material in the container is siphoned into the nozzle area where it mixes with the steam.

Procedures for using the Lucas spray are similar to those used for

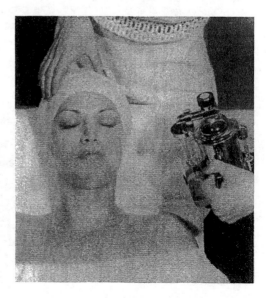

16.8—Pulverisator *(Courtesy of Sothys, USA, Inc.)*

the spray machine, as discussed earlier. However, care should be taken since boiling water and steam are present.

THE GALVANIC CURRENT MACHINE

The galvanic current machine, like the vacuum-spray machine, has two uses. Depending on the polarity set, it is used for disincrustation or for iontophoresis. The galvanic current machine is equipped with:

- an on-off switch,
- a polarity reversing switch to change the current on the working electrode from positive to negative,
- a rheostat to regulate the amount of current,
- and an ammeter for measuring the amount of current being delivered.

Two electrodes attach to the machine—a passive electrode that is held by the client during the treatment and a working electrode that is used by the esthetician (Fig. 16.9).

The process of disincrustation helps soften hardened sebum in the pores so it can be removed more easily. The working electrode is set as the negative pole. The passive electrode is the positive pole. In this polarity condition, it will stimulate the skin and increase the circulation. The current works in conjunction with an alkaline disincrustation solution that penetrates and dissolves the oily deposits.

The process of iontophoresis allows the penetration of water soluble treatment products into the skin where they can work more effectively than they can by remaining on the surface. The working electrode is set as the positive pole. The passive electrode is the negative pole. In this polarity condition, it will soothe the skin and decrease circulation. Any desired treatment product can be used as long as it is water soluble and is on the acidic side.

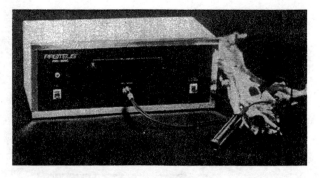

16.9—Galvanic current machine (*Courtesy of Proteus, Inc.*)

The procedure for iontophoresis is similar to that for disincrustation. The client holds the passive electrode, which is now the negative pole. The treatment product is applied to the client's face. It is not necessary to cover the working electrode with gauze.

Unlike disincrustation, which is used only on oily, clogged skin, iontophoresis can be used on any type of skin. As before, however, the machine should not be used on pregnant women or clients with pacemakers, high blood pressure, or heart conditions.

THE HIGH-FREQUENCY MACHINE

The high-frequency machine generates a rapidly oscillating current that is transmitted to the client's skin through glass electrodes. This current produces heat deep in the dermal layer of the skin and stimulates the skin and improves circulation. The high-frequency current also increases the absorption rate of skin creams and acts as a germicide to kill harmful bacteria (Fig. 16.10).

The machine generally has an on-off switch, an intensity control, and an insulated electrode holder. Some models incorporate a timer to regulate the length of treatment. The electrodes are usually made of glass and come in a number of shapes. The most commonly used electrode is mushroom shaped. The electrodes are sealed and are filled with a gas, such as neon. When the electrode is inserted into the holder and current flows through, the gas glows with a characteristic violet to reddish-orange color.

The high-frequency current can be applied either directly or indirectly. The current is used over the treatment cream or oil. The high-frequency machine can also be used for sparking. As with all machinery, follow the manufacturer's instructions for the proper use of the machine.

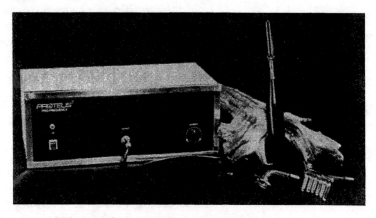

16.10—Large high-frequency machine *(Courtesy of Proteus, Inc.)*

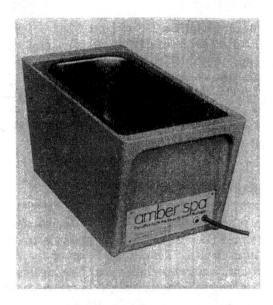

16.11—Large paraffin bath *(Courtesy of Amber Products Co.)*

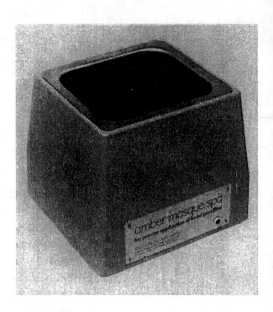

16.12—Small paraffin bath *(Courtesy of Amber Products Co.)*

PARAFFIN BATH

Paraffin bath tanks melt and hold paraffin wax at the proper temperature for use in hand and foot treatments or for paraffin facial masks (Fig. 16.11 and Fig. 16.12).

The larger tanks are designed to let the client dip hands or feet into the molten paraffin, letting it coat the extremity and trapping heat and moisture inside the wax glove thus formed. These tanks hold the paraffin at a temperature of about 134°F. The smaller tank, used for paraffin facial masks, is designed to hold the molten wax in a state during which it can be transferred to the client's face by brush. Because some heat is lost during the transfer, this tank operates at a slightly higher temperature, about 136°F.

REVIEW QUESTIONS

1. Why should the esthetician use specialized equipment for a facial?
2. Why should the facial chair be comfortable?
3. When is the magnifying lamp used?
4. What is the operating principle of the Wood's lamp?
5. Under the Wood's lamp, what does an orange fluorescence indicate?
6. What are two benefits of using steam during the facial?

7. What is ozone?
8. Why shouldn't tap water be used in the vaporizer?
9. Why is the rotary brush used?
10. Why is the vacuum side of the vacuum/spray machine used?
11. Why is the spray side of the vacuum/spray machine used?
12. When should the vacuum treatment be done?
13. What is the electric pulverisator?
14. In what two ways is the galvanic current machine used?
15. What is disincrustation?
16. What is iontophoresis?
17. For what type of skin is disincrustation used?
18. Why is the high-frequency machine used?
19. What are three methods of applying high-frequency current?
20. What is the benefit of the paraffin bath?

1 Glossary of Terms

abiotic—Nonliving factors that make up an ecosystem.

acid—A chemical that gives up hydrogen in solution with water and reacts with metals to produce hydrogen.

afferent nerve—A sensory nerve that transmits information from sensory receptors to the brain.

AIDS—Acquired Immune Deficiency Syndrome, a disease that destroys the immune system, leaving the body vulnerable to disease.

alcohol—A hydrocarbon derivative formed by replacing one or more hydrogens with a hydroxo group.

aldehyde—A class of chemical compounds made by oxidizing primary alcohols.

algae—Members of the phylum Thallophyta. Unicellular or multicellular plants that have no roots, stems or leaves.

alkali—Another word for a base.

alkali metal—A family of active metallic elements in group 1A on the periodic table.

alkaline earth metal—A family of active metallic elements in group 2A on the periodic table.

allergen—A substance that causes an allergic reaction.

allopathic—A form of medicine that relies on synthetic drugs as therapeutic agents.

alveoli—Structures in the lungs that exchange oxygen and carbon dioxide gases during respiration.

amino acid—The building block of the body, produced by the digestion of proteins.

ampere—A measure of the intensity of an electrical current.

anabolism—The part of metabolism in which nutrients are converted to chemicals that build up tissue.

anatomy—The study of gross structures, i.e., those that can be seen by the unaided eye.

animalia—The biological kingdom of animals, i.e., multicellular organisms whose cells contain chromosomes.

anion—A particle with a negative charge because of an excess of electrons.

antibodies—Bodies produced in the immune system to attack antigens.

antigen—an organism that causes an immune system response.

antiseptic—An agent that kills germs and protects against infection.

aromatherapy—A branch of herbal medicine that utilizes the essential oils derived from plants.

atom—The smallest unit of matter.

atomic number—The number of protons contained in the nucleus of an atom.

atrophy—The withering away of an organ or tissue through disuse.

autonomic nervous system—The system responsible for functions under involuntary control.

B-lymphocytes—Immune system cells that produce antibodies.

bacilla—A species of rod shaped bacteria. The most numerous form of bacteria.

bacteria—Microscopic, single-celled organisms of the kingdom Monera.

balneotherapy—Methods of water therapy that utilize fresh water.

base—A chemical that gives up hydroxide ions in solution with water.

biology—The scientific study of living organisms.

biotic—Living factors that make up an ecosystem.

blepharoplasty—A cosmetic surgical procedure to correct flaws in the upper and lower eyelids.

bone—A hard combination of living and nonliving matter that forms the skeletal system, which supports the body.

botany—The study of plants.

Boyle's Law—The scientific law that states volume of a gas will vary inversely with pressure as long as temperature remains constant.

brow lift—A cosmetic surgical procedure to smoothe out furrows and lines in the forehead.

buffer—A solution that reacts with acids and bases to limit changes in pH.

calorie—The fuel value of a given nutrient, measured by the heat given off when the nutrient is oxidized.

carbohydrate—A class of nutrient that supplies most of the body's energy. Sugars, starches and cellulose.

carcinogen—A substance that can cause cancer.

cartilage—A specialized form of connective tissue that helps support the body.

catabolism—The part of metabolism in which nutrients are broken down to supply energy.

catalyst—A substance that increases the yield of a chemical reaction without becoming part of the reaction product.

cation—A particle with a positive charge because of a deficiency of electrons.

cell—The basic unit of living organisms.

cellulite—A term used by some in the beauty industry to describe rough, orange-peel appearing fat deposits around the thighs.

cellulose—A form of carbohydrate that is indigestible by humans.

chelation—A chemical bonding of a mineral with an amino acid to allow the mineral to be digested.

chemical peel—A procedure to remove fine wrinkles and smooth skin by chemically burning off the outer layer of skin.

chemistry—The branch of the physical sciences concerned with changes in the various states of matter.

chlorophyll—A green pigment that gives color to plants and gathers light energy from the sun to allow photosynthesis.

cholesterol—A chemical product of nutrition used in a number of physiological processes.

chromosome—A chromatin-containing organelle in the cell nucleus, containing the sex characteristics of the organism.

chyme—The food mass, after it has been liquified in the stomach.

cilia—A series of short, hair-like filaments around some microorganisms. Cilia undulate to allow motility.

cocci—A species of round bacteria that grow in pairs, chains, or clusters.

coelom—The body cavity of the higher animal forms.

collagen—Inelastic, flexible white fiber bundles found in connective tissue.

collagen injection—A semi-permanent procedure for smoothing out wrinkles by injecting soluble collagen under the skin.

colloid—A liquid in which very small undissolved particles are suspended.

compound—Two or more elements joined together chemically to create a new substance.

conductor—A substance that allows the free movement of electrons, i.e., lets electricity flow readily.

cortex—The center layer of the hair shaft.

cuticle—The outer layer of the hair shaft.

cystine—A sulfur-containing amino acid.

cytology—The study of cells at the microscopic level.

cytoplasm—Living matter that surrounds the nucleus of a cell.

decoction—A herbal preparation made by boiling a herb in water.

deionization—A process of removing metallic mineral ions from water to purify it.

demographics—The characteristics of a given population.

dermabrasion—A procedure for smoothing skin by abrading the outer layer of skin.

dermaplaning—A procedure for smoothing skin by shaving off the outer layer of skin.

dermatome—A razor-like device for dermaplaning.

dermis—The innermost layer of skin.

diatomaceous earth—A porous silica composed of the remains of diatoms, used in facial masks as an absorbing and tightening agent.

disinfectant—A chemical substance used to kill germs.

distillation—A process of boiling water and condensing the steam on plates to purify it.

DNA—Deoxyribonucleic acid. A nucleotide found in the cell nucleus. Takes the form of a double stranded helix. With RNA carries genetic information.

echo—The reflection of sound from a smooth surface.

ecology—The study of the relationships between living organisms and their environment.

ectoderm—The outer embryonic germ layer.

edema—The swelling of tissues.

efferent nerve—A motor nerve that transmits signals from the brain to the muscles.

effleurage—In massage, gentle stroking movements.

elastin—A component of elastic fibers found in connective tissue.

electrolyte—A conductor of electricity.

electron—A negatively charged atomic particle rotating around the nucleus of an atom.

element—The simplest form of matter. There are currently 105 known elements.

embryology—The study of the embryo, the period between the fertilization of the egg and the completion of the body structure.

emulsifier—An agent that allows immiscible liquids to be mixed together.

endocrine gland—A ductless gland of the endocrine system, which injects secretions directly into the bloodstream.

endoderm—The inner embryonic germ layer.

endorphin—A natural painkilling chemical substance produced by the body.

endoskeleton—An internal skeleton that provides support for an animal body.

endothermic—A chemical reaction that absorbs heat.

energy—The capacity of an object to do work.

enzyme—A substance produced in the body that acts as a catalyst in the various chemical reactions of the body processes.

epidermis—The outermost layer of skin.

equilibrium—The point in a chemical reaction when the reaction stops.

ester—A class of chemical compounds made by reacting a carboxylic acid with an alcohol.

esthetics—The branch of cosmetology that treats the skin using nonmedical methods, to normalize and maintain the beauty and the health of the skin.

estrogen—The hormone that gives females their sex characteristics.

eunuch—A castrated male, castrated before the onset of puberty.

exocrine gland—A ducted gland that transports secretions through a system of ducts.

exoskeleton—An external skeleton that provides support for an animal body.

exothermic—A chemical reaction that gives off heat.

fat—A class of nutrient that provides a concentrated source of energy.

fatty acid—The chemical compound that gives fat its characteristic taste and texture.

fibroblast—A long, irregularly shaped cell that synthesizes protein for tissue growth. A typical cell in connective tissue.

flagella—A single, long, hair-like appendage that allows motility in a microorganism.

fomentation—A herbal preparation made by soaking a towel in a hot infusion.

frequency—The number of complete vibrations that occur in a given unit of time.

friction—A force that opposes free motion of objects moving over other objects.

Fuller's earth—Aluminum magnesium silicate used in facial masks as an absorbing and tightening agent.

fumigant—A vaporized chemical substance whose fumes kill germs.

fungi—The biological kingdom of plantlike organisms that do not obtain nutrients through photosynthesis.

fuse—A safety device to interrupt electrical flow during an overload in a circuit.

genetics—The study of heredity and the gene structures of organisms.

glucose—The chemical produced by the action of enzymes on carbohydrates to produce energy for immediate use.

glycogen—The chemical produced from glucose and stored in the liver for later use.

Golgi apparatus—An organelle that stores and transports materials used by other parts of a cell.

ground substance—Nonliving intercellular material. Also called matrix.

herb—A plant material, generally used as a medicine or as a spice.

hertz—The common unit of frequency expressed in cycles per second.

heterogeneous—Mixtures that are not uniform throughout.

HIV—The AIDS virus.

homeopathic—A form of medicine that relies on natural substances as theraputic agents.

homeostasis—The process that regulates the internal environment of an organism so it remains constant.

homogenous—Mixtures that are uniform throughout.

hormone—A chemical substance that retards or stimulates the function of another organ.

hue—A color, i.e., red, green, etc.

hydrocarbon—An organic compound containing hydrogen and carbon.

hypothesis—A tentative explanation of a scientific law.

immiscible—The quality that does not allow two liquids to mix readily.

indicator—A substance that changes color to determine the acidity or alkalinity of a solution.

inertia—The tendency of an object at rest to stay at rest or for an object in motion to stay in motion.

infusion—A herbal preparation made by steeping a herb in boiling water.

insulator—A nonconductor of electricity.

integument—The outer covering of a human being. The skin.

intensity—The brightness or dullness of a color.

International System Unit—A basic metric unit used in scientific discussion because of its precision and uniformity.

invertebrate—A member of the animal kingdom that does not have a backbone.

ion—A charged atomic particle.

iridology—A controversial diagnostic technique utilizing nerve endings in the iris of the eye.

isotope—A form of an element in which the number of neutrons varies. The atomic number stays the same but the atomic weight changes.

joint—An articulation at the junction of two or more bones.

kaolin—A yellowish-white clay used in facial masks as an absorbing and tightening agent.

kelp—A form of seaweed.

keratin—A sulfur-containing protein that is the major component of the epidermis, nails and hair.

ketone—A class of chemical compounds made by oxidizing secondary alcohols.

ki—The body's vital energy force constantly circulating through the meridians.

Kieselguhr—Diatomaceous earth.

lanolin—A natural animal oil derived from sheep wool, used in cosmetics and skin care products as a lubricant.

law—A generalized statement that describes and summarizes observed scientific phenomena.

Law of Conservation of Energy—A scientific law that states that energy can neither be created nor destroyed.

Law of Conservation of Mass—A scientific law that states that matter can neither be created nor destroyed.

Law of Intensity of Illumination—A scientific law that states light intensity varies directly with the candlepower of the source and inversely with the square of the distance.

Law of Machines—A scientific law that states the output of work must equal the input of work.

Law of Motion—A set of scientific laws that characterize the physical response of objects in motion or at rest.

Law of Universal Gravitation—Newton's law that states every object in the universe attracts every other object with a force directly proportional to the product of their masses and inversely proportional to the square of their distance apart.

lesion—A circumscribed, well-defined change in a body part caused by injury.

lipid—A fatty substance that is one of the components of living cells.

litmus—An indicator used to determine the acidity or alkalinity of a solution.

lymphocyte—A cell in the lymphatic system that attacks disease-causing microorganisms.

malar implant—A cosmetic surgical procedure to add shape to the cheeks through the use of surgical implants.

mass—The amount of matter an object contains.

matter—Any substance that has mass and occupies space.

medulla—The inner layer of the hair shaft.

melanin—The pigment that gives skin its characteristic color.

mentoplasty—A cosmetic surgical procedure to correct flaws in the chin.

meridian—A channel in the body along which the vital energy force, ki, flows.

mesoderm—The middle embryonic germ layer.

metabolism—The complex biochemical activities that sustain life in an organism, by which nutrients are converted to either tissue or to energy.

mineral—An inorganic element. In nutrition, inorganic nutrients that let vitamins work.

miscible—The quality that allows two liquids to be mixed together.

mitosis—The process of cell division.

mixture—Two or more elements intermingled physically but not chemically.

molecule—A combination of atoms bound tightly together.

momentum—The tendency of an object in motion to resist changes in its motion.

monera—The biological kingdom of single-celled organisms without an organized nucleus, i.e., bacteria.

morphology—The study of the structures of living organisms.

nephron—The structural unit of the kidney that performs the filtration function.

neuron—The basic unit of the nervous system.

neurotransmitter—A chemical particle that transmits electrical impulses across the gap between neurons.

neutron—A neutrally charged atomic particle in the nucleus of an atom.

nucleic acid—DNA or RNA, responsible for carrying genetic information.

nucleus—The largest organelle in a cell.

Ohm's Law—A scientific law that characterizes the relationship of electrical intensity to voltage and resistance.

ointment—A herbal preparation made by mixing a herb with a hot fat or petroleum jelly to make a thick cream.

organ—A group of tissues formed to provide specialized functions.

organelle—A part of a cell.

otoplasty—A cosmetic surgical procedure to correct protruding ears.

paleontology—The study of ancient and extinct life forms through the examination of fossils.

parasite—An organism that takes nourishment from living organic matter.

Pascal's Law— A scientific law that states pressure in an enclosed liquid is transmitted undiminished throughout the entire liquid.

pathogenic—An agent that causes disease.

papain—An enzyme found in papaya, used in skin care products to dissolve dead surface cells.

perennial—A plant that grows throughout the year.

Periodic Table—A graphic representation for classifying elements by their atomic number and their familial characteristics.

peristalsis—A rippling, wave-like motion of the muscles of the esophagus or of the intestines, which moves food through the alimentary canal.

petrissage—In massage, kneading and pulling motions.

petrolatum—A jelly-like substance derived from petroleum, used in cosmetics and skin-care products as a lubricant.

pH—A measurement of the degree of acidity or alkalinity of a solution on a scale of 1 to 14.

photosynthesis—The process in which plants convert sunlight into nutrients.

physics—The science that studies physical changes in matter.

physiology—The study of the parts of an organism and how they function.

phytohormone—A plant hormone.

pitch—A characteristic of sound determined by the frequency.

plantae—The biological kingdom of plants, i.e., multicellular organisms that manufacture food by photosynthesis and contain cellulose in their cell walls.

polymerization—A chemical process of bonding hydrocarbon molecules into long chains.

poultice—A herbal preparation made by mixing a crushed herb with a hot liquid or gum to make a paste.

power—In physics, the work divided by the time it takes to do the work.

primate—The highest order of mammal. Man is a primate.

product—The substance formed as the result of a chemical reaction.

pronator—A muscle that turns the forearm and hand palm down.

protein—A nutrient that supplies materials for building tissue and for producing hormones and enzymes.

protista—The biological kingdom of single-celled organisms with an organized nucleus, i.e., amoebae.

proton—A positively charged atomic particle in the nucleus of an atom.

protoplasm—Living matter.

rare gas—A family of elements in group 8A of the periodic table. Also called inert gases.

reactant—An original or starting substance in a chemical reaction.

reflex—An automatic response to a stimulus triggered directly from the spinal cord.

refraction—The tendency of a light ray to bend as it passes from one transparent medium to another.

resistance—The ability of a metal to conduct electricity.

reticulin—A protein that, along with collagen and elastin, gives the skin its elasticity, resilience and strength.

rhinoplasty—A cosmetic surgical procedure to remove flaws in the nose.

rhytidectomy—A cosmetic surgical procedure to tighten loose skin on the face and neck. A face lift.

RNA—Riboneucleic acid. A nucleotide found in the cell cytoplasm. With DNA, carries genetic information.

saliva—A secretion in the mouth that moistens food and begins breaking it down into simple sugars.

saprophyte—An organism that takes nourishment from dead organic matter.

schizomycete—The biological phylum to which bacteria belong.

seaweed—A multicellular form of algae found in ocean waters. It contains valuable minerals and nutrients.

silicone injection—A permanent procedure for smoothing out wrinkles by injecting silicone under the skin.

sinus—A space in a bone around the nasal cavity that reduces weight of the bone and supplies mucus to the nasal cavity.

skin pigmentation procedure—The injection of dyes into the skin for permanently darkening it.

solution—A mixture that is uniform throughout.

somatic nervous system—The system responsible for functions under voluntary, or conscious, control.

species—A group of organisms related by their ability to produce fertile young.

SPF—Skin Protection Factor. A rating given to sunscreen agents to indicate safe exposure to the sun.

spirilla—A species of motile, spiral shaped bacteria.

spirochete—A species of highly motile bacteria that are long and curved and move in a corkscrew motion.

spore—An almost indestructible dormant form of cell by which certain organisms survive when conditions for growth are disrupted.

starch—A form of carbohydrate that is converted to sugar during digestion.

supinator—A muscle that turns the forearm and hand palm up.

synovial fluid—A lubricating liquid found in joints.

system—A group of organs working together to perform specific functions.

tapotement—In massage, tapping or other percussion movements.

taxonomy—The study of organisms as a whole and their classification into groups that are similar in structure.

testosterone—The hormone that gives males their sex characteristics.

thalassotherapy—The technique of using sea water and sea products as theraputic agents.

theory—A generalized explanation of a scientific law.

tincture—A herbal preparation made by soaking a herb in alcohol.

tissue—The structural material of the body formed by cells grouped according to specialization.

transition metal—A family of metallic elements grouped in the center of the periodic table.

triglyceride—A class of fat and oil that contains three groups of hydrocarbon chains.

tsubo—A specific pressure point along a meridian where pressure is applied during a shiatsu or accupressure massage.

valence—The capacity of an atom to combine chemically with other atoms. The charge of a single ion.

value—The lightness or darkness of a color.

vector—A graphic representation of a force, indicating size and direction.

vertebrate—A member of the animal kingdom that has a backbone.

virus—An infectious, nonliving parasite.

vitamin—An organic catalyst that allows nutrients to work.

voltage—The measure of the difference in the electrical charge between two poles.

watt—The measure of electrical power, the rate at which electrical energy is used.

wavelength—The distance between two corresponding points along a wave during one complete vibration.

weight—The effect on an object of the earth's gravitational pull.

white blood cells—Lymphocytes. The bodies that fight disease in the body.

work—In physics, the product of the force applied to an object multiplied by the displacement.

yang—In eastern philosophy, the masculine component of the whole.

yeast—A unicellular form of fungi.

yin—In eastern philosophy, the feminine component of the whole.

zooflagellate—A species of animal-like protozoa. Members of the biological kingdom protista.

zoology—The study of animals.

Suggested Readings

Abehsera, Michael. *The Healing Clay.* Brooklyn: Swan House Publishing Co., 1979.

Abravanel, Eliot D. *Dr. Abravanel's Body Type Diet And Lifetime Nutrition Plan.* New York: Bantam Books, 1984.

Ardell, Donald B. *High Level Wellness.* New York: Bantam Books, 1981.

Asimov, Isaac. *On The Human Body And The Human Brain.* New York: Bonanza Books, 1985.

Bach, Edward. *The Bach Flower Remedies.* New Canaan: Keats Publishing, Inc., 1979.

Ballentine, Rudolph. *Diet And Nutrition: A Holistic Approach.* Honesdale: Himalayan International Institute, 1978.

Beck, Mark. *The Theory And Practice Of Therapeutic Massage.* Albany, NY: Milady Publishing Co., 1988.

Berkeley Holistic Health Center. *The Holistic Health Handbook.* Berkeley: And/Or Press, 1978.

Binnick, Steven A. *Skin Diseases: Diagnosis And Management In Clinical Practice.* Menlo Park: Addison-Wesley Publishing Co., 1982.

Bodanis, David. *The Body Book.* Boston: Little, Brown and Co., 1984.

Bolemon, Jay. *Physics, An Introduction.* Englewood Cliffs: Prentice-Hall, Inc., 1985.

Boxer, Arabella, and Back, Philippa. *The Herb Book.* London: Octopus Books, 1984.

Brody, Jane. *Jane Brody's Nutrition Book.* New York: W. W. Norton, 1981.

Brown, Theodore L., and LeMay, H. Eugene. *Chemistry, The Central Science.* Englewood Cliffs: Prentice-Hall, Inc., 1977.

Bruun, Ruth D., and Bruun, Bertel. *The Human Body.* New York: Random House, 1982.

Buchman, Dian Dincin. *The Complete Herbal Guide To Natural Health and Beauty.* Garden City: Doubleday and Co., 1973.

Buchman, Dian Dincin. *Herbal Medicine.* New York: Gramercy Publishing Co., 1980.

Cho, Emily. *Looking, Working, Living Terrific 24 Hours A Day*. New York: G.P. Putnam's Sons, 1982.

Clark, Kenneth. *Feminine Beauty*. London: Weidenfeld and Nicolson, 1980.

Cruickshank, Alexandra. *The New Beauty Book*. New York: Mayflower Books, 1982.

Dox, Ida; Melloni, Biagio J.; and Eisner, Gilbert M. *Melloni's Illustrated Medical Dictionary*. Baltimore: The Williams and Wilkins Co., 1979.

Dvorine, William. *A Dermatologists' Guide To Home Skin Treatment*. New York: Charles Scribners and Sons, 1983.

Edwards, Gabrielle I. *Biology The Easy Way*. Woodbury: Barron's Educational Series, Inc., 1984.

Gawain, Shakti. *Creative Visualization*. New York: Bantam Books, 1982.

Gerson, Joel. *Standard Textbook For Professional Estheticians*, 6th Ed. Albany, NY: Milady Publishing Co., 1989.

Gewirtz, Herman. *Essentials Of Physics*. Woodbury: Barron's Educational Series, Inc., 1974.

Gior, Fino. *Modern Electrology*. Albany, NY: Milady Publishing Co., 1987.

Goodman, Thomas. *The Skin Doctor's Skin Doctoring Book*. New York: Sterling Publishing Co., Inc., 1984.

Haberman, Frederick, and Fortino, Denise. *Your Skin*. New York: PBJ Books, Inc., 1983.

Hosler, Ray. *Massage Book*. Mountain View: Runners World Books, 1982.

Jensen, Bernard. *Iridology Simplified*. Escondido: Iridologists International, 1980.

Kaye, Anna, and Matchan, Don C. *Reflexology For Good Health*. North Hollywood: Wilshire Book Co., 1978.

Kirschmann, John D., and Dunne, Lavon J. *Nutrition Almanac*, 2nd Ed. New York: McGraw-Hill Book Co., 1984.

Kloss, Jethro. *Back To Eden*. Santa Barbara: Woodbridge Press Publishing Co., 1981.

Kunz, Kevin, and Kunz, Barbara. *Hand And Foot Reflexology: A Self-Help Guide*. Englewood Cliffs: Prentice-Hall, Inc., 1984.

Lawrence, D. Baloti, and Harrison, Lewis. *Massageworks*. New York: Putnam Publishing Co., 1983.

Lidell, Lucinda, et al. *The Book Of Massage*. New York: Simon and Schuster, 1984.

Luscher, Max. *The Luscher Color Test*. New York: Washington Square Press, 1969.

Lust, John. *The Herb Book*. New York: Bantam Books, 1974.

Madry, Bobby Ray. *Student's Illustrated Cosmetology Dictionary*. Albany, NY: Milady Publishing Co., 1990.

Milady's Standard Textbook of Cosmetology. Albany, NY: Milady Publishing Co., 1991.

Mindell, Earl. *Vitamin Bible*. New York: Warner Books, 1985.

Montagna, William, and Parakkal, Paul F. *The Structure And Function Of The Skin*, 3rd Ed. New York: Academic Press, 1974.

Montagu, Ashley. *Touching, The Human Significance Of The Skin*, 2nd Ed. New York: Harper and Row, 1978.

Namikoshi, Toru. *The Complete Book Of Shiatsu Therapy*. Tokyo: Japan Publications, Inc., 1981.

Null, Gary, and Null, Steve. *The Complete Handbook Of Nutrition*. New York: Dell Publishing Co., 1972.

Null, Gary. *Food Combining Handbook*. New York: Jove Books, 1983.

Pearson, Durk, and Shaw, Sandy. *Life Extension*. New York: Warner Books, 1982.

Pearson, Durk, and Shaw, Sandy. *The Life Extension Companion*. New York: Warner Books, 1984.

Place, Stan Campbell. *The Art And Science Of Professional Makeup*. Albany, NY: Milady Publishing Co., 1989.

Restak, Richard M. *The Brain*. New York: Bantam Books, 1984.

Reviva Labs. *The Cosmetic Ingredient Manual*. Haddonfield: Reviva Labs, Inc., 1980.

Rodgers, C. Leland. *Essentials Of Biology*. Woodbury: Barron's Educational Services, Inc., 1974.

Sauer, Gordon C. *Manual Of Skin Diseases*, 4th Ed. Philadelphia: J. B. Lippincott Co., 1980.

Schoen, Linda A., ed. *The AMA Book Of Skin And Hair Care*. New York: Avon Books, 1978.

Schrader, Constance. *Makeovers*. Englewood Cliffs: Prentice-Hall, Inc., 1979.

Shepard, Stephen P. *Healing Energies*. Provo: Hawthorne Books, 1981.

Steen, Edwin, and Montagu, Ashley. *Anatomy And Physiology*, Volumes 1 and 2, 2nd Ed. New York: Barnes and Noble, 1984.

Tenney, Louise. *Today's Herbal Health*. Provo: Woodland Books, 1983.

Tierra, Michael. *The Way Of Herbs*. New York: Washington Square Press, 1983.

Tisserand, Robert B. *The Art Of Aromatherapy*. New York: Inner Traditions International, Ltd., 1979.

Valnet, Jean. *The Practice Of Aromatherapy*. New York: Destiny Books, 1982.

Vannini, Vanio, and Pogliani, Guiliano, ed. *The Color Atlas Of Human Anatomy*. New York: Beekman House, 1980.

Winter, Ruth. *A Consumer's Dictionary Of Cosmetic Ingredients*. New York: Crown Publishers, Inc., 1984.

3 Answers to Chapter Review Questions

Chapter 1
Introduction to Esthetics

1. Esthetics is the nonmedical care of the skin, to maintain its health and beauty.
2. The three elements of a successful skin-care program are cleanliness, nutrition, and attitude. All three must work together.
3. Attitude is important because skin care requires a commitment to make the effort required to care for the skin.
4. Esthetics is a health care field as well as a beauty-care field. It utilizes many of the aspects of holistic medical practice, such as herbals and aromatherapy. However, the esthetician is *not* a medical doctor and can neither diagnose nor treat illnesses.
5. Esthetics is both a science and an art. It requires the knowledge, study and understanding of the scientist, along with the talent, experience and intuition of the artist.
6. Beauty is a perception on the part of the viewer, not an absolute value. It is an emotional value, stemming from the ancient Greek concepts of symmetry and proportion, which make the object pleasing to the eye.
7. The classical measure of proportion is the length of the head. The well-proportioned body is 7½ head lengths tall.
8. A person cannot feel beautiful without being healthy. Good health promotes the well-being needed for beauty.
9. The esthetician must have a basic understanding of the physical sciences, physiology, skin structure and function, skin disorders, skin-care products and machinery, nutrition, massage techniques, psychology, and salesmanship.
10. The attributes a professional esthetician needs are: appearance, manner, knowledge, talent, confidence, creativity, empathy, and trustworthiness.

Chapter 2
Introduction to the Facial

1. The facial is the key to skin care in the salon. It is the basis of the day-to-day work of the esthetician.
2. A facial is a multi-step process for cleaning the client's skin, alleviating minor disorders and normalizing its function.

3. The esthetician must know how to perform the procedures in a facial and which products and equipment to use. He or she must also know skin-care theory and must be able to identify skin types.
4. Facials can be given without machinery, but it is always necessary to use some kind of chemical product.
5. The proper equipment makes a facial more efficient and more effective.
6. The two basic parts of the facial are deep-pore cleansing and normalization and treatment.
7. Deep-pore cleansing removes impurities from the skin. Normalization and treatment put nutrients back into the skin.
8. The esthetician must first consult with the client and analyze the client's skin.
9. The general steps in a facial are: application and removal of cleanser, application of toner or astringent, massage, steaming, disincrustation, vacuum application, manual extraction, mask, iontophoresis, high-frequency current and application of moisturizers and nutrients.
10. No, the steps will vary in each facial depending on the client's skin type and needs.

Chapter 3
Bacteriology and
Sanitation

1. Cleanliness is important in the salon to prevent the spread of disease.
2. The two types of bacteria are saprophytes and parasites.
3. Saprophytes take nourishment from dead organic matter; parasites take nourishment from living hosts.
4. Bacteria thrive under dark, warm, damp, and dirty conditions where there is a lot of food.
5. Spirochetes and eubacteria are of most interest to the esthetician because they are the bacteria that cause disease.
6. The three classes of eubacteria are bacilli, rod shaped; cocci, round shaped; and spirilla, spiral shaped.
7. Staphylococci cause pus-forming infections, such as boils and abscesses.
8. Viruses are infectious parasites, but are not living organisms. They can only exist inside living cells.
9. DNA-viruses are responsible for diseases such as herpes simplex, venereal herpes, shingles, and warts.
10. The immune system is the body's watchdog that protects it from disease.
11. Lymphocytes are the basic units of the immune system.
12. The esthetician can avoid the spread of infectious diseases by avoiding contact with infected persons and maintaining scrupulous cleanliness and sanitation standards.
13. AIDS is Acquired Immune Deficiency Syndrome, a disease that destroys the body's immune system.
14. The esthetician can help prevent the spread of AIDS by wearing rubber gloves and a surgical mask during manual extraction and other procedures.
15. Louis Pasteur was the scientist who proved that germs cause disease and who made a number of discoveries that advanced the cause of sanitation.
16. The two phases of sanitation are sterilization, killing germs; and prevention, keeping germs from regrowing.

17. Four ways to sterilize implements are heat, ultraviolet light, gamma radiation, and chemicals.
18. Antiseptics are generally milder than disinfectants and can be used safely on the skin.
19. The esthetician must handle waste materials properly to prevent contamination.
20. The most important part of sanitation is common sense.
21. Sanitation is especially critical during manual extraction because it is the step where the client's skin is most exposed to germs and during which the esthetician is most likely to come into contact with the client's blood and debris from the skin.
22. Metallic comedone extractors should never be used because they exert too much force and can damage the skin.
23. A lancet is a medical device, like a razor or needle, that can be used to help remove blemishes from the skin.
24. The esthetician must be aware of safety because he or she comes into contact with a number of potential hazards, such as heat, water, steam, and electricity.
25. Safety is a matter of awareness—of being safety conscious and using common sense.
26. Electrical circuits are protected by fuses or circuit breakers.
27. The rules for safe use of fuses include: use fuses of the right size. Never bypass a fuse by putting a metal object into the the fuse holder. Use a new fuse of the proper rating for the circuit.
28. Two kinds of electrical current are Alternating Current (AC) and Direct Current (DC).
29. The purpose of most government agencies is to protect the public.
30. The FDA is the agency responsible for assuring the safety and efficacy of products in the marketplace.
31. OSHA is the agency responsible for assuring safety in the workplace.
32. Material Safety Data Sheets are documents that describe chemicals and inform users of any possible hazards and use requirements for the product.

Chapter 4
Biology for the Esthetician

1. Biology is important to the esthetician because he or she works with living matter and should understand how it works. In addition, a knowledge of biology helps the esthetician better understand nutrition and sanitation.
2. 1-b, 2-j, 3-d, 4-i, 5-g, 6-a, 7-e, 8-f, 9-h, 10-c.
3. The sun provides energy to the plant, which provides food to the herbivore, which provides food to the carnivore, whose leavings provide food for the scavenger. Decomposers put minerals back into the soil, where they are used by plants.
4. Biology is the science of life.
5. The life functions include: nutrition, transport, respiration, excretion, synthesis, regulation, growth and reproduction. These are known as the metabolic processes.
6. 1-h, 2-i, 3-e, 4-c, 5-f, 6-a, 7-j, 8-d, 9-b, 10-g.
7. Living organisms are classified according to species.
8. In order, organisms are classified by kingdom, phylum, subphylum, class, order, family, genus, and species.

9. The five kingdoms are: monera—single celled organisms without a nucleus; protista—single celled organisms with a nucleus; fungi—plant-like organisms without chlorophyll; plantae—organisms with chlorophyll; animalia—organisms whose cells contain chromosomes.
10. Dead diatoms become diatomaceous earth and are used in some facial masks.
11. Chlorophyll is a green pigment that gives plants their color and gathers energy from the sun for photosynthesis.
12. Photosynthesis is the process by which light energy is converted to chemical energy to provide nutrients for plants.
13. Algaes contain beneficial minerals and nutrients and are used in a variety of skin-care products, including facial masks and body packs.
14. All animal species must obtain food from other sources than themselves. All animal species are more responsive to their environment than plants. And all have some form of support for their bodies.
15. The two classifications of animals are: invertebrates—animals without a backbone, and vertebrates—animals with a backbone.
16. The arthropoda, which includes spiders, crustaceans and insects, has more than 800,000 species.
17. Mammals are the most highly developed class of animals.
18. Man is a primate of the order homo sapiens.

Chapter 5
Physiology for the
Esthetician

1. Physiology is the branch of science that studies the functioning of living organisms.
2. Physiology is important to the esthetician because it is necessary to understand the functions of the body that affect the health of the skin.
3. All of the organs and systems are important to skin health, either directly or indirectly.
4. A cell is the basic unit of living organisms.
5. Cells reproduce by a process called mitosis, or cell division, in which the cell splits into two identical cells.
6. Tissues are the structural materials of the body, and are made up of specialized cells grouped together.
7. There are five kinds of tissue—epithelial tissue, muscular tissue, connective tissue, nerve tissue, and liquid tissue.
8. Epithelial tissue is a sheet-like tissue that makes up the outer covering of the body. The skin.
9. Organs are groups of tissues formed into specialized body parts, such as the brain and heart.
10. Skin is both a tissue and an organ. It is the largest organ of the body.
11. Systems are groups of organs working together to perform specific functions.
12. There are nine systems—skeletal, muscular, nervous, endocrine, circulatory, respiratory, digestive, excretory, and reproductive.
13. The skeletal system is the supporting structure of the body. It consists of the bones, cartilage, and ligaments.
14. The esthetician is most concerned with the bones of the skull, arms and hands, and the foot.
15. There are three kinds of muscle tissue—striated, smooth and cardiac.
16. Skeletal muscles control the movement of the body.

17. There are eighty muscles in the face. They allow the formation of more than 7,000 different expressions.
18. The factors that stimulate or soothe muscles are massage, chemical solutions, electrical current and heat.
19. The nervous system is the electrical control system for all body functions.
20. Nerves affect the muscles and the skin. Various operations conducted during a facial affect the nerves.
21. Afferent, or sensory, nerves transmit information from the senses to the brain. Efferent, or motor, nerves transmit impulses from the brain to the muscles.
22. The twelve pairs of cranial nerves are: first—olfactory; second—optic; third—oculomotor; fourth—trochlear; fifth—trigeminal; sixth—abducent; seventh—facial; eighth—vestibulocochlear; ninth—glossopharyngeal; tenth—vagus; eleventh—accessory; and twelfth—hypoglossal.
23. The fifth—trigeminal, seventh—facial, and eleventh—accessory nerves are of most importance to the esthetician.
24. The endocrine system is the chemical control system of the body.
25. A hormone is a chemical that retards or stimulates the functions of another organ. They control most basic life functions.
26. Proper circulation affects the health of the skin.
27. The four chambers of the heart are the left and right atria, the upper chambers, and the left and right ventricles, the lower chambers.
28. The respiratory system brings oxygen to the body so nutrients can be burned and converted to energy.
29. The digestive system processes and distributes nutrients derived from food throughout the body.
30. The digestive system consists of the alimentary canal and the accessory glands, which include the salivary glands, the liver, gallbladder and pancreas.
31. The excretory system removes waste materials and keeps the body from being poisoned.
32. It is important to remember that all systems work together and are interrelated. All have an effect on the skin, either directly or indirectly.

Chapter 6
Skin Structure and Function

1. The skin has two layers, the epidermis and the dermis. The subcutaneous layer is not considered part of the skin.
2. The cutaneous appendages consist of the hair and hair follicles, nails, sweat and oil glands, blood and lymph vessels, nerve endings, and muscles.
3. The epidermis has five layers: the stratum corneum, stratum lucidum, stratum granulosum, stratum spinosum, and stratum germinativum.
4. The Malpighian layer is the name given to the stratum spinosum and stratum germinativum layers collectively.
5. It takes approximately twenty-eight days for cells to migrate through the epidermal layers.
6. The outermost layer, the stratum corneum, is the thickest layer of the epidermis.
7. The stratum corneum provides protection for the rest of the skin.
8. The dermis has two layers, the papillary layer and the reticular layer.

9. Most sensory receptors are found in the reticular layer.
10. Collagen is the supportive component of the skin and is present in the largest amount.
11. Mast cells help heal injury to the skin.
12. The subcutaneous layer is a bed of loose fatty tissue that cushions the skin and gives shape to the body.
13. The only muscles in the skin are the arrector pili muscles attached to hair follicles, which cause hair to stand erect.
14. Sebum is an oily, waxy substance, made of lipids, secreted from the sebaceous glands.
15. The two types of sweat glands are the apocrine and eccrine glands.
16. Apocrine secretion is stimulated by emotional stress. Eccrine secretion is stimulated by both heat and emotional stress.
17. Eccrine glands serve as thermal regulators for the body.
18. 1-b; 2-d; 3-a; 4-e; 5-c.
19. The physiological functions of the skin are protection, regulation, and sensory reception.
20. The chemical functions of the skin are production of sweat, sebum, glucose, lipids, keratin, and melanin.
21. The psychological functions of the skin are communication, arousal, and comforting.
22. Skin type is determined by appearance, texture, pore size, coloration, and gland functioning.
23. The clients' skin type determines the treatments and products chosen.
24. The six basic skin types are: normal, oily, dry, couperose, blemished, and mature.
25. 1-c; 2-a; 3-d; 4-b.

Chapter 7
Skin Disorders

1. The esthetician can work to normalize skin functions and help alleviate certain skin disorders, as well as teach clients how to care for their own skins.
2. The factors harmful to skin are sunlight, smoking, drugs and alcohol, poor nutrition, chemicals, and time.
3. The sun is a problem to skin because it generates ultraviolet radiation, which can damage skin structure.
4. The three bands of the ultraviolet spectrum are: the UV-A band, from 400 to 320 nanometers; the UV-B band, from 320 to 290 nanometers; and the UV-C band, from 290 to 200 nanometers.
5. The UV-A band is the tanning region; the UV-B band is the burning region; and the UV-C band is the germicidal region.
6. Tanning is a defense mechanism in which the skin darkens on exposure to ultraviolet radiation in order to protect itself from damage.
7. Smoking is bad for the skin because it decreases blood circulation and deprives the skin of oxygen and nutrients. Smoke clogs the pores and nicotine stains the skin.
8. Medications can produce side effects that show up as various skin disorders.
9. Common household chemicals, such as laundry detergents, bleaches, and drain cleaners can cause dermatitis.
10. The effects of age on the skin include wrinkles, lines, cracks, dryness, poor circulation, roughness, and itching.

11. With proper techniques and products, the esthetician can retard the effects of aging on the skin.
12. 1-d; 2-f; 3-a; 4-j; 5-g; 6-i; 7-b; 8-c; 9-e; 10-h.
13. Pruritis is the medical term for itching.
14. Blackheads are black plugs of accumulated sebum and other materials in the openings of follicles.
15. Whiteheads are plugs of sebum and other materials trapped below the surface of the skin.
16. Males are more prone to acne than females because acne is related to the production of androgens, male hormones. Females have fewer androgens than men.
17. Rosacea can be helped by proper cleansing and normalization of skin functions.
18. Papulosquamous disorders are scale forming disorders resulting from the excessive accumulation of keratin on the surface of the skin.
19. The two papulosquamous disorders of most importance to the esthetician are seborrheic dermatitis and psoriasis.
20. In cases of dermatitis, the esthetician should refer the client to a physician.
21. Warts are viral infections characterized by round, rough bumps on the skin.
22. Actinic keratoses are premalignant skin tumors.
23. The most common tumors found on the body are moles, or beauty marks.
24. Basal cell carcinomas are malignant tumors starting in the basal cell layer of the skin. They are the most common form of skin cancer.
25. The most dangerous form of skin cancer is the malignant melanoma.
26. Two types of pigment disorders are hyperpigmentation and hypopigmentation.
27. The esthetician should have some knowledge about cosmetic surgery procedures because he or she will encounter clients who have undergone such treatments.
28. Before giving a facial to someone who has had cosmetic surgery treatments, the esthetician should contact the client's doctor and find out if it is safe to give the facial.
29. Dermabrasion is a technique for smoothing the skin and removing scars by sanding the skin surface with a metal brush or file.
30. Rhinoplasty is an operation to remove humps and straighten the nose.
31. Mentoplasty is an operation that changes the shape of the chin.
32. A rhytidectomy is the name given to a complete face and neck lift.

Chapter 8
Nutrition

1. Nutrition is important to the skin because the skin relies on a regular supply of nutrients to function properly.
2. With poor nutrition, the skin appears dull and lifeless, with poor color and improper functioning.
3. The three points of the nutritional triad are ingestion, digestion, and elimination.
4. Good nutrition starts with the proper choice of food.
5. Proper elimination is vital so the body rids itself of waste materials before they putrefy and spread toxins throughout the body.

6. The two phases of metabolism are anabolism, where nutrients are converted chemically to build up tissue and body chemicals; and catabolism, where nutrients are broken down to supply energy.
7. The fuel value of a nutrient is expressed as calories.
8. Carbohydrates supply most energy needs for the body.
9. The main carbohydrates are sugar, starch and, cellulose.
10. Proteins build tissues.
11. The essential amino acids are the eight amino acids that must come from food.
12. Complete proteins contain all eight essential amino acids; incomplete proteins lack one or more of them.
13. Vitamins are catalysts that help nutrients work.
14. The two types of vitamins are fat soluble and water soluble.
15. Vitamin A is necessary for proper growth of the bottom layer of skin.
16. Vitamin C is important to the maintenance of collagen and the formation of connective tissue.
17. Vitamin D is synthesized in the body through the action of sunlight on the skin.
18. Minerals are important because they let vitamins work.
19. Minerals cannot be synthesized in the body.
20. The minerals most important to life are calcium, iodine, iron, magnesium, phosphorus, and zinc.
21. Calcium is present in the body in the largest amount.
22. Copper helps pigment the skin and helps form elastin.
23. Sulfur keeps the skin smooth and youthful and helps tissue respiration.
24. Water is important because it carries the other nutrients through the body.
25. The seven guidelines to good nutrition are:
    1. Eat a variety of foods.
    2. Maintain an ideal weight.
    3. Avoid too much fat, saturated fat, and cholesterol.
    4. Eat foods with adequate starch and fiber.
    5. Avoid too much sugar.
    6. Avoid too much sodium.
    7. Drink alcohol only in moderation, if at all.

Chapter 9
Massage Theory

1. Massage relaxes the client, stimulates and soothes the skin, and prepares the client's skin for the steps to come.
2. Massage is important because it is the most emotional part of the facial and it forges the trust between the client and the esthetician.
3. Massage is either structure-based or energy-based.
4. Swedish massage is used to stimulate circulation, improve muscle tone, and relieve soreness.
5. Shiatsu is an energy-based system of massage that involves pressure on accupressure points combined with stretching of the spine and limbs.
6. "Ki" is the vital life force of the body, which flows along twelve energy meridians.
7. The esthetician uses elements from many types of massage to deliver the most beneficial treatment to clients.
8. Psychologically, massage brings relaxation and a sense of well-being to the client.

9. Massage helps feed the body by improving blood circulation and increasing the amount of nutrients and oxygen delivered throughout the body.

10. Massage helps cleanse the body by helping remove waste products.

11. Endorphins are the natural painkillers of the body, released during massage.

12. Massage revitalizes the body by balancing the nervous system and bringing the energy flow into balance.

13. Yin is feminine, passive, dark, moist, and cool. Yang is masculine, active, light, dry, hard, and hot.

14. Energy flows upward in yin meridians and downward in yang meridians.

15. When yin and yang are in balance, energy flow is unobstructed and the body is healthy. When they are not in balance, energy flow is obstructed and the body is ill.

16. The three planes of the aura are the etheric, astral, and mental.

17. Effleurage is the name given to the stroking movements that are the most basic massage movements. They are given with light to moderate pressure.

18. Feathering is used as a light touch to break contact with the body to avoid unpleasantness as a result of sudden loss of touch between the client and the esthetician.

19. Friction movements increase circulation and promote warmth in deeper muscle tissues.

20. Petrissage movements are good for oil-dry skin because they stimulate sebum production.

21. Stretching movements relieve tightness, improve flexibility in the joints, and are soothing and relaxing.

22. Tsubos are pressure points along the meridians.

23. Pressure on pressure points relieves tension, eases fatigue, and removes energy blockages to help clear the skin and improve its functions.

24. As a science, massage relies on knowledge of physiology and manipulation of energy fields. As art, it relies on empathy, sensitivity, and an intuitive feel for the movements.

25. There is no one right way to give a facial massage. Instead of following rote procedures, the esthetician should work in a logical sequence and work rhythmically.

26. When breaking contact with the client's skin, the hands should be removed slowly, with pressure gradually diminishing until it is feather-light.

27. Massage should not be given if the skin is infected or if there is a skin disease.

28. If a client has had cosmetic surgery within a year, the esthetician should first consult the surgeon and obtain permission to give the massage before starting.

**Chapter 10
Hair Structure and
Removal Methods**

1. Hair is a filamentous keratin thread that covers most of the body. It is an appendage of the skin.

2. The pilary system is made up of the hair and the follicles.

3. A follicle is a tubular structure of the epidermis that extends from deep in the dermis to the skin's surface.

4. The three phases of hair growth are the anagen phase, where it is actively growing; the catagen phase, where it separates from the papilla and falls out; and the telogen phase, where the follicle is inactive.

5. The three layers of the hair shaft are the outer layer, the cuticle; the center layer, the cortex; and the inner layer, the medulla.

6. Vellus hairs are very short, soft, unpigmented hairs distributed over most of the body.

7. The four methods of removing unwanted hair are shaving, chemical depilatories, waxing, and electrolysis.

8. Waxing and electrolysis are valid hair removal services in the skin-care salon.

9. Only electrolysis offers permanent hair removal.

10. Chemical depilatories chemically burn off the hair.

11. Waxing pulls hair out by the roots without damaging the papilla. The results last longer than shaving and it leaves the skin smooth.

12. The esthetician should not wax over pustules, pimples, lesions, or moles.

13. The two types of electrolysis machines are the conventional needle type and the tweezer type.

14. The tweezer type is more gentle than the needle type, but takes longer and the results may not be as permanent.

15. Hair should not be removed from inside the nose, ears or eyelids, or from moles.

Chapter 11
Chemistry for the
Esthetician

1. Chemistry is concerned with matter, the fundamental materials of the world.

2. Chemistry is the science that studies changes in matter and the interaction of different materials.

3. A knowledge of chemistry is important to the esthetician because the products he or she uses are chemicals and it is necessary to understand the components, how they interact, and why they have the effects they do.

4. According to the ancient Greeks, nature was composed of four elements—fire, earth, air and water.

5. The scientific method is a method of study in which careful observations and measured results of experiments are used to develop generalized statements that describe observed phenomena.

6. A theory is a generalized explanation of a scientific law.

7. Matter is any substance that has mass and occupies space.

8. The three states of matter are gases, liquids, and solids.

9. Elements are the simplest form of matter.

10. The three most common elements in the body are carbon, oxygen, and hydrogen.

11. A mixture consists of two or more elements intermingled physically but not chemically.

12. A compound consists of two or more elements joined chemically to create a new substance.

13. An atom is the smallest unit of an element that can combine with other elements.

14. The parts of an atom are protons, neutrons, and electrons.

15. The Periodic Table is an aid to classifying elements by their atomic numbers and family characteristics.
16. Molecules are combinations of atoms bound tightly together.
17. For a chemical equation to balance, there must be an equal number of atoms of each reactant and each product.
18. A catalyst is a substance that increases the output of a chemical reaction without changing or becoming part of the product.
19. The two types of chemical reactions of most importance to the esthetician are oxidation-reduction reactions and neutralization reactions.
20. Acids and bases are important to the esthetician because many products used in skin care have acidic or basic properties.
21. Indicators are substances, such as litmus, that change color to indicate the acidity or alkalinity of a solution.
22. pH is a measure of the degree of acidity or alkalinity.
23. The pH of skin ranges from 3 to 9, depending on skin type.
24. A solution is a homogenous mixture in which the molecules of the components are uniformly intermingled. A solution can be a gas, liquid or solid.
25. There are two parts to a solution, the solute, the substance being dissolved, and the solvent, the substance that dissolves the solute.
26. The most common solvent is water.
27. Immiscible liquids are liquids that do not mix together readily, such as oil and water.
28. An emulsifier is an agent that keeps immiscible liquids from separating into their component phases.
29. Organic chemistry is the branch of chemistry that is concerned with substances that contain carbon, which is found in all life forms.
30. The four groups of hydrocarbons are alkanes, alkenes, alkynes, and aromatics.
31. The body can be considered as a type of chemical factory because it utilizes plant and animal materials to produce energy and chemical products for life processes.
32. Amino acids are the building blocks of the body.
33. Enzymes are proteins that act as catalysts in the biochemical reactions of the body.
34. RNA and DNA are important because they carry the genetic information that determines how the body will grow.

Chapter 12
Skin-Care Products

1. The esthetician must know about skin-care products because skin-care treatments cannot be given without the use of some type of chemical product. The ability to choose the right products will determine the success or failure of the treatment.
2. It is important to use the correct product formulation for the client's skin type because using the wrong formulation is ineffective at best, and may worsen the client's skin problems.
3. The esthetician should ask the client about food or drug allergies because some product ingredients may have unwelcome side effects.
4. When the esthetician is not sure about using a product on a client, he or she should first conduct a patch test.
5. The most likely ingredient to cause an allergic reaction in a skin-care product is the fragrance.

6. Creams tend to be thicker in viscosity than liquids and are generally emulsified.

7. A properly designed package keeps the product clean, indentifies the product and the ingredients, allows easy access to the product, and attracts the customer's attention.

8. Ampoules are small hermetically sealed glass tubes that contain a concentrated active ingredient.

9. An active ingredient is an ingredient that works directly on the skin.

10. Ingredients in skin-care products derive from plant materials, animal products, vitamins, minerals, and synthetic chemicals.

11. An antioxidant is a substance that prevents spoilage caused by exposure to oxygen.

12. FD&C colorants are certified by the FDA to be safe for use on food, drugs and cosmetics.

13. An emollient is an active ingredient used to soften and soothe the skin.

14. The three levels on which a fragrance operates are the top-note, the body-note and the bottom-note.

15. A humectant is an ingredient that retards moisture loss in the product.

16. A sequestering agent is an ingredient that retards changes in the appearance of a product, especially its color or texture.

17. A vehicle is the carrier for the other ingredients, most commonly water.

18. According to the FDA labeling law, all cosmetic products must list all ingredients on the label in descending order, according to the amount contained in the product.

19. The esthetician works with cleansers, toners, moisturizers, night creams, masks, and a variety of treatment products.

20. A moisturizer helps prevent loss of moisture from the skin and helps protect the skin.

Chapter 13
Facial Masks

1. The mask is a transition step between the cleansing aspects and the normalization aspects of a facial.

2. Masks are used to remove impurities from the skin, to absorb oils, to tighten, to nourish, to soothe, or to stimulate the skin.

3. Two reasons estheticians should use commercially available masks are to lessen the risk of contamination and of infections or adverse reactions and to lower the risk of liability suits.

4. Masks can be classified as tightening, or hardening, and conditioning.

5. Hardening masks are used for cleansing and toning up skin.

6. Tightening masks improve skin tone and texture and temporarily remove fine lines and wrinkles.

7. Conditioning masks nourish the skin and draw out impurities.

8. Some commonly use ingredients in masks are clays, gums, herbs, lubricants, minerals, moisturizers, and nutrients.

9. Clays are used as absorbing and tightening agents in masks.

10. Some of the most commonly used herbs in masks are aloe vera, camphor, chamomile, comfrey, sage, and witch hazel.

11. Sulfur is used in masks as an antiseptic for blemished skin.

12. Masks should be used after most cleansing operations are finished because it is at this stage that the skin is most receptive to the action of the mask.

13. Algae masks nourish and remineralize the skin.
14. Collagen masks are super-moisturizing masks in the form of dried sheets of collagen.
15. Contour masks firm and tighten skin and remove fine lines and wrinkles.
16. Herb-based cream masks are generally used on dry, mature, and sensitive skins.
17. Paraffin masks remove wrinkles because trapped moisture is reabsorbed into the skin, plumping the skin and filling in fine lines and wrinkles.
18. A wide variety of fruits, vegetables, and herbs may be used in masks at home.
19. Pineapple and papaya are effective ingredients in masks because they contain enzymes that help dissolve dead surface cells and remove surface impurities.
20. When suggesting homemade masks, the esthetician should warn the client to use them carefully and to avoid ingredients to which the client may have an allergic reaction.

**Chapter 14
Supplemental
Techniques**

1. The esthetician must be aware of many advanced techniques in skin care to be able to take full care of the client's needs.
2. The medical uses of herbs include detoxification, normalization, and building.
3. Normalizing herbs help correct imbalances in bodily functions so that the body can heal itself.
4. Herbs are prepared as infusions, decoctions, poultices, fomentations, tinctures, or ointments.
5. Infusions are made by steeping herbs in boiling water.
6. Tinctures are made by soaking herbs in alcohol.
7. Except for serving herb teas as refreshments, the esthetician must never administer any herbal preparation internally to any client.
8. Aloe vera heals and soothes skin and reduces inflammation.
9. The active ingredient in birch bark is salicylic acid, the major component of aspirin.
10. Chamomile softens and heals skin. It is also an astringent.
11. Aromatherapy is a branch of plant medicine that utilizes essential oils derived from plants.
12. A phytohormone is a plant hormone.
13. The four basic properties that make essential oils important in skin care are: germicidal, stimulating or calming, penetrating, and containing phytohormones.
14. All essential oils are natural antiseptics, with the ability to kill bacteria and fungi.
15. Benzoin soothes the skin and helps promote healing.
16. Geranium oil is especially good on congested, oily skin.
17. Thalassotherapy is the technique of using sea water and sea products for the care of the skin.
18. A thalassotherapy tub is a theraputic tub filled with hot sea water, in which the client relaxes while air bubbles gently massage the lymphatic system and water jets massage deeper tissues.
19. All spa treatments promote detoxification of tissues and remineralize the body.

20. The composition of sea water is identical to the composition of the natural fluids of the body.
21. Peloids are a blend of mud and oyster secretions that are rich in trace elements and minerals.
22. Seaweed and algaes stimulate circulation and aid nutrition and detoxification of cells.
23. Peloids soothe and calm the skin and help decongest pores.
24. Iridology is the analysis of the iris of the eye to determine the health of the individual. It is a controversial topic that has not been accepted by the medical community.

Chapter 15
Physics for the Esthetician

1. Physics is important to the esthetician because the laws of physics explain the operating principles of much of the equipment used in the practice of skin care.
2. Physics focuses on the physical, rather than the chemical, changes in matter.
3. 1-d; 2-e; 3-g; 4-f; 5-b; 6-c; 7-a.
4. Energy is the capacity of an object to do work.
5. The Law of Conservation of Energy is the physical law that states that energy can neither be created nor destroyed.
6. Friction is a force that opposes free motion of objects moving over other objects.
7. A screw is an inclined plane wrapped around a cylinder.
8. Pascal's Law is the physical law that states that pressure in an enclosed liquid is transmitted undiminished throughout the entire liquid.
9. Pascal's Law is important because it is the principle behind the operation of the hydraulic chair.
10. Boyle's Law is the physical law that states that with constant temperature, the volume of a gas varies inversely with pressure.
11. Boyle's Law is important because it is the principle behind the operation of the vacuum/spray machine.
12. Newton's Third Law of Motion states that for every action, there is an equal and opposite reaction.
13. The two temperatures in common use are Farenheit and Celcius.
14. Heat is transferred through convection, conduction or radiation.
15. The speed of light is 186,000 miles per second.
16. We see an object because light reflected from the object reaches our eyes.
17. Candlepower is the measure of intensity of a light source.
18. The colors of the visible spectrum are red, orange, yellow, green, blue, indigo, and violet.
19. The spectra on either side of the visible spectrum are the infrared, to the left of red, and the ultraviolet, to the right of violet.
20. An object's color is determined by the wavelength of the light reflected from it.
21. The primary colors in pigments are red, yellow, and blue.
22. Complementary colors are mixtures of equal quantities of two primary colors.
23. Color is discussed in terms of hue, value, and intensity.
24. The esthetician should understand color to be able to advise clients on cosmetic and fashion colors that enhance their skin and hair tones.

25. Green has a soothing and tranquilizing effect, making it ideal for use in treatment rooms.
26. Soundwaves are characterized by wavelength, amplitude, and frequency.
27. Frequency is the number of complete vibrations that occur in a given unit of time.
28. Music is characterized by pitch, loudness, and quality.
29. The most important form of energy for the esthetician is electrical energy.
30. The intensity of an electrical current is measured in amperes, with an ammeter.
31. An insulator is a substance through which current will not flow.
32. Ohm's Law states that the intensity of an electrical current varies directly with voltage and inversely with resistance.

Chapter 16
Skin-Care Equipment

1. The esthetician should use the specialized equipment for a facial because it makes the procedures more efficient and more effective.
2. The facial chair should be comfortable because the client spends an hour or more in it during the facial and it is important to the relaxed feel necessary to a successful facial.
3. The magnifying lamp is used during analysis and during manual extraction.
4. The operating principle of the Wood's lamp is that different skin conditions fluoresce differently under ultraviolet light.
5. Orange fluorescence under the Wood's lamp indicates oily skin with clogged pores and comedones.
6. Two benefits of using steam during the facial are that it relaxes the pores and helps moisten and revitalize the skin.
7. Ozone is a form of oxygen that acts as a disinfectant.
8. Tap water shouldn't be used in the vaporizer because it contains minerals that form deposits and will clog the nozzle.
9. The rotary brush is used for deep cleansing, surface peeling, and light massage.
10. The vacuum side of the vacuum/spray machine is used to help remove excess oil and dirt from the skin.
11. The spray side of the vacuum/spray machine is used to apply lotions and other products in a fine, even mist.
12. The vacuum treatment is done after steaming and disincrustation.
13. The electric pulverisator is a hand held spray machine capable of combining herbs or other products with water and applying them in a spray.
14. The galvanic current machine is used for disincrustation and for iontophoresis.
15. Disincrustation is a process to soften hardened sebum so it can be removed more easily.
16. Iontophoresis is a process that allows the penetration of treatment products into the skin.
17. Disincrustation is used on oily, clogged skin.
18. The high-frequency machine is used to produce heat deep in the dermal layer of the skin to stimulate the skin, improve circulation and provide germicidal properties.
19. High-frequency current can be applied directly, indirectly, or by sparking.
20. The paraffin bath holds the wax at a constant temperature.

Index